Buerger's Disease
Pathology, Diagnosis and Treatment

ISBN: 9784815801502

Buerger's Disease
Pathology, Diagnosis and Treatment

SHIGEHIKO SHIONOYA, M.D.

Professor of the First Department of Surgery
Nagoya University School of Medicine
Nagoya, Japan

The University of Nagoya Press

Buerger's Disease
©THE UNIVERSITY OF NAGOYA PRESS
ISBN 4-8158-0150-9
Printed in Japan

All rights reserved. No part of this publication may be reproduced or transmitted in any form or by any means, electronic or mechanical, including photocopy, recording, or any information storage and retrieval system, without permission in writing from the publisher.

November 1990

Published by
THE UNIVERSITY OF NAGOYA PRESS
1 Furo-cho, Chikusa-ku, Nagoya, 464-01 Japan

PREFACE

Buerger's disease was a disease of misconceptions. Although the concept of the disease originated in an interesting group of patients with characteristic clinical features which the Germans had described under the name "spontaneous gangrene," the concept was obliged to come to look different from what it used to be in the course of time. During a long period of researching the disease, its characteristic clinical features were ignored and the identity was mainly criticized from the pathohistological standpoint of view. Disagreement over the concept of definition of vascular inflammation had added fresh fuel to the discussion and led to confusion. Young scholars stretched the concept of the disease in one's favor and the disease was transformed into a mysterious creature which affected all the vascular system in the whole body.

During about thirty years between Winiwarter's first report and Buerger's first description, several clinical and pathohistological investigations on "spontaneous gangrene" were published in Japan. As diagnosis and treatment of the disease was one of the most importnat problems in the field of surgery in our country at that time, the pathologists and surgeons groped their way toward an understanding of the pathogenesis of the intractable disease and development of a remedy for it.

A contoversy regarding the existence of Buerger's disease after the Second World War threw new light upon the pathogenesis of peripheral arterial occlusive disease and the disease has been regenerated. Abundant proofs of the existence of a peculiar form of occlusive disease of the peripheral arteries in young smokers were brought forward.

While the incidence of new patients with Buerger's disease is recently decreasing in Europe and USA, the disease is still quite prevalent in Asia including Japan. In 1973 the Buerger's Disease Research Committee of the Ministry of Health and Welfare of Japan started with a three-year-project, and the extensive studies were accomplished in the field of epidemiology, pathology, diagnosis and treatment of the disease. Subsequently to it, other research teams succeeded to the previous studies, and the nationwide research teams have obtained excellent results.

At the First Department of Surgery, Nagoya University School of Medicine, Makoto Saito, one of the pioneers of angiography in the world, investigated angiographic features of the patients with Buerger's disease in detail at the begining of 1930s, and it followed that a lot of clinical and experimental studies on etiology, pathology, diagnostics and treatment of the disease have been carried out in the author's department. It appears to us that making a survey of our own experiences pertinent to the subject, with a particular emphasis upon pathology, diagnosis and treatment, based on the current of studies on Buerger's disease, would be of interest.

I wish to express my gratitude to Dr. K. Kamiya for his encouragement and criticism throughout a thirty-year-period. Under his guidance I have set about making inquiries into Buerger's disease. I pay my respects to senior doctors at our department and scholars in the Research Teams of the disease whose splendid results I quoted in various parts of the book. Among our faculty colleagues at the Department of Surgery, Nagoya University Branch Hospital and the First Department of Surgery, Nagoya University School of Medicine, who were helpful, I am particularly indebted to Dr. I. Ban, Dr. Y. Nakata, Dr. T. Yano, Dr. J. Matsubara, Dr. M. Hirai, Dr. T. Ohta and Dr. T. Sakurai for their cooperative studies. I thank Dr. M. Hirai especially for his clinical and pathophysiological investigations. Without their contributions, this book would not have been published. I must thank Miss F. Takeuchi and Miss C. Mizuno for collecting the literatures, Miss I. Mizutani and Mrs. K. Hasegawa for typing and retying the mauscript, Mr. K. Ito for analyzing the data, and Mrs. E. Hayakawa for taking photographs of angiograms and things.

To the staff of our Publisher, The University of Nagoya Press, I am deeply grateful for their interest in and support for this undertaking.

Nagoya, November 1990

Shigehiko Shionoya

CONTENTS

PREFACE i

CHAPTER I HISTORICAL REVIEW OF STUDIES OF
BUERGER'S DISEASE 1
    before 1908 1/1908–1945 9/After 1950s 18/References 24

CHAPTER II EPIDEMIOLOGY 28
    USA and Europe 28/Asia 29/Buerger's disease in women 33/Blackfoot disease 35/References 35

CHAPTER III ETIOLOGY 38
    Cold injury 38/Infection 38/Ergotism 39/Hyperadrenalinemia 40/Metabolic abnormalities 40/Changes in the blood 41/Allergy 42/Autoimmune mechanism 43/Smoking 44/References 52

CHAPTER IV PATHOLOGY 57
    Acute stage 57/Intermediate stage 61/Chronic stage 61/Site of the initial lesion 63/Interpretation of pathologic findings 63/Skip lesion 65/Lesions outside the extremities 69/Venous involvement 71/Nerve lesions 73/Aneurysm formation 74/A peculiar form of the lesion 76/Characteristic of pathologic findings 76/References 77

CHAPTER V PATHOPHYSIOLOGY 80
    Critical limb ischemia 80/Blood flow velocity 81/Vasospasm 84/Vasomotion 86/Hypercoagulable state 88/Blood viscosity 89/Muscle circulation 90/Distribution of perfusion 95/References 97

CHAPTER VI CLINICAL MANIFESTATIONS 101
    Initial symptom 101/Coldness 102/Paresthesia 102/Skin color changes 102/Edema 104/Intermittent claudication 104/Rest pain 105/Pain of ischemic neuropathy 106/Thrombophlebitis migrans 106/Gangrene and ulceration 107/Other trophic changes 110/Involvement of the upper extremity 110/Mental symptoms 111/Clinical correlations 112/References 116

CHAPTER VII ANGIOGRAPHIC FINDINGS 118
    A. *The dawning of angiography* 118
    B. *Angiographic characteristics in Buerger's disease* 122
        Description of arteriographic features 125
    C. *Typical arteriographic figures of occlusive lesions* 128
        Sites of initial lesions 128/Occlusion 131/Stenosis and irregularity 135/Dilatation 137/Diffuse smooth narrowing 138/Fine thread 139/Accordion-like appearance 139/Early venous filling 142/Figures at venous phase 143/Collaterals 144/References 149

CHAPTER VIII CLINICAL COURSE 151
    A. *Pattern of arterial occlusion* 151
        Site of arterial occlusion 151/Pattern of crural arterial occlusion 152/Crural arterial occlusion pattern and necrotic lesion 155/Affection of the popliteal

artery 156/Manner and rate of progression 156/Progression of arterial occlusion and trophic lesion 157/Initial pattern of arterial occlusion and the course of the disease 158
B. *Correlation between the vessel involved and its clisical course* 158
Involvement of the arteries of the upper extremities 159/
Involvement of the foot arteries 161/Femoropopliteal involvement 160/
Aortoiliac involvement 164
C. *Extraperipheral arterial involvement* 171
Cerebral involvement 171/Coronary involvement 174/Visceral involvement 176/Generalized involvement 182/References 185

CHAPTER IX DIAGNOSIS 189

Clinical diagnostic criteria 189/Smoking 189/Age at onset 190/Sex 190/Infrapopliteal arterial occlusive lesions 190/Migrating phlebitis 191/Absence of atherosclerotic risk factors 192/A point of diagnostic importance 192/Differential diagnosis 193/References 197

CHAPTER X TREATMENT 199

A. *Prerequisites for treatment* 199
Tobacco abstinence 199/General regimen 201
B. *Conservative treatment* 201
Physical method of enhancing the circulation 202/Pharmacologic measures 204/Bridging treatment 209/Local treatment 209
C. *Surgical treatment* 212
1. Regional sympathetic denervation 212
   Sympathetic ganglion block with drugs 212/Sympathectomy 212
2. Peripheral nerve division 215
3. Arterectomy 217
4. Adrenalectomy 217
5. Muscle revascularization by vascular implantation 217
6. Omental transplantation 218
7. Arterial reconstruction 219
   Thromboendarterectomy (TEA) 219/Bypass grafting 220/
   Special measures of arterial reconstruction 229
8. Amputation 231
9. Selection of patients for treatment 233
   References 234

CHAPTER XI NATURAL HISTORY 242

Present ischemic symptoms 242/Outcome as to life and limb 243/Employment conditions 245/Natural history of patients with Buerger's disease 246/
References 246

CHAPTER XII WHAT IS BUERGER'S DISEASE ? 248

Epidemiology 248/Etiology 249/Pathology 249/Pathophysiology 250/Clinical manifestations 250/Clinical course 251/Diagnosis 251/Treatment 252/
Natural history 253/Summary 253

INDEX 255

CHAPTER I
HISTORICAL REVIEW OF STUDIES ON BUERGER'S DISEASE

Before 1908

Besides gangrene due to trauma, ergotism, arteriosclerosis, thrombosis or embolism, the existence of a group of cases characterized by gangrene occurring in young males had been known under the name "spontaneous gangrene," but it is obscure what time the prevalence of the disease dated from. It is difficult to identify the first case with spontaneous gangrene in the world.

In 1850 Skegg[1] reported a 35-year-old man with gangrene of the right foot. The patient complained of pain, swelling and weakness of the affected foot and no pulsation was noticed in the diseased limb. He died two days after limb amputation, but no pathohistological study was carried out. Exposure to extreme coldness was regarded as an exciting cause of gangrene. In 1865 Jaesche[2] reported a about 30-year-old man who suffered from pain in the lower extremity and underwent toe amputation because of necrotic lesion, but below knee amputation was later performed on account of proximal progression of necrosis. The pulsation of the femoral artery was not palpable. In 1866 Larivière[3] described the case of a 46-year-old officer who had been exposed to repeated colds and acquired spontaneous gangrene of the left foot. In spite of weak pulsation of the femoral artery, below knee amputation resulted in cure. Arteries and veins in the amputated leg were strikingly narrowed. He considered that the extreme cold induced an inflammation in the superficial arteries and fibrin congelation was organized, followed with occlusion of the small arteries and gangrene.

In 1867 Burrow[4] reported a 40-year-old man who had a rheumatism-like pain in the right foot for several weeks and underwent above knee amputation because of failure of toe and transmetatarsal amputation. He directed his attention to characteristic clinical features, namely, intractable pain, chronic but continuous progression and bad demarcation. He was right in his way of looking at the disease. In the days of only observation of the peripheral pulses, he was harassed by the question about the determination of site of arterial occlusion and amputation level. Later Baumgarten[5] studied microscopically the amputation specimen by Burrow and emphasized the occlusive lesion was different from that due to arteriosclerosis or syphilitic arteritis.

In 1876 Friedländer[6] took notice of connective tissue rich in cells in the intima of the small and medium-sized arteries, leading to complete occlusion of the lumen, surrounded by various pathological processes, namely, cicatrization, cicatricose ulceration, and chronic inflammation etc. The proliferative tissue resembled a granulation tissue and changed to a sclerotic connective tissue in certain circumstances. The entire process had a likeness to the organization of thrombus. He called the lesion as arteritis obliterans, though the term "endarteritis obliterans" also was used, and primary arteritis obliterans was regarded as rare, contrary to the secondary one. The obstructive process of the Ductus Botalli and the umbilical artery was considered as a physiological one.

In 1878 Winiwarter[7] reported a case of a 57-year-old man who underwent below knee amputation because of gangrene of the right foot. The patient complained of a rheumatism-like pain in the lower extremities for twelve years since the age of 45 and suffered from frostbite of the big toe eight years ago. The big toe became gangrenous with a purulent infection four months ago. Billroth, Winiwarter's teacher, expected a spontaneous demarcation without surgery, but the gangrene progressed to the instep and sole of the foot and foot salvage was judged hopeless. Billroth asked Winiwarter to make macro-and microscopic examination on the amputated limb in 1877. Perhaps Billroth suspected that the gangrene might have been caused by some unusual vascular lesions, because he managed the patient for two months and was interested in pathogenesis of spontaneous gangrene. The posterior tibial artery was separated from the accompanying thrombosed veins with difficulty, and its lumen was occluded with soft and loose tissue. Although the popliteal and the anterior tibial arteries were patent, severe necrosis of the almost entire foot seemed to be unusual compared with other senile gangrene.

Microscopically characteristic finding was a proliferation of the intimal cells of the arteries and veins , and the lumen was narrowed or occluded with the proliferative process of the intima, but not with thrombus or atheromatous degeneration of the intima. While Skegg, Jaesche, Larivière and Burrow had previously reported similar cases as Winiwarter's one, they made no microscopic studies. Winiwarter considered the intimal proliferation not as secondary but as primary process, and thought the process could be advanced before gangrene developed.

He presumed the cause of the process to be repeated exposure to cold and humidity, and gangrene was regarded as a secondary phenomenon brought about by occlusion of the lumen due to proliferation of the intimal cells. The concept of endarteriitis and endophlebitis proposed by Winiwarter deserved an estimation, and he did not disappoint his mentor.

Felix von Winiwarter was born in 1852 and received his M. D. from the University of Vienna in 1876. He had a brother, Alexander, four years older than he, and both brothers were Billroth's assistants. Alexander became later professor of surgery at the University of Liège in Belgium. He was a chain smoker and died at the age of 69 years with chronic ischemic leg ulceration through the irony of chance. He was frequently mistaken for his brother, Felix. Although Felix's single case report attracted the medical profession's attention, he accepted the appointment of hospital director in Hollabrunn, north to Vienna, at the age of 29 years in 1881.[8] In the same year, Billroth was successful in the first case of gastrectomy in the world.[9]

While he stayed in the hospital as diredtor until his death in 1931, he published only three case reports on gastroenterological surgery for fifty long years (Fig. I-1). Why did he lose an interest in vascular disease, notwithstanding that his paper on the resistance of the vascular walls in the normal state and during inflammation appeared in the journal in 1873[10], when he was still a medical student in the department of physiology at the University of Vienna?

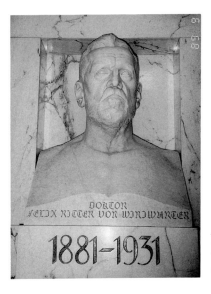

Figure I-1. A bust of Winiwarter in the Hollabrunn hospital. 1881-1931 represents his period of service in the director of the hospital.

According his business report on a 30-year result in the hospital in 1906,[11] the number of the patients who were treated at the hospital was remarkably increased and the financial condition of the hospital was also improved. While he devoted himself to management of the hospital, he performed operations mainly in the digestive organs: there was yet long time before the dawn of vascular surgery. However, it came home to him that medical and surgical treatment was helpless against most of diseases at that time. The maxim mounted at the Vienna General Hospital by the Emperor Joseph was his motto: heal the sick and comfort patient's mind. Out of recognition of the miserable status of medical service at that time, however, Winiwarter worked hard to console a patient in his sorrow at most, if the disease will yield to no remedy. Hospital should be provided with humanity, technique, convenience and luxury to improve lives of patients : patients are entitled to receive clear air through beautiful garden, kingly bed, deluxe clothes, nutritive food and good service, in addition to the first class physicians and nurses : even the most poor patient has a right to be treated just like the most richest person. Therefore, it was a duty for him as director of the hospital to strive for replenishment of equipment and improvement in medical knowledge. He wound up his report with following words : I wish from the heart the regional government and bank their continuous help for the hospital and expect that my dream will be realized at the era of my successor.

Looking unconcernedly on heated discussion on the pathogenesis of spontaneous gangrene triggered by Winiwarter, he should have lost a interest in scientific achievement, though he was very enthusiastic about perfection of the hospital and health care for the provincial people. The street in front of the hospital in Hollabrunn is named as Winiwarter street. Winiwarter built a milestone in the research of spontaneous gangrene, but he finished his life as a faithful surgeon to the starting point of medical science (Fig. I-2).

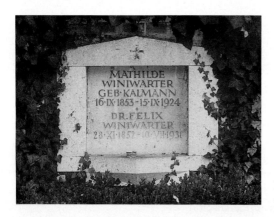

Figure I-2. A grave of Winiwarter and his wife in Hollabrunn.

Billroth[12] described the clinical features of spontaneous gangrene as follows : Premonitory symptoms are pallor of the extremity, coldness, feeling of oppression, paresthesia, claudication and fatigue, and an accidental pressure or incision brings about an atonic and necrotic ulceration. The gangrene is very painful and wet, and accompanied with inflammatory phenomenon and chronic sepsis. It is dangerous to wait for spontaneous demarcation of the lesion, because it frequently recurs in spite of a transient remission. Apart from the indication of amputation, his symptomatology of the disease was almost perfect.

In 1882 Israel[13] considered "endarteritis obliterans" as a factor leading to spontaneous gangrene due to insufficient blood flow, in addition to arteriosclerosis. In 1886 Will[14] described the case of a 52-year-old man with upper extremity involvement with the disease. The patient had been healthy during last 10 years and a bloody blister occurred in the left midfinger without trauma and it became painful. The pulsation of bilateral radial and ulnar arteries and left brachial artery was not palpable. Because of necrosis of the finger, exarticulation of the midfinger was carried out, but gangrenous lesion progressed to the forearm and the right arm also became gangrenous, and the patient died of sepsis. The lumina of the arteries of the upper extremities were occluded with grayish red tissue and calcification was sporadically seen in the media. Microscopic examination showed proliferation of the intimal cells, namely, "endarteriitis obliterans" by Winiwarter. He recognized no influence of cold and moistness in the patient's environment.

In 1888 Riedel[15] described the case of a 36-year-old female who underwent above knee amputation because of gangrene. Pulsation of the posterior tibial and popliteal arteries was not palpable and the femoral artery was occluded at the amputation level. He gave a name " endarteriitis circumscripta " to the microscopic features of the occlusive lesions, because of a localized plaque due to endarteriitis in the femoral artery. In the same year, Hadden[16] described three cases of obliterative arteritis: two 19-year-old males and one 35-year-old female. They showed spontaneous ischemia of the right finger and obstruction of the forearm arteries. Because of thrill or pulsatile swelling of the subcalvian artery, thoracic outlet syndrome or subclavian artery aneurysm was suspected.

In 1889 Haga[17] in Tokyo, first in Japan, reported clinical features of 10 cases and pathohistological findnings of 13 specimens. As 7 of 10 patients suffered from a veneral disease and he found round cell infiltration mostly around the vasa vasorum in the adventitia and often in the thickened intima and the media of the leg arteries, a gumma-like lesion after Baumgarten, he considered syphilis as an etiological factor. It is interesting that pulsation of the radial artery was not palpable or very weak in 5 of the 10 cases. Judging from that the occlusive lesion progressed to the femoropopliteal or the iliac segment according to palpation of the arteries in 8 cases in his series, the majority of the patients seemed to be already in the advanced stage at their visit to the hospital. Nine years later,[18] he contributed his paper with additional cases of spontaneous gangrene to Virchow's Archiv, and Virchow commented on the significance of syphilitic lesion in the vessel.

In 1891, at the 20th Congress of German Society for Surgery, Zoege-Manteuffel[19], professor of surgery in Dorpat, objected to the concept of endarteriitis obliterans by Winiwarter and pointed out arteriosclerotic changes in the affected vessels, on the basis of his experiences of six patients with spontaneous gangrene, ranging from 34 to 49 years in age. He summarized the clinical characterisitics as follows:
Spontaneous gangrene is defined as a kind of gangrene which is similar to the senile one but mainly attacks the lower extremity in the prime of life with no affection of diabetes, ergotism, syphilis or frostbite. The majority of the patients with the

disease suffer from a rheumatism-like pain in the extremity before onset of gangrene. In spite of a hot-spring cure, elevation of the affected limb and so on, the pain becomes so severe that patients can't stand the pain without narcotics. By and by a blue and hemorrhagic blister occurs near the nail of a toe, but the lesion is mistaken as paronychia, and under black discoloration of the lesion, a diagnosis of spontaneous gangrene is correctly made at last. His clinical diagnostic criteria of spontaneous gangrene was almost the same as Billroth's one. At the same Congress, Braun[20] in Königsberg commented Zoege-Manteuffel's speech, on the ground of his own experience, and pointed out the importance of cold weather as an etiological factor. He thought obstruction of the arterial lumen was due to proliferation of the intimal and medial cells.

In 1882 Widemann[21] described two cases with gangrene of the foot or hand due to endarteriitis obliterans, pointing out round cell infiltration and fibrosis in the adventitia: the intimal lesion was considered as a secondary phenomenon following the adventitial lesions. In 1895 Weiss,[22] Zoege-Manteuffel's surgical assistant, in opposition to Winiwarter's concept, emphasized that the arterial lumen was occluded with thrombus formed on the ordinary arteriosclerotic lesions of the vessel wall, on the basis of pathohistological study on Zoege-Manteuffel's six cases with spontaneous gangrene.

On the ground of the studies by his school, Zoege-Manteuffel[23] presumed the pathogenesis of the disease as follows:

Arteriosclerosis might be induced by thermal, chemical, neurovasomotic stimuli or acute or chronic infection, but the intimal thickening itself does not occlude the lumen. However, occlusive thrombus owes its inception to the formation of a parietal white thrombus on the rough surface denuded of the endothelium and it will be soon organized by proliferation of the intimal cells, a picture resembling an obliterative endarteriitis. Acute aggrevation of ischemic symptoms in the extremity supports an acute obstructive process by thrombosis based on the longstanding arteriosclerotic lesions. In the lower extremity, the oldest occlusive lesion was found most frequently in the popliteal artery, at its bifurcation, and the thrombotic obstruction progressed into both proximal and peripheral region.

He rated Rokitansky's theory on the pathogenesis of arteriosclerosis high, marked incorporation of components in blood into the intima, and fortified his case with Rokitansky's concept. Zoege-Manteuffel thought that degenerative metamorphosis of cellular components including destruction, necrosis and calcification should be regarded as a terminal stage or complications of arteriosclerosis, and genuine arteriosclerosis consisted of somewhat uniform proliferation of the intima, namely, a formation of connective tissue, and connective tissue fibres were derived from protoplasma rich cells with a large nucleus, analogous to the process of scar formation. Although atheromatous ulceration and calcification occur at last in consequence of degenerative metamorphosis of arteriosclerosis, it itself does not obstruct the arterial lumen. In case of superposition of another harmful stimuli, however, some new phenomena would appear without atheromatous changes.

Judging from his original illustrations of the occlusive lesion, it consisted of proliferation of the intimal cells and parietal white or platelet thrombus at the site of desquamation of the endothelium, and the lumen was completely obstructed with additional red thrombus. Therefore, he emphasized that it was unreasonable to decide a lesion of nonarteriosclerotic origin, based on absence of atheromatous changes or calcification in the sections. On the other hand, he based his counterargument to Winiwarter's concept on Thoms's theory. In 1883 Thoma,[24] who later moved from Heidelberg into Dorpat, posed a problem if the disturbance of circulation could be related with the intimal thickening named as fibrous endarteriitis and found a correlation between blood flow and diameter of the vessel: decrease in blood flow was accompanied with intimal thickening, namely, adaptative thickening of the intima. If blood flow became stagnant in the arteries and veins, it brought about hyperemia of the vasa vasorum and formation of connective tissue, and the blood velocity was returned to the previous level more or less: the process was named as compensatory endarteriitis.[25]

In case of arteriosclerosis without complications such as obstruction, atheroma or gangrene, Zoege-Manteuffel observed only a simple proliferation of the intimal cells and he insisted that the term "inflammation" should not be used to a process belonging to physiological in common with pathological phenomenon. While Winiwarter's new interpretation was criticized by Zoege-Manteuffel and his school from the viewpoint of a concept of arteriosclerosis, controversy between Winiwarter and Zoege-Manteuffel seems to be derived from confusion of the concept of proliferation of the intimal cells, in other words, the definition of inflammation or arteriosclerosis. I would like not to go deep into the subject.

In 1897 Borchard,[26] a disciple of Braun, reported that proliferation of the endothelium was able to obstruct completely or almost the lumen, but there were sometimes coagula on the surface of the hollow and edge of the thickend intima which were organized. In 1898 Watsuji and Kuroiwa[27] noticed proliferation of epithelioid cells, new vessels and sometimes hemosiderin pigments in the occluding tissue but no granulomatous round cell infiltration in the vessel wall, in the specimens obtained from six cases of spontaneous gangrene, contrary to Haga's report. In 1900 Sternberg,[28] assented to Winiwarter's concept, regarded an influence of various harmful factors on the vascular system being constitutionally weak as important to occurrence of endarteriitis obliterans. In the same year, Bunge[29] in Königsberg reported organized thrombus was easily differentiated from an intimal sclerotic proliferation by means of elastic staining: scanty elastic fibres in the thrombus but abundant new ealstic fibres in the intima. He considered the pathogenesis of the disease as ascending or descending thrombus originated at the narrowing of the lumen due to primary multiple arteriosclerotic intimal thickening and proposed a term "arteriosclerosis obliterans" : the name "endarteriitis obliterans" should be restricted to such a physiological endarteriitis as spontaneous occlusion of the Ductus Botalli. In short, Zoege-Manteuffel and Bunge denied a peculiar cell-rich proliferation of the intima. According to them, the intimal thickening observed in the arteries of the lower extremities in the juvenile people was rich in elastic fibres but scanty of vessels and showed sometimes hyalin or fatty degeneration or calcification : arterial occlusion always originated at the site of an early sclerotic lesion of the arteries.

In 1901 Tanaka and Tanaka,[30] based on histological study of the amputated legs, reported that thickening of the intima was a secondary phenomenon following ascending occlusive thombus formed in the necrotic lesion and disturbance of vasomotor nerve might be a primary etiological factor. In 1903 Kojima[31] in Nagoya, concluded that the arterial lumen was occluded with intimal thickening and secondary thrombus and its features were the same as usual arteriosclerotic changes, though the onset was in the prime of life, based on his own clinicopathological study of two cases with spontaneous gangrene.

In 1903, at the 5th Annual Meeting of Japanese Society of Surgery, Tanaka[32] reported a clinical aspect of 128 patients with spontaneous gangrene collected in Japan : 115 males and 13 females. His clinical criteria of spontaneous gangrene were onset in the prime of life, frequent occurrence of gangrene in the lower extremity and absence of diabetes mellitus, ergotism, heart disease and intoxication. Fifty-eight % of the patients were farmer : syphilis was recognized in 35 cases. He attributed the cause of rare occurrence of gangrene in the upper extremity in spite of frequent absence of pulsation of the arm arteries to a rarity of stagnant blood flow and keeping the upper limb clean. He emphasized that the disease did not endanger patient's life. At the same Congress, Katsura[33] reported that the disease was due to a presenile arteriosclerosis and the lumen was occluded with thrombus originated in the sclerotic intima, based on pathohistological study of 5 amputated legs. Taking a general view of Japanese reports before Buerger's first paper, intimal sclerosis and thrombus formation was the essential feature of occlusive lesions in the affected legs and the majority of them subscribed to Zoege-Manteuffel's opinion. While they presumed that the intimal thickening would occur under the influence of usual etiological factors of arteriosclerosis in the prime of life, they did not discuss why particular subjects were liable to be sensitive to such stimuli in their manhood.

At the beginning of founding the concept of spontaneous gangrene, controversy continued regarding pathological interpretation of the occlusive lesion : endarteriitis or arteriosclerosis ? However, there was no divergence of opinion about the existence of an interesting group of patients characterized by typical clinical symptoms which had been described under the name "spontaneous gangrene." With an increase in the number of cases of the disease in time, its clinical characteristics were almost established until the beginning of the 20th century. In the early days of investigations of the disease, surgeons and pathologists in mainly German-speaking countries were actively engaged in its etiology, pathology and treatment, though determinating the time of operation and the amputation level was surgeons' greatest concern.

1908-1945

At the Meeting of the Association of American Physicians, Washington, D.C., May in 1908, Buerger[34] read a paper entitled "thrombo-angiitis obliterans: a study of the vascular lesions leading to presenile spontaneous gangrene," on the basis of pathohistological studies on the vessels obtained from eleven amputated limbs.

Leo Buerger was born in Vienna in 1879, one year after Winiwarter's first paper. The Buerger family moved to New York while he was quite young, so his schooling and medical education were both in that city, where he spent most of his life, apart from a relatively short period in Los Angeles, as professor of urology.[35] He received his medical degree from the College of Physicians and Surgeons in New York City in 1901. He was associated surgical pathologist at Mount Sinai Hospital in New York from 1906 to 1913 and associated surgeon at the same institution from 1914 to 1920.[36] It was at his age of 29 years old when he wrote the epoch-making paper on the subject.

In the first paper, he described clinical characteristics of the disease as follows: 1) onset between 20-40 years; 2) attacks of ischemia, namely, indefinite pains in the foot, the calf, or the toes, and particularly of a sense of numbness or coldness whenever the weather is unfavorable; 3) one or both feet are markedly blanched, almost cadaveric in appearance, cold to the touch, and when the foot becomes warm some color gradually returns; 4) absent ankle pulses; 5) rheumatic pain in the leg; 6) intermittent claudication; 7) trophic disturbances after months or years; erythromelalgia, a bright red blush of the toes and the foot in the pendent position, a blister, hemorrhagic bleb, or ulcer near the tip of the toe, usually on the big toe, under the nail and severe pain; and 8) cyanotic discoloration and gangrene.

In short, after longer or shorter periods, charcterized by pain, coldness of the foot, ischemia, intermittent claudication, and erythromelalgic symptoms, evidences of trophic disturbances appear which finally pass over into a condition of dry gangrene. The symptomatology of the disease was covered in a well-rounded fullness in his article.

Gross pathology:
There is an extensive obliteration of the larger arteries and veins, the periarteritis and the arteriosclerosis of varying degree. The vessel is filled with a grayish or yellowish mass that can be distinctly differentiated from the annular wall of the vessel. Such obturating tissue is firm in consistency, and does not at all resemble the crescentic or semilunar occlusing masses typical of arteriosclerosis. The vessel itself is usually contracted, so that its wall appears somewhat thickened. This picture is characteristic of arteries or veins which are the seat of a very old obstructive process, and is to be found most frequently in the peripheral portions of the vessels. Tracing the obliterating vessels upward, it becomes softer, more brownish in color, and terminates abruptly in the lumen of an apparently normal vessel; at other times the brownish tissue gives way to soft reddish masses which are evidently the results of recent thrombosis. Veins share equally with arteries in the lesion of occlusion. There is often an involvement of some of the smaller branches, such as metatarsal and tarsal, but the smallest arteries are free. The beginnings of the obliteration are not to be sought in the capillaries nor in the finest branches. There is a sudden cessation of the process, and some 5 or 10 cm of vessel's length is closed and the portions above and below are apparently normal. The apparently normal condition of the vessel above and below the occluding masses, and the transition into thrombosed areas, all speak in favor of the view that we are dealing with a thromboarteritis or thrombophlebitis, rather than with a proliferative or obliterating process derived from the intima of the arteries and veins.

Besides the lesion of occlusion there are two other striking changes, namely a certain amount of arteriosclerotic thickening and periarteritis. A very slight degree of whitening or thickening of the intima is noted here and there in the patent portions of the vessels, and in a very few cases small atheromatous patches are present. A much more interesting and more important change is the fibrotic thickening of tissues immediately about the vessels. Wherever the vessels are occluded there is apt to be an agglutinative process which binds together the artery and its veins, and sometimes also the accompanying nerve, so that liberation of the individual vessels by dissection is difficult: the vascular structures make up one dense rigid cord. Macroscopic features of the affected vessels were exhaustively described in his article.

Histology:
1) The lesions of arteriosclerosis

The arteries and veins show varying degrees of thickening of the intima with marked hypertrophy of the internal elastic lamina without much proliferation of new elastic tissue in the thickening of the intima. Although the very small arteries may also be the site of thickening of the intima, this change is never sufficiently great to lead to complete or even marked obliteration of the lumen of the vessel. In the popliteal artery the formation of nodular thickening is most extensive, but even here these are of moderate size.

2) The periarteritis

The perivascular changes manifest themselves in a proliferaion of connective tissue, in and around the adventitia. Here and there small perivascular foci of lymphoid cells are found, but these do not seem to take an important part in the formation of connective tissue. In the old variety the fibrotic process appears to have come to a standstill, and the vessels and nervess are encased by dense bands of fibrous tissue, sometimes of a hyaline nature.

3) The old obliterating process

Although the whole picture is similar to endarteriitis obliterans, the new-formed tissue occluding the original lumen is not derivatives of the intima, but owes its origin to organization of obliterating red thrombi. In the occlusing tissue, a fairly large number of capillaries, some blood pigments, and fibrous tissue are seen. The internal elastic lamina is thrown into marked folds. The striking lesion of the media is the presence of capillaries with or without a small amount of lymphoid infiltration in their immediate vicinity. The fine vessels come in from the adventitia, pass through the media, and penetrate the internal elastic lamina in order to vascularize the obturationg mass.

4) The differentiation from arteriosclerotic changes

While arteriosclerotic thickening of the intima is rich in elastic fibres, the elastic fibres are absent or found only around the larger canalizing vessels, particularly about those which are thick-walled and old, in the occluding masses of the disease.

5) The various stages of the occluding process

Transitions from areas of red thrombosis into the older stages are found. Miliary foci, not unlike miliary tubercles, make their appearance near the periphery in the thrombus, and there are evidences of organization such as the formation of capillary sprouts, fine capillaries and fibroblasts. The miliary foci present a central area of fibrin and one or more giant cells (probably phagocytic in nature) with cells not unlike endothelial cells in a peripheral zone. Such giant cell foci are early stages in the process of organization. The miliary foci gradually become lost, the vascularizaion of the clot becomes marked, the fibrin is almost absent, and numerous small round cells are scattered throughout as time goes on.

The fine vessels in the thrombus soon change their character: some of them become dilated, forming large spaces with well defined walls; at times there are numerous sinuses giving a fenestrated appearance. The recanalizing vessels become very large and thick walled, and become affected by the same thrombotic changes that had previously occurred in the parent vessel. The changes in the media are dependent upon vascularization of the clot and are not primary.

In short, the occlusion of the vessel is effected by red obturating thrombi;

certain changes in the perivascular tissues, in the adventitia, media and intima, regularly accompany the occluding process. There is moderate thickening of the intima, but this is never sufficient to cause marked narrowing of the lumina of the vessels. The intensity of the cellular and vascular change seems in general to depend upon the activity of the organization of the clot; however, it seems to be sufficiently marked to make it appear that the same agent which calls forth the coagulation of the blood is also effective in producing the mesarterial lesion. The occluding masses frequently terminate abruptly in apparently normal vessels. The changes in the media never extend into the walls of the patent portions of the vessels; usually they terminate before the end of the obturating tissue or thrombus is reached.

Contrary to Zoege-Manteuffel's view that parietal white thrombi first lodged in the popliteal artery and gradually extended downward, and were rarely mixed with small red clots of recent origin, he emphasized the large territories filled with red thrombi and the frequent absence of any change in the upper parts of the anterior and poterior tibial arteries when very distal parts were occluded, and further, the presence of pulsation in the popliteal artery in some of the cases in which that vessel could not be examined, and he gained the impression that the obturation ascended rather than descended. As the cause of the extensive thrombosis of the arteries and veins, he denied the changes in the intima, because the independency of arteriosclerotic thickening and obliterating thrombosis was well illustrated.

Etiology:

While he thought it was important to determine what role syphilis might play in the production of the lesion, he was able to demonstrate neither spirocheta pallida nor pathogenic bacteria in any of sections.

He concluded as follows: Taking the the true nature of the lesion into consideration, I would suggest that the names "endartariitis obliterans" and "arteriosclerotic gangrene" be discarded in this connection, and that we adopt the term "obliterating thrombo-angiitis" of the lower extremities when we wish to speak *of the disease under discussion*. His detailed observation and desciption about clinical and pathohistological features of the disease was so perfect and beyond compare that the disease has been called Buerger's disease after that time. The crucial words "*of the disease under discussion*" came to be ignored, however,and Buerger's advice that the term "arteriosclerotic gangrene" be abandoned was remembered, out of its intended context with the result that all cases of lower-extremity gangrene at any age came to be diagnosed thromboangiitis oblitrerans.[35]

In his first paper, he laid more emphasis on thrombosis than on changes of the vessel wall. In 1909 he[37] emphasized the importance of frequent association of migrating thrombophlebitis (thrombo-phlebitis of superficial veins of the arms and legs) with thrombo-angiitis obliterans, and recommended that in the presence of migrating phlebitis or cutaneous nodosities we should carefully search for evidence of thrombo-angiitis obliterans, in the form of pulseless vessels, erythromelia (he used the word for erythromelalgia), blanching of the leg in the elevated posture, cold and blue toes, pain in the calf of the leg brought on by walking, and other typical phenomenon. He assumed that the same determining causative factor might be responsible for the lesions of both the superficial and deep vessels.

In the same year, Buerger[38] commented on a new surgical procedure to divert the arterial stream into patent veins by arteriovenous anstomosis and asked surgeons to pay attention to the patency of the superficial and deep veins for the sake of successful operation, based on the fact of frequent occlusion of the accompanying and superficial veins in eight cases of thromboangiitis obliterans. He still presumed the vascular lesions apparently initiated by the formation of occlusive thrombi, followed by organization or healing, with an attempt at the production of sufficient collateral circulation. Although he suspected syphilis as an etiological factor at first in 1910,[39] he held that the disease was probably not of luetic origin, because of negative reaction in complement fixation tsets for syphilis in his own 29 cases of thromboangiitis obliterans.

In 1914, on the basis of pathohistological study of 40 amputated limbs, 2 amputated forearms and 25 extirpated veins from 18 patients, Buerger[40] published his idea about the etiology of the disease: thromboangiitis obliterans is an infectious disease in which a specific type of organism is at work, though it has not been possible to demonstrate either bacteriologically or morphologically the presence of the offending agent. He emphasized "miliary giant-cell foci" as "specific" morphological alterations in the thrombus and he considered foci of pus-cells in the periphery of the red clot as the precursors of the "miliary giant-cell foci." Because the typical foci could even be discovered in "daughter" canalizing vessels of arteries that were already in the healing stage and such changes had never been seen elsewhere, it was regarded as the peculiar appearance caused by some specific microbial process. He thought that the giant-cells and endothelioid cells were the expression of abortive attempts on the part of the angioblasts at organizing or healing a focus which is infectious. He noticed the lesion involved deep veins in about 40%, and the superficial veins of the upper and lower extremity in 20%, of the cases.

In the same year in another journal, he[41] stated that an inflammatory phlebitis and periphlebitis (or arteritis and periarteritis) were the inital lesions, synchronous with the phenomenon of complete vascular occlusion by clot; some specific agent, parasitic or bacterial, was responsible for the disease. While he said at first that the determining cause which leaded to the thrombosis also evoked the changes in the media, adventitia, and perivascular connective tissue, his view of an initial scene of the disease underwent a change during these a few years. Because of no discovery of the causative agent in the specimens, however, we can understand his suffering from his previous statement[40] that thromboangiitis obliterans is a disease in which an acute inflammatory lesion and occlusive thrombis of arteries and veins are the characteristic lesions, but the thrombotic occlusion is the most important phenomenon, from the mechanical point of view and from the standpoint of symptomatology; the thrombosis is probably preceded, and certainly accompanied by an acute inflammatory or exudative stage. A which-came-first-thrombosis-or-angiitis question remains to be resolved even at the present, and he finally made a noncommittal expression that an acute inflammatory stage might be an initial manifestation of the pathology of the disease, thrombo-angiits obliterans.[41]

In 1915 he[42] investigated the symptomatology of the disease thoroughly, especially concerning vasomotor and trophic disturbances of the upper extremities, based on his series composed of 200 cases during the last eight years (1906 to 1914). As he noticed that the disease affected the upper extremity, where thromboangiitis obliterans was most frequently mistaken for such other affections as Raynaud's disease, scleroderma or acrocyanosis, he stressed the need of differentiating thromboangiitis obliterans from such vasospastic disorders. It is well said "if we do not overestimate the importance of single manifestations of vasomotor irritation, but regard as more important the clinical course and the symptoms in their totality, we will not fail to separate very clearly in our mind the true vasomotor neuroses from the organic vascular disease attended with vasomotor phenomenon."

In 1927 Constam[43] reported four cases of primary involvement of the upper extremities in Buerger's disease in the Mayo Clinic. As the lower limbs also were sooner or later affected, he stressed that protective measures to the lower extremities were indicated in all cases of Buerger's disease of the hands, even if clinical evidence of their involvement was lacking.

In these days, Buerger devoted himself to popularize the idea of thromboangiitis obliterans as a clinicopathological entity through his lectures at many Meetings of Medical Societies. With the years, he brought the characteristic clinical features of the disease in relief. He emphasized that the clinical diagnosis of thromboangiits obliterans should be depended upon: 1) the racial (Hebrew) and sex (male) prediction; 2) the early involvement of the lower extremities; 3) the early symptoms of pain or intermittent claudication; 4) the presence of migrating phlebitis; 5) the evidence of pulseless vessels; 6) the presence of blanching of the extremity in the elevated position; 7) the existence of rubor in the dependent position; 8) the relation of hyperemic phenomena to posture; 9) the absence of simultaneous, symmetrical involvement; and 10) the slow, progressive chronic course terminating in gangrene.[42] His clinical study was in no way inferior to his pathological one, and the symptomatology of the disease was perfect except in respect of smoking.

In 1916 Weber[44] described his own cases of thomboangiitis obliterans and rated

Buerger's contribution to the symptomatology and pathohistology of the disease high. He noticed that all the arteries appeared small (hypoplastic) in relation to the patient's size and in some cases there appeared to have been a certain degree of congenital hypoplasia or deficient development, of the affected arteries. While he did not regard the cigarette-smoking as more than a contributory factor in inducing the disease, he pointed out the fact that he had never come across an instance of the disease in a woman, nor yet in a man who was not, or had not been, a free cigarette-smoker, in the additional note of the same paper.

In 1917 Buerger[45] collected more than 300 cases with thromboangiitis obliterans, namely, 20-30 new cases a year on the average, and he made the investigation of all phases of the pathological and clinical course of the disease possible. The lesions in thromboangiitis obliterans were in chronological order: 1) an acute inflammatory lesion with occlusive thrombosis, the formation of miliary giant-cell foci; 2) the stage of organization or healing, with the disappearance of the miliary giant-cell foci, the organization and canalization of the clot, the disappearance of the inflammtory procedures; and 3) the development of fibrotic tissue in the adventitia that bound together the artery, vein and nerves.

Having learned that the incipient lesion of thromboangiitis obliterans is an acute inflammatory one, involving the arterial and venous walls, he would expect an occlusive thrombosis as the immediate sequence: the patients afflicted with thromboangiitis obliterans do not suffer directly from the disease itself but from the disastrous occlusive thrombosis which signalizes Nature's method of healing a vascular lesion, that has long since disappeared. The patient in its earlier stages might offer no objective evidences suggestive of the true nature, or of the site of the lesion: it was but in a very few cases of his own series that he felt justified in ascribing certain symptoms to the incipient stage of the disease. Under the difficult circumstances, handicapped by the inadequacy of anatomical material of the deep vessels for study and by no obvious initial symptoms at the onset, it was a great help to him that he perceived the association of migrating thrombophlebitis of the superficial veins with the disease.

In 1920[46] Buerger said that what is clinically recognized as thromboangiitis obliterans is, as a rule, no longer a syndrome produced by the disease itself, but a combination of subjective and objective phenomena dependent upon impoverished circulation; and that, with all the well-known manifestations, such as intermittent claudication, skin color changes, trophic disorders and gangrenous lesions, we may still be dealing with arteries that are healed so far as the disease thromboangiitis obliterans is concerned. Although he recognized harmful effects of tobacco on the arterial wall, he thought that the use of tobacco might render the vessels more susceptible to special agents, be they toxic or infectious, and was opposed to the opinion that tobacco was the only and exciting cause. In 1921, bassed on clinicopathological studies of patients with thromboangiitis obliterans in Japan, Koyano[47] concluded that the occurrence of the associated thrombophlebitis of the superficial veins was rare among Japanese patients with the disease, and he threw doubt on the specifity of purulent foci or giant-cell foci in the thrombus, because similar lesions were found in the cases with gangrene due to a different cause, influenza.

In 1924 Buerger[48] published a monograph entitled "The circulatory disturbances of the extremities including gangrene, vasomotor and trophic disorders." This voluminous book, 628 pages, contained anatomy and physiology of vascular system, arterial obstructive disease, aneurysm, thrombo-embolism and vasospastic diseases, and about one fourth of the whole volume was spared to thromboangiitis obliterans. This was a comprehensive survey of his studies on circulatory disturbances of the extremities, and his accurate observation on clinical features based in insight into the pathophysiology of peripheral circulation was the best part of the book. In 1925 Buerger[49] analysed symptomatology of arterial occlusive diseases of the extremities in the light of their pathology. One of the questions puzzling him was an initial symptom at the onset of the inflammation in the deep vessels, and he assumed that non-localizable shooting pains in the calf or foot, attended with difficulty in walking, with possibly tender muscles of the calf, with or without vasomotor symptoms, and with or without absence of the dorsalis pedis and posterior tibial pulses might be the only symptoms. According to him, a distinct differentiation must be made between the symptoms referable to the malady itself, and those that are attributable to the results of vascular occlusion, but such a discrimination seems to be unattainable in practice. It was noticeable that he already found the acute lesion as thromboangiitis obliterans in the spermatic artery, though he recognized that the disease had a prediction for the vessels of the extrmeities.

In 1925 Perla[50] described 41 cases of thromboangiitis obliterans, including a case involving the coronaries and the aorta, and four out of the sixteen cases studied pathologically showed definite arteriosclerotic changes. He considered that the two disorders were unrelated, though arteriosclerotic changes were often associated with the disease. In the same year, Meleney and Miller[51] surveyed their twenty-four cases of thromboangiitis obliterans in China, and regarded the disease as occurred widely throughout China, though only 60% of their cases used tobacco. A new inflammatory process superimposed upon an old thrombotic process was considered as the most characteristic feature of the disease. In 1926 Gemmill[52] reported the first case of thromboangiitis obliterans occurring in a negro. In 1947 Davis and King[53] were the first to report Buerger's disease in the female negro, confirmed by pathological studies of the tissues.

Buerger turned his attention to the reproduction of the acute lesions of thromboangiitis obliterans, having failed to discover a micro-organism. For about ten years, he had occasion from time to time to inoculate the veins of monkeys with emulsion of a coagulum taken from veins involved in the process of acute migrating phlebitis of thromboangiitis obliterans variety but without success. Since 1926 he[54] repeated these experiments using human veins, with the full consent of those whose veins were employed, precautions having been taken as follows: first, the vein of the forearm was tied off centrally and distally, including between the ligatures from one-half to an inch or more of its length, second, all tributaries were also ligated, and, third, only persons who had thromboangiitis obliterans many years before, but in whom symptoms were quiescent, were inoculated. He inoculated the clot harvested from a portion of an acutely inflamed and thrombosed vein of the patient with acute migrating phlebitis of thromboangiitis obliterans, presumely less than a week after the onset of the lesion, into the lumen of the isolated recipient's vein, but all these experiments were failures. Nothing daunted by failure, a new method was devised: he placed an incision at least 1 cm in either side and parallel to the course of the recipient's vein and the clot was introduced partly underneath, partly on the side or over the vein. In two out of eight veins excised from nine to twelve days after the implantation, lesions practically identical with those of acute thromboangiitis obliterans were found; namely, a diffuse polymorphonuclear infiltration of the wall of the vein and a clot containing typical miliary giant cell foci (in 1929). Although his experiment on a human body is of course open to criticism, his effort that went into the research should be recognized.

In 1930 Buerger became professor of urologic surgery at the College of Medical Evangelists in Los Angeles, and the publication of his papers on thromboangiitis obliterans came to a halt thereafter. In 1939, at the age of 60 years, he[55] issued a paper entitled "thromboangiitis obliterans: concept of pathogenesis and pathology." He pointed out that the cases reported by investigators or commentators did not belong to the group to which the medical profession has given the name Buerger's disease and that thromboangiitis obliterans was a pathological but not a clinical entity in the formal sense, and the clinical course in toto rather than over a short period of its existence often furnished adequate data for diagnosis. He was against a new fashion in medicine at that time that a modern hyperergic or allergic hypothesis might apply to thromboangiits obliterans, on the ground of a morphological similarity of the lesions, and mentioned that neither focal infections, nor general infections or infectious diseases, seemed to have any causal connection with that type of arterial and venous lesion which was pathognomonic of thromboangiits obliterans. He appended a note that Buerger's disease might affect not only arteries and veins of the upper and lower extremities but has been demonstrated to occur in the cerebral, ocular, spermatic, renal, mesenteric, coronary vessels and even in the spermatic cord. He squarely first used "Buerger's disease" as a synonym of thromboangiitis obliterans in this paper.

Judging from his extensive, epoch-making reports, he should have been absorbed in his study with its patient single-mindedness for 30 years: he remained a bachelor until the age of 59 and died in 1943 at the age of 64.[35] In spite of his warning against misunderstanding thromboangiits obliterans, the following studies of the disease resulted in confusion, and the disease became a monsterious one. If he were alive more than 10 years, the future dispute about the existence of Buerger's disease would have changed a lot.

Immediately after Buerger's first report in 1908, similar cases were reported under the name "thromboangiits obliterans." However, the term "erythromelalgia" also was still used to describe the condition at that time, because the term "erythromelalgia" was so expressive of the clinical feature, namely, rubor and pain, and some suggested that it would be better to postpone the use of a histological nomenclature until a discovery of the actual cause of the vascular changes[56]. On the contrary, it was said that nothing would be gained by introducing the symptomatic term as erythromelalgia or intermittent claudication.[56]

From 1930s to 1940s, a lot of clinical studies on thromboangiitis obliterans were reported, based on their own experiences at the institutions. While the etiology of the disease remained unknown yet, there was no controversy regarding the existence of a distinct clinical entity from other arterial occlusive diseases of the extremity. It was a matter for regret that no clinical diagnostic criteria of the disease was established in those days, and the diagnosis was decided by excluding senile, embolic, traumatic, diabetic or vasospastic gangrene; labeled as a basket diagnosis.

After 1950s

After the end of the second world war, about 50 years after Buerger's first contribution, came what might be called the Harvard indictment. In 1957 Fisher,[57] neurologist, based on reconsideration of cerebral thromboangiitis obliterans, considered the type I of Spatz and Lindenberg as the result of stagnation of blood flow consequent to the proximal occlusion, and concluded that Buerger's disease represented atherosclerotic occlusion of the aortic, iliac or femoral vessels associated with distal thrombosis due to slowed collateral blood flow with subsequent organization of the thrombus. In 1958 Gore and Burrows[58] reconsidered the pathogeneis of Buerger's disease, based on pathological findings obtained from three autopsy cases. The basic lesion was said to be arterial thrombosis, which originated in distal small arteries and progressed by means of retrograde extension to the larger proximal channels and no evidence of primary arterial inflammation was observed and the large visceral channels manifested advanced degree of atherosclerosis. They concluded that the process that occluded small and medium-sized muscular arteries produced mural thrombi in large channels, and such thrombi were incorporated into the intima and thereby accounted for augumented atherosclerosis. The aim of their study was to ascertain whether or not visceral arteries were involved in Buerger's disease and the death cause in their series was myocardial infarction in two and cardiac failure in one. This refutation was a modernized revival of the skepticism from the viewpoint of atherosclerosis, like Zoege-Manteuffel.

In 1960 Wessler and his colleagues[59] brought forth a counterargument against Buerger's statement on a large scale. They selected 84 patients with onset of arterial insufficiency before the age of 45 years, from all patients with peripheral arterial occlusive disease admitted to the Beth Israel Hospital in Boston from 1928 through 1956, regardless of sex or the recorded diagnosis of the patients' vascular disease. Among the 84 patients, clinical evidence of heart disease or atherosclerosis was present in 36, and analysis of the various clinical factors believed by many to show a high correlation with Buerger's disease revealed no significant difference between these 36 patients and the remainder: males in 96% in the latter and 95% in the former, use of tobacco in 95% and 96%, Jews in 85% and 85%, and phlebitis in 41% and 62%, respectively. Futhermore, the relation between continued smoking and clinical progression of arterial insufficiency was not as invariable as had been reported. They concluded that the clinical demonstration of the absence of heart disease or atherosclerosis could be of no assistance in the clinical diagnosis of Buerger's disease.

Thirty-five amputation specimen from 18 patients were available for examination: arterial thrombosis was found in all the specimens, and in 10 of all the cases obliterative peripheral atherosclerosis was also seen; among the 8 patients without peripheral atherosclerosis in the resected limbs, 3 demonstrated systemic arterial emboli at autopsy, and the other five had clinical evidence of heart disease or organic arterial disease in the residual stump, or both. Some of the thrombi in the resected legs were recent and invariably lacked significant inflammatory reaction; other thrombi corresponded to the late stage of organization described by Buerger. Many of the deep veins were frequently thrombosed, and there was a variable amount of perivascular fibrosis, but in no case was a specific acute arterial or deep venous lesion found. For comparison with this group of 35 amputation specimens, 66 lower limbs amputated for atherosclerotic gangrene were also examined: arterial thrombosis was found in 85%, inflammation in arterial wall in 52%, venous thrombosis in 39%, inflammation in venous wall in 28%, perivascular fibrosis in 73% and fibrosis involving nerve in 49%; it was a matter of course that these specimens came from patients considerably older than those in the pathological study group. Fourteen superficial vein biopsies from 14 patients were included in the study material: ten of these biopsies showed normal veins free of thrombi, 2 of the 4 remaining specimens contained fresh thrombi with minimal inflammatory reaction and the other 2 biopsies showed the typical acute specific venous lesion described by Buerger. To obtain some frame of reference within which to interpret the superficial venous lesions, 71 unselected specimens of thrombosed peripheral veins were reviewed: an inflammatory reaction was seen in a greater or less degree in 4 of 11 fresh thrombi, in 25 of 36 organizing thrombi, in 1 of 7 old thrombi, in 7 of and 17 mixed thrombi; multinucleated giant cells were noticed in 7 of all the cases.

Judging from the above described finding, they concluded as follows: The disease originally described by Buerger was indistinguishable from atherosclerosis, systemic embolization or peripheral thrombosis singly or in combination. Adequate data were never presented to indicate that the patients Buerger and his contemporaries studied had a clinically, pathologically or etiologically distinct morbid process. Under these circumstances, it appeared that thromboangiitis obliterans could not be considered an entity in either the clinical or pathologic sense, and they therefore recommended that the term be discarded.

In the August issue of the New England Journal of Medicine, two months after the Wessler's paper, de Takats[60] recognized an early acute phase of the disease in persons below the age of forty who exhibited distal or terminal arterial occlusion, with or without ascending periphlebitis, with intact peripheral pulses, which gradually disappeared, and in the absence of gout, diabetics, rheumatic infection, hypertension or polycythemia: this is obviously a diagnosis by exclusion. According to him, there would be no particular purpose, however, in hanging on to a vague, ill defined syndrome, unless it responded to therapy, but abstinence from tobacco, administration of sodium thiosulfate in the acute phase and sympathectomy in the healing stage of endarteriitis obliterans have been of such help in patients with sensitization angiitis, that one would deprive a definite number of patients from intensive treatment by eliminating this diagnosis. He concluded that unless Wessler and his associates could obtain autopsy studies in this early phase—and not just in an early age group—they have not proved their point.

In the same issue Wessler et al.[61] replied to de Takats's letter, but they only repeated their opinion described in the original paper and they did not answer to the core of his question. In October of the same year, the editorial[62] of the Lancet entitled an exciting subject "Does Buerger's disease exist?" appeared: having agreed with Wessler's statement, it concluded writing with "Can we discard altogether the concept of thromboangiitis obliterans?"

In the same year, one month after the editorial, Dible[63] contributed a letter to the editor of the Lancet. He was against the conclusion of Gore and Burrow as well as Wessler et al. He pointed out that a group of cases in young males in which the histological changes in the small peripheral vessels of the lower extremity marked them off from the commoner senile or diabetic gangrene due to atherosclerosis and thrombosis, and posed question "if we are asked to assume that atherosclerosis of the proximal vessel is the cause of these peripheral changes, how is it that it produces this peculiar picture of arterial and venous thrombo-angiitis in the young and not equally in the elderly?" He concluded that the histological descriptions given by Buerger were not wholly accurate, but this did not invalidate the whole conception, and therefore, it might be as well to discard the eponymous title and to use the term thromboangiitis obliterans for this syndrome which described it accurately—at any rate in the lower extremity.

In 1961 Wessler[64] stressed again the elimination of Buerger's disease, in the leading article of Circulation. In the January 1961 number of the Lancet, Lewes,[65] encouraged by Dible's letter to the editor in the Journal, a medical specialist, wrote his personal case-history as a patient with Buerger's disease: his disease process was completely arrested after abstaining from smoking. He emphasized that the smaller arteries were principally involved and the claudication was confined to the sole of the foot in Buerger's disease. The story of his experiences, as a doctor as well as a patient, was impressive.

In the January 1961 issue of British Medical Journal, Corelli[66], an italian authority on Buerger's disease, refuted the Wessler's indictment with the belief that the cause of Buerger's disease is tobacco smoke and the disease is well distinguished from arteriosclerotic occlusive disease, judging from clinical cure of the disease with malaria treatment and complete refraining from voluntary and involuntary smoking. In the February 1961 issue of the same Journal, Oldhalm[67] agreed with Corelli's opinion and emphasized the differnce in clinical features between Buerger's disease and arteriosclerotic group: as the former started near the periphery, rest pain and necrotic lesions of the digits were the common presenting symptoms, whereas the great majority of the latter complained first of intermittent claudication; the ill effects of smoking were infinitely worse in the former than in the latter.

In the same year, Horwitz[68] disproved Wessler's opinion from the standpoint of clinical view, quoting the definition of a disease from Dorland's Illustrated Medical Dictionary: a definite morbid process having a characteristic train of symptoms; it may affect the whole body or any of its parts, and its etiology, pathology, and prognosis may be known or unknown." According to this definition, he said, that we were presently unconcerned about the findings of the pathologists in establishing Buerger's disease as a disease. Further he listed his points of disagreement as follows: 1) it is impossible to consider all patients with peripheral arterial obstruction before the age of 45 as arteriosclerosis, systemic embolization of peripheral thrombosis; 2) it has not been their experience that in individual patients no clear correlation can be predicted between the continuation of smoking and the progression of the arterial insufficiency; and 3) while the number of patients with Buerger's disease has decreased, arteriosclerosis is flourishing. If these patients with Buerger's disease had arteriosclerosis, why have they become practically nonexistent? The very fact that such patients are seen less frequent in their hospital where arteriosclerosis continues to prevail strongly suggests the existence of a different disease process. In the same year, Ishikawa and Kawase[69] recognized the same acute lesions as Buerger described in 5 of 12 cases at early phase: biopsy of the radial artery within 10 days to 4 months after the onset of such symptoms as red swelling of the skin over the artery revealed the typical acute inflammatory lesions with giant cell foci.

In 1962 Barker[70] advocated that the diagnostic category "thromboangiitis obliterans" should be retained: the superficial thrombophlebitis, the involvement of the upper as well as the lower extremities, and the localization of the occluded segments, at least during the early course of the disease, in the small and medium-sized arteries and veins were the distinctive clinical manifestation. As to the association of arteriosclerosis, he said, it might be true that the patients under consideration had early atherosclerotic lesions in the aorta even though these were not detectable clinically or radiographically at the time of onset of the vascular lesions in the extremities, and a relationship of this early aortic atherosclerosis to the peripheral arterial and venous occlusive lesions was highly improbable, however, since such aortic lesions developed in almost all adults during the third and fourth decades of life.

In the same year, McKusick and his colleagues[71] maintained that Buerger's disease must be considered a separate and distinct entity, based on the study of their own cases and the cases in korea and Japan. According to them, the nosologic questions are two: Is there a distinct etiologic and pathogenetic entity which gives clinical picture of the Buerger syndrome and therefore can legitimately be termed Buerger's disease? If so, is this entity primarily an angiits? Failure to differenciate between these 2 issues has led, when histologic support for angiits could not be discovered, to the non sequitur, that Buerger's disease does not exist as separate entity. They summarized as follows: 1) Buerger's disease of classic type occurred relatively frequently in korea and Japan, despite the rarity of atherosclerosis and of thromboembolic disease; 2) the arteriographic findings in Bueger's disease, particularly the involvement of the arteries of the upper extremities and the focal changes, were distinctive; and 3) depending on study at the proper site and at the proper time in the evolution of the disease, characteristic histopathologic changes were demonstrable. The impression they gained from the study of the vessels in all stages of the lesions was that the site of the acute primary alteration was in the thrombus itself rather than in the vessel wall, though a primary alteration of the wall of the vessel could not be excluded as the factor in the thrombus.

In 1963 Kamiya and Shionoya[72] emphasized the existence of Buerger's disease as a clinicopathological entity, based on the histological study by sections of 52 specimens obtained from 202 patients with the disease : an unitary interpretation of all the vascular lesion in the whole body was deemed to be a strained one and a coexistence of thromboangiitic and arteriosclerotic lesions was considered as a natural consequence. In the same year, Abramson and his colleagues,[73] on the basis of the observed clinical differences between 182 patients with thromboangiitis obliterans and 199 patients with arteriosclerosis obliterans, concluded that the term thromboangiitis obliterans should be used to indicate a rare, chronic, recurrent, segmental phlebitis and arteritis affecting vessels in all four limbs predominantly in young men who manifested no signs of diabetes mellitus. In 1964 Inada and his colleagues[74] reported an autopsy case of Buerger's disease who died of operative complications : they laid emphasis on the role of thrombus formation in the pathogenesis of the disease, because of concomitant arteriosclerotic occlusive lesions in the iliofemoral region in addition to typical lesions in the peripheral arteries.

Further, a few voices of notably experienced students of peripheral vascular disease have been raised in protest. At the 19th Congress of the European Society of Cardiovascular Surgery in Warsaw in 1970, the symposium on Buerger's disease was held.[75] The conclusion was that Buerger's disease did exist as a distinct entity, though the symposiasts' diagnostic criteria of the disease were not always the same. As Buerger's disease in the strict sense was a disease that on anatomical ground was not amenable to direct reconstructive surgery and surgery was ousted by Corelli's malariotherapy, "what are surgeons to do at present, faced by Buerger's disease" was their question.

While the clinical and pathological studies by Buerger were so outstanding to deserve terming the disease after his name, the excellence of his work seems to consist rather in symptomatology than in pathology. Because of lack of the specimens at acute stage which revealed the characteristic features, his histological description did not to be persuasive, though it was to his credit that he perceived the association of migrating thrombophlebitis and it was also a great to him. His closing remarks in the first paper in 1908 "Taking the true nature of the lesion into consideration, I would suggest that the name "endarteriitis obliterans" and "arteriosclerotic gangrene" be discarded in this connection and that we adopt the term "obliterating thromboangiitis" of the lower extremities when we wish to speak *of the disease under consideration.*" However, the crucial words, *of the disease under consideration*, came to be ignored. Buerger's advice that the term "arteriosclerotic gangrene" be abandoned was fulfilled, out of its intended contex with the result that all cases of lower extremity gangrene at any age came to be diagnosed as Buerger's disease, as stated before.

Although Buerger already pointed out the coexistence of arteriosclerotic lesions in cases of thromboangiitis obliterans in his first paper, the future opponents attributed the cause of the occlusive process to arteriosclerosis, especially the proximal arteriosclerotic lesions, if arteriosclerotic changes were seen in any parts of the systemic arteries. The overdiagnosis and the dogged unitary interpretation of the systemic vessels resulted in the misunderstanding and misconception of the disease. However, evidences that Buerger's disese is a distinct clinical and pathological entity have been assembled from all parts of the world.[76-80]

REFERENCES

1. Skegg R. Brand eines Fusses mit Verstopfung der Schenkel-Arterien. Lond med Exam Sept 1850 (quoted from Schmidt's Jahrbücher der In- und Ausländischen Gesammten Medicin 1851; 70: 73-4).
2. Jaesche G. Einiges über die Gliederabsetzung beim freiwilligen Absterben derselben. Arch klin Chir 1865; 6: 694-711.
3. Larivière. J de Bord 3 Sér I.9: 463; Sept. 1866 (quoted from Schmidt's Jahrbücher der In- und Ausländischen Gesammten Medicin 1871; 149: 28-9).
4. Burow jun. Spontane Gangrän am Fusse, Amputation des Oberschenkels, Heilung. Arch path Anat 1867; 38: 569-71.
5. Baumgarten. Sitzungsbericht des Königsberger Vereins. Berl klin Wschr 1883; 20: 507.
6. Friedländer C. Über Arteriitis obliterans. Zbl med Wiss 1876; 14: 65-71.
7. Winiwarter F. Über eine eigenthümliche Form von Endarteriitis und Endophlebitis mit Gangrän des Fusses. Arch klin Chir 1878; 23: 202-26.
8. Lie JT, Mann RJ, Ludwing J. The brothers von Winiwarter, Alexander (1848-1917) and Felix (1852-1931), and thromboangiitis obliterans. Mayo Clin Proc 1979; 54: 802-7.
9. Wyklicky H. Vor hundert Jahren Billroths erste Pylorusresektion, seine diesbezüglichen Publikationen in der "Wiener Medizinischen Wochenschrift" und ein Rückblick auf seine Zeit. Wien med Wschr 1981; 131: 1-13.
10. Winiwarter F. Der Widerstand der Gefässwände im normalen Zustande und während der Entzündung. Akademie Wiss (Wien) 1873; 68: 30-4.
11. Winiwarter F. Bericht über die Leistungen der Anstalt in den 30 Jahren ihres Bestandes. Oberhollabrunn, 1906: 27-35.
12. Billroth T̂. Chirurg Klinik Wien 1871-1876: 512 (quoted from Tanaka N. Über Spontane Gangrän. J. Jpn Surg Soc 1903; 5: 120-43).
13. Israel J. Sitzungsbericht der Hufeland'schen Gesellschaft. Berl klin Wschr 1882; 19: 705-6.
14. Will A. Ein Fall von Gnagrän an beiden oberen Extremitäten in Folge von Arteriitis obliterans. Berl klin Wschr 1886; 23: 268-9.
15. Riedel. Endarteriitis circumscripta Art. femoralis mit nachfolgender Gnagrän des Beines bei einer 36 jährigen Frau. Zbl Chir 1888; 15: 554-6.
16. Hadden WB. Note on three cases of obliterative arteritis. Lancet 1888; 1: 268-9.
17. Haga E. Spontanenous gangrene in Japan. J Tokyo Med Ass 1889; 3: 419-22, 560-65, 630-33, 1217-21, 1346-53 (in Japanese).
18. Haga E. Über spontane Gangrän. Arch path Anat 1898; 152: 26-60.
19. Zoege-Manteuffel W. Über angiosclerotische Gangrän. Arch klin Chir 1891; 42: 569-74.

20. Braun. Sitzungsbericht. Verh dtsch Ges Chir 1891 ; 20 : 166.
21. Widenmann A. Zur Entstehung und Behandlung der Gangrän der Extremitaten. Beitr Klin Chir 1892 ; 9 : 218-32.
22. Weiss E. Untersuchungen über die spontane Ganrän der Extremitäten und ihre Abhängigkeit von Gefässerkrankungen. Dtsch Z Chir 1895 ; 40 : 1-42.
23. Zoege-Manteuffel W. Über die Ursachen des Gefässverschlusses bei Gangrän. Dtsch Z Chir 1898 ; 47 : 463-75.
24. Thoma R. Über die Abhängigkeit der Bindegewebsneubildung in der Arterienintima von den mechanischen Bedingungen des Blutumlaufes. Die Rückwirkung des Verschlusses der Nabelarterien und des arteriösen Ganges auf die Structur der Aortenwand. Arch path Anat 1883 ; 93 : 443-505.
25. Thoma R. Über die compensatorische Endarteriitis. Arch path Anat 1888 ; 112 : 10-6.
26. Borchard. Beiträge zur primären Endarteriitis obliterans Dtsch Z Chir 1897 ; 44 : 131-178.
27. Watsuji H, Kuroiwa F. Endarteriitis obliterans in spontaneous gangrene. Tokyo Med New J 1069 : 2529-34, 2632-37 (in Japanese).
28. Sternberg C. Endarteriitis und Endophlebitis obliterans und ihr Verhältnis zur Spontan-Gnagrän. Arch path Anat 1900 ; 161 : 199-252.
29. Bunge. Zur Pathogenese und Therapie der verschiedenen Formen der Gangrän an den unteren Extremitäten. Arch klin Chir 1900 ; 62 : 179-87.
30. Tanaka U, Tanaka K. Histologic changes of the arteries in spontaneous gangrene. Chugai Med J 1901 ; 516 : 1225-33 (in Japanese).
31. Kojima U. Sontaneous gangrene. Chugai Med J 1903 ; 552 : 361-81 (in Japanese).
32. Tanaka N. Sontaneous gangrene. J Jpn Surg Soc 1903 ; 3 : 120-43 (in Japanese).
33. Katsura S. Vascular changes in spontaneous gangrene. J Jpn Surg Soc 1903 ; 5 : 144-202 (in Japanese).
34. Buerger L. Thrombo-angiitis obliterans : A study leading to presenile spontaneous gangrene. Am J Med Sci 1908 ; 136 : 567-80.
35. Eastcott HHG. Buerger's disease. In : Bergan JJ, Yao JST eds. Evaluation and treatment of upper and lower extremity circulatory disorders. Orlando : Grune & Stratton 1984 : pp 483-97.
36. Juergens JL : Thromboangiitis obliterans (Buerger's disease, TAO) In : Juergens JL, Spittell JA, Jr, Fairbairn JF II, eds. Peripheral vascular diseases 5th ed. Philadelphia : W.B. Saunders, 1980, pp 468-91.
37. Buerger L. The association of migrating thrombophlebitis with thromboangiitis obliterans. Internat Clin 1909 ; 19 : 84-105.
38. Buerger L. The veins in thromboangiitis obliterans : with particular reference to arteriovenous anastomosis as a cure for the condition. JAMA 1909 ; 52 : 1319-25.
39. Buerger L. Kaliski DJ. Complement-fixation tests in thromboangiitis obliterans. Med Rec 1910 ; 78 : 665-9.
40. Buerger L. Is thrombo-angiitis obliterans an infectious disease? Surg Gynecol Obstet 1914 ; 19 : 582-8.
41. Buerger L. Recent studies in the pathology of thrombo-angiitis obliterans. J Med Res 1914 ; 26 : 181-94.
42. Buerger L. Concerning vasomotor and trophic disturbances of the upper extremities ; with

particular reference to thrombo-angiitis obliterans. Am J Med Sci 1915 ; 149 : 210-29.
43. Constam GR. Primary involvement of the upper extremities in thrombo-angiitis obliterans (Buerger's disease). Am J Med Sci 1927 ; 174 : 530-6.
44. Weber FP. Thrombo-angiitis obliterans (non-syphilitic arteritis obliterans of Hebrews). Q J Med 1916 ; 9 : 289-300.
45. Buerger L. The pathological and clinical aspects of thrombo-angiitis obliterans. Am J Med Sci 1917 ; 154 : 319-29.
46. Buerger L. The pathology of thromboangiitis obliterans. Med Rec. 1920 ; 97 : 431-7.
47. Koyano K. Clinical and experimental studies in thromboangiitis obliterans. Acta Scholae Med Univ Imp Kioto 1921 ; 4 : 501-10.
48. Buerger L. The circulatory disturbances of the extremities : including gangrene, vasomotor and trophic disorders. Philadelphia : W.B.Saunders Company 1924.
49. Buerger L. Symptomatology of the diseases of the vessels of the extremities in the light of their pathology. Ann Clin Med 1925 ; 4 : 54-61.
50. Perla D. An analysis of forty-one cases of thrombo-angiitis obliterans : with a report of a case involved the coronaries and the aorta. Surg Gynecol Obstet 1925 ; 41 : 21-30.
51. Meleney FL, Miller GG, A contribution to the study of thrombo-angiitis obliterans. Ann Surg 1925 ; 81 : 976-93.
52. Gemmill WF. Thrombo-angiitis obliterans : report of a case occurring in a negro. Atl Med J 1926 ; 29 : 244-5.
53. Davis HA, King LD. A comparative study of thromboangiitis obliterans in white and negro patients. Surg Gynecol Obstet 1947 ; 85 : 597-603.
54. Buerger L. Thrombo-angiitis obliterans : experimental reproduction of lesions. Arch Path 1929 ; 7 : 381-90.
55. Buerger L. Thrombo-angiitis obliterans : concepts of pathogenesis and pathology. J Internat Chir 1939 ; 4 : 399-426.
56. Weber FP. Thrombo-angiitis obliterans (non-syphilitic arteritis obliterans in Hebrews) affecting three limbs. Proc Roy Soc Med 1916 ; 10 : 1-3.
57. Fisher CM. Cerebral thromboangiitis obliterans (including a critical review of the literature). Medicine 1957 ; 36 : 169-209.
58. Gore I, Burrow S. A reconsideration of the pathogenesis of Buerger's disease. Am J Clin Path 1958 ; 29 : 319-30.
59. Wessler S, Ming SC, Gurewich V, Freiman DG. A critical evaluation of thromboangiitis obliterans. The case against Buerger's disease. N Engl J Med 1960 ; 262 : 1149-62.
60. de Takats G. Classification of Buerger's disease (letter to the editor). N Engl J Med 1960 ; 263 : 412.
61. Wessler S, Ming SC, Gurewich V, Freiman DG. A reply to de Takats's letter. N Engl J Med 1960 ; 263 : 412.
62. Editorial. Does Buerger's disease exist? Lancet 1960 ; 2 : 969-70.
63. Dible JH. Does Buerger's disease exist? Lancet 1960 ; 2 : 1138-9.
64. Wessler S. Thrombo-angiitis obliterans : fact or fancy. Circulation 1961 ; 23 : 165-7.
65. Lewes D. Does Buerger's disease exist? Lancet 1961 ; 1 : 170-1.
66. Corelli F. Buerger's disease. Br Med J 1961 ; 1 : 209.
67. Oldham JB. Buerger's disease. Br Med J 1961 ; 1 : 503.

REFERENCES

68. Horwitz O. Buerger's disease retrieved. Ann Int Med 1961 ; 55 : 341-4.
69. Ishikawa K, Kawase S. Occlusive arterial disease of the extremities and angiitis. Igakunoayumi 1961 ; 37 : 253-60 (in Japanese).
70. Barker NW. The case for retention of the diagnostic category "thrombo-angiitis obliterans." Circulation 1962 ; 25 : 1-4.
71. McKusick VA, Harris WS, Ottesen OE, Goodman RM, Shelley WM, Bloodwell RD. Buerger's disease : a distinct clinical and pathologic entity. JAMA 1962 ; 181 : 5-12.
72. Kamiya K, Shionoya S. Reconsideration of Buerger's disease : from the standpoint of histology. Geka 1963 ; 25 : 1343-54 (in Japanese).
73. Abramson DI, Zayas M, Canning JR, Edinburg JJ. Thromboangiitis obliterans : a true clinical entity. Am J Cardiol 1963 ; 12 : 107-18.
74. Inada K, Morimoto K, Ohmoto T, Seki S. Inquires about the true nature of Buerger's disease : centering around an autopsied case. Geka 1964 ; 26 : 387-97 (in Japanese).
75. Vink M, Malan E. Symposium on Buerger's disease at 19th Congress of the European Society of Cardiovascular Surgery. J Cardiovasc Surg 1973 ; 14 : 1-4, 50-51.
76. Prusik B, Reinis Z. Does Buerger's disease exist ? Angiologica 1964 ; 1 : 94-102.
77. Brown H, Sellwood RA, Harrison CV, Martin P. Thromboangiitis obliterans. Br J Surg 1969 ; 56 : 59-63.
78. Kummer A, Widmer LK, Da Silva A, Hug B, Thromboangiitis obliterans-zum Morbus Winiwarter-Buerger. VASA 1977 ; 6 : 384-91.
79. Shionoya S. What is Buerger's disease ? World J Surg 1983 ; 7 : 544-51.
80. Lie JT. Thromboangiitis obliterans (Buerger's disease) revisited. Pathol Ann 1988 ; 23 : 257-91.

Chapter II
EPIDEMIOLOGY

Buerger's disease was initially thought to occur primarily in Jews, but further investigations have shown that the disease was not restricted to Jews, for it has been described in many ethnic groups throughout the world. However, it is interesting that the Ashkenazim made up the bulk of cases of Buerger's disease in Israel: the Ashkenazim, who originally settled in Germany, spread from Germany to Poland, Russia and other countries in Europe and they also form the majority of the present day communities of North and South America, England and South Africa[1].

USA and Europe

It is an established fact that the number of new patients with Buerger's disease in Europe and the United States has been decreased mainly through the reexamination of the diagnostic criteria of the disease. The actual conditions of the overdiagnosis of Buerger's disease were given in the report by Herman[2] at the Mount Sinai Hospital, in which Buerger worked for a long time: while 205 cases were diagnosed as Buerger's disease at the Hospital from 1933 through 1963, only 33 out of the 205 cases were compatible with the present criteria, and the diagnosis was questionable in 28 cases and incorrect in 144 cases.

At the Mayo Clinic[3], the annual patient registration has almost doubled, from 119, 337 in 1949 to 204,000 in 1978. However, the rate of patients with the diagnosis of Buerger's disease has steadily declined from 104 per 100,000 patient registration in 1949 to 10 per 100,000 patient registration in 1978, a greater than 10-fold decrease; the reason for this dramatic decline was obscure but the decline seemed genuine. Among approximately 2,000 patients with peripheral arterial disease seen by Eastcott between 1950-1965, there were forty probable cases of Buerger's disease, most of which were subsequently confirmed at arteriography. In an analysis of 1,000 femoral arteriograms at St Mary's Hospital, London, there were forty cases of Buerger's disease; the remaining 96 per cent were obviously atheromatous[4]. At the Aggertalklinik, a special hospital for peripheral vascular disease in Germany, Buerger's disease was diagnosed in 30 out of 700 males with peripheral arterial occlusive disease in 1967[5].

At the Hospital de S. Joao in Portugal, the annual rate of patients with Buerger's disease among all patients with vascular disease ranged from 2.0 to 4.5 per cent for the period from 1982 to 1986.[6]

At the International Symposium on Buerger's disease in Bad Gastein, Austria in 1986, Cachovan[7] reported the rate of Buerger's disease among peripheral arterial occlusive disease in Europe and other countries: 1-3% in Switzerland, 0.5-5% in West-Germany, 1.2-5.6% in France, 4% in Belgium, 0.5% in Italy, 0.25% in United Kingdom, 3.3% in Poland, 6.7% in East-Germany, 11.5% in Czechoslovakia, 39% in Jugoslavia, 80% in Israel (Ashkenazim), 45-63% in India and 16-66% in korea and Japan. Although the percentage was below about 5% in Europe on the average, that in Jugoslavia was exceptionally high, but it is obscure whether the variance might be due to a racial difference.

At the same Symposium, Pirnat and Simič[8] reviewed epidemiology and geographic distribution of 335 patients with Buerger's disease examined from 1975 to 1984 in Jugoslavia. Forty-eight (14.3%) of the 335 patients were muscular laborers; 31 (9.2%), metalists; 66 (19.7%), machinemen; 23 (6.8%), carpenters; 30 (8.9%), woodmen; 15 (4.4%), mountain folks; 21 (6.2%), farmers; 22 (6.6%), taxi-drivers and 79 (23.9%), clerks. Forty-eight of the 335 patients (14%) were female, and the percentage of the female patients in their previous series of 158 cases from 1967 to 1975 was 2.5%. It remains unknown whether the apparent increase in prevalence of Buerger's disease among women in Jugoslavia might be related to their increased use of tobacco or not. They noticed no climatic or endemic influence on the occurrence of the disease. The above-mentioned rates of Buerger's disease among peripheral arterial occlusive disease were derived from patients presenting themselves at specialized institutions rather than from the population as a rule. No nationwide epidemiologic studies have been carried out in these countries.

Asia

In the Middle, Near and Far East, a much higher proportion of patients with limb ischemia show the peripheral, four-limb, youthful type of picture than in Europe and the United States. In India, the pattern of limb ischemia has been sporadically reported. A study[9] from Calcutta in 1952, reported an incidence of 0.6% for Buerger's disease out of the total, annual, surgical, hospital admissions and the disease was the commonest cause of limb ischemia. Another study[10] from Calcutta in 1966, also observed the frequent occurrence of the disease as a cause of limb ischemia in West Bengal. However, one study[11] from Varanasi in 1967, indicated a higher incidence of arteriosclerosis obliterans (55%) as compared to Buerger's disease (45%) being a cause of limb ischemia, though the pathological lesions of 54 patients with peripheral arterial occlusive disease in Ceylon were often atherosclerotic in the larger arteries but usually thrombotic more peripherally; this was unlike Buerger's disease in that there was no episode of superficial phlebitis[12]. In 1980 Nigam et al.[13] in Delhi reported that Buerger's disease accounted for 63% (107 cases), arteriosclerosis obliterans for 15% (25 cases) and miscellaneous for 22% (37 cases) out of 169 cases of limb ischemia during the three year period. At the Christian Medical College Hospital in Vellore, South India, 186 of 352 patients with peripheral arterial occlusive disease were diagnosed as Buerger's disease (53%); the other 166 as arteriosclerosis obliterans obliterans (47%) in 1989.[14]

In China, Whyte,[15] a missionary surgeon in Swatow, reported the clinical features of two patients with Buerger's disease in 1917, and he called attention to the occurrence of the disease in natives of that country. Although it is now well known that the disease occurs widely throughout China, there is no report about the incidence rate of Buerger's disease among peripheral arterial occlusive disease in that country.

In 1920 Ludlow,[16] a missonary surgeon at Severance Union Medical College in Seoul, Korea, who had seen five typical cases of Buerger's disease in that country before 1917, described the profile of four patients with the disease treated at his hospital from 1917 to 1919. In 1931, reviewing the data of 50 cases of the disease, Ludlow[17] reported that the ratio of patients with Buerger's disease to the total number of inpatients was 1 : 400 and the ratio to the number of male inpatients was 1 : 250. In 1961 McKusick and Harris[18] reported 28 cases of Buerger's disease reexamined at the Presbyterian Medical Center in Chonju, Korea : all patients were male and smokers. Twenty-three of the 28 patients were farmers or farm laborers, and all the 23 patients were of the lowest socioeconomic status. The five non-farmers were machine operator in a rice mill, operator of a lumber shop, government clerk, clerk and foreman in a construction company, and a seamen-fisherman. They noticed that the Korean farmers worked long hours, much of it with feet and hands in the cold waters of the rice paddy and the rubber shoes customarily worn by the Koreans afforded little protection against cold, especially when water got insides.

In 1973 Hill and his colleagues[19] reported 106 patients with Buerger's disease in Java, Indonesia : all the patients were cigarette smokers and only one was a woman. Twenty-nine patients were rice farmers, 63 were outdoor workers and only 14 had indoor jobs during the immediate 3-year period prior to the onset of the illness. In general all the patients were from the poorer section of the community and there were no patients who could be judged middle class even by Indonesian standards. Thirty of 106 patients had had some form of cold injury and this was in general associated with working with feet immersed in water over long periods of time (trench foot). Forty-two patients claimed that they had had various forms of dermatomycoses before the onset of their disease : only 16 of the controls, when compared with the onset age of their matched patients, had had tinea pedis; the difference was highly significant (p<0.001). They concluded that the environmental factors of significance in this disease as it presented in Java appeared to be tobacco, cold injury and a past history of mycotic infection.

In 1931 Noble[20] reported 15 cases of Buerger's disease in Bangkok, Thailand: 14 males and one female. The majority of the patients had an outdoor occupations; 6 were farmers, 4 coolies, and 2 outdoor vendors, while a teacher, a civil servant, and a rice-miller accounted for one each. All except one were heavy smokers; one exception was the female patient, and she habitually chewed betel-nut. No report on the present situation of the patients with the disease in Thailand is available.

In 1976 the Buerger's Disease Research Committee of the Ministry of Health and Welfare of Japan studied 3030 patients with the disease from all over Japan (2930 men; 104 women) and estimated its incidence to be about 5 per 100,000 population[21] (Fig. II-1). The patients were reported from all the provinces of Japan, though the incidence varied with the prefecture. As to occupations of the patients, muscular laborers including farmer, industrial worker, driver and the like, ranked high, but there were no grounds to regard the disease as an occupational disease. A familial occurrence was recognized in 1% of the series, but no evidence of a familial disorder was seen.

An epidemioloigcal investigation of Buerger's disease by case-control study in 1983 took a side view of the patient's living environment and eating habits: 91 male patients with the average age of 46.5 ± 8.49 years; 91 control males with the average age of 46.5 ± 8.37 years[22]. The majority of the patients were heavy smokers, but not heavy drinkers; they had a lower intake of beans, vegetables, fruits, fishes, water and green tea, but a higher coffee intake compared with the control group. As a rule, the patients had a tendency to have an unbalanced diet and an irregular mealtime; they weighed light at birth and had a simple meal during the period of development.

In 1986 the Epidemiology of Intractable Diseases Research Committee of the Ministry of Health and Welfare of Japan estimated the number of patients with the disease who were managed at the institutions in Japan during the prevoius year at 8858, or about 5 per 100,000 population: there was no significantly high prevalence in muscular laborers[23](Fig. II-2). Judging from the tendency of the number of new patients with Buerger's disease and arteriosclerosis obliterans at the Department of Surgery, Nagoya University School of Medicine, 1967 to 1988, the diagnosis of arteriosclerosis obliterans has steadily increased year by year, especially from 1980s, but the number of new patients with Buerger's disease per annum remained almost unchanged. Although we must not jump at conclusions, a westernized diet and a prolongation of the average life span of the Japanese might be concerned with the increase in the patients with arteriosclerosis obliterans in Japan of late years. At the author's institution, the current ratio of new patients with Buerger's disease

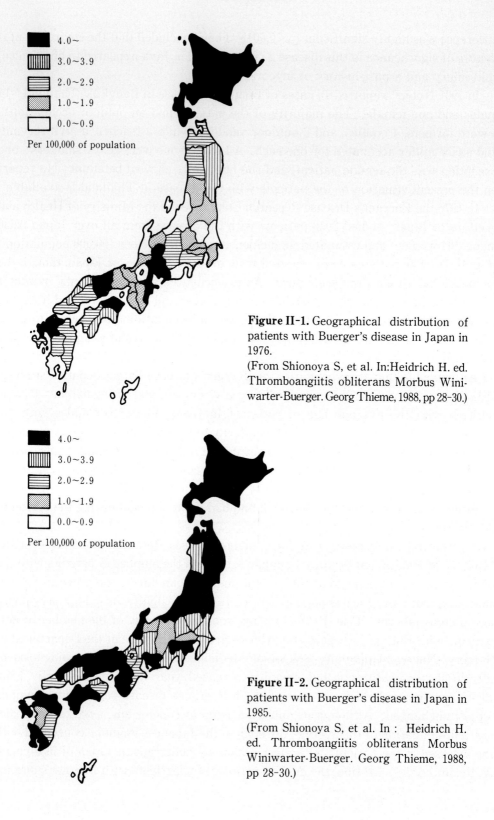

Figure II-1. Geographical distribution of patients with Buerger's disease in Japan in 1976.
(From Shionoya S, et al. In:Heidrich H. ed. Thromboangiitis obliterans Morbus Winiwarter-Buerger. Georg Thieme, 1988, pp 28-30.)

Figure II-2. Geographical distribution of patients with Buerger's disease in Japan in 1985.
(From Shionoya S, et al. In : Heidrich H. ed. Thromboangiitis obliterans Morbus Winiwarter-Buerger. Georg Thieme, 1988, pp 28-30.)

to new patients with arteriosclerosis obliterans is about 1 : 3, so that Buerger's disease is still quite prevalent: the number of the patients with the disease under the care of a physician remains almost unchanged due to recurrence of the disease.

Buerger's disease in women

Buerger's disease was exceedingly uncommon in women. Earlier published series indicated that about 1 per cent of affected patients were women[24]: the prevalence of women with Buerger's disease was 0.4% (2 of 500 cases) in Buerger's series,[25] 1.5% (10 of 700 cases) in Horton and Brown's series[26], 2.6% (2 of 77 cases) in LeFevre and Burn's series[27], 1.6% (25 of 1,600 cases) in Silbert's series[28], 0.9% (1 of 106 cases) in Hill's series[17], 0.9% (1 of 107 cases) in Nigam's series[11], and 0% (0 of 50 cases) in Ludlow's series[15].

While the prevalence of female patients with the disease was 0.8% (1 of 120 cases) in Koyano's series[29] in 1921, 99(11.5%) of 860 cases reported from six institutions in Japan from 1935 to 1955[30-36] were women; the prevalence was much higher in Japan than that documented in other countries. However, it is undeniable that not a few questionable cases were included in the reported cases of women patients with Buerger's disease in former times.

In 1959 Cutler found the diagnosis to be acceptable clinically in 52 of 69 women with Buerger's disease reported from 1922 to 1959 and only 10 of these had histological confirmation.[37] In 1973 Morris-Jones and Jones[38] indicated that the diagnosis was considered as probable, taking into clinical and angiographic criteria, in only 8 of the 22 histologically acceptable female patients with Buerger's disease reported over a period of 50 years.

However, recent published series after restudying of the diagnostic criteria of Buerger's disease showed higher prevalence of women with the disease compared with that previously documented. At the Mayo Clinic from 1981 to 1985, 12 of 109 patients with the disease were female (11%)[3]; 5 of 26 patients with the disease followed for up to 10 years at 1987 at the Oregon Health Sciences University were female (19%)[39]; 48 of 335 patients with the disease from 1975 to 1984 in Jugoslavia were female (14%)[20]; 5 of 27 cases in 1981 in Vellore were women (19%)[40], and out of 53 biopsy or amputation materials at Zürich University from 1968 to 1984, 41 were male and 12 were female[41]. Judging from the high rate of limb loss of 67% in Mayo's[3] and 31% in Oregon's[39] series, it is surprising that many females had already lapsed into an advanced stage.

The epidemiologic investigation[21] for 1976 in Japan disclosed that 3.4% of the collected patients with the Buerger's disease were women: the repeated examination for 1985[23] presumed the prevalence of women with the disease 5.4%. While it remains to be resolved whether the increase in the prevalence of women with

Buerger's disease might be related to the increased habit of smoking among young women, the prevalence of women with the disease in Japan is low compared with the rate of smokers in them.

As a possible explanation for the low prevalence of women with the disease, Horton and Brown[26] thought that women might have the disease in a much milder form, and the disease was overlooked because of the failure of development of gangrene or the more serious sequelae: if more women were examined as a routine measure for pulsations in the peripheral arteries, the absence of pulsations in one or more vessels, without symptoms, would be found in a certain small percentage.

In diagnosing the female patients with ischemia of the extremities as Buerger's disease, it is essential to differentiate them from collagen disease. Since the long-term outlook for patients with Buerger's disease is favorable, especially if they stop smoking, it is important to establish the correct diagnosis for young female

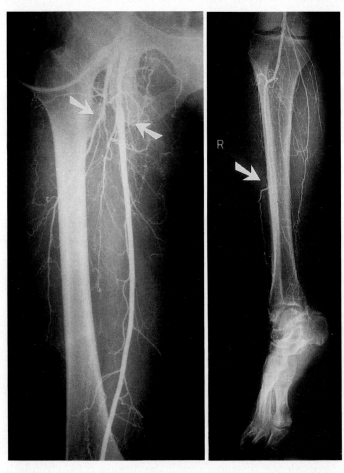

Figure II-3. Right femoral arteriograms of a 47-year-old female with Buerger's disease.
A: The superficial femoral artery shows a poststenotic dilatation at its proximal region, and the deep femoral artery is occluded below the descending branch of the lateral circumflex femoral artery (arrows).
B: The posterior tibial and the peroneal artery are occluded at the origin and the anterior tibial artery shows a tapering occlusion at the middle of the leg (arrow).

smokers[42,43](Fig. II-3). In addition, therapy for disorders that can present in a similar fashion, such as vasculitis and collagen vascular disease, is not benign and can have avoidable deleterious side effects if administered to patients with Buerger's disease.[43]

Blackfoot disease

An endemic peripheral vascular disease involving a relatively large number of inhabitants has been noted in a limited area on the southern coast of Taiwan, and it has been called "blackfoot disease" because of the characteristic black discoloration of dry gangrene of the extremities.[44] Symptoms and findings of blackfoot disease are similar to those of Buerger's disease. However, major leg amputation rate was 65.5%, and a 10-year cumulative mortality was 32.1% ; the main death causes were cardiovascular disorder and cancer.[45] The ratio of men to women was 1.85 : 1, and it increased with age. Sixty-two per cent of patients of both sexes and 93 per cent of female patients were nonsmokers.[46] About three-fourths of the occlusive arterial lesions showed pathologically changes of obliterating arteriosclerosis, though the remaining lesions were compatible with thromboangiitis obliterans.[44] Although a high concentration of arsenic in the artesian drinking water has been noticed in this area,[45] attention is riveted to fluorescent substances as an important etiological factor of the disease, based on its deleterious influence on endothelial cells.[47]

REFERENCES

1. Goodman RM, Elian B, Mozes M, Deutsch V. Buerger's disease in Israel. Am J Med 1965 ; 39 : 601-15.
2. Herman BE. Buerger's syndrome. Angiology 1975 ; 26 : 713-6.
3. Lie JT. Thromboangiitis obliterans (Buerger's disease)in women. Medicine 1987 ; 64 : 65-72.
4. Eastcott HHG. Arterial surgery. London : Pitman Medical. 1969 ; p 95.
5. Schoop W. Personal communication. 1987.
6. Roncon A. Personal communication. 1987.
7. Cachovan M. Epidemiologie und geographisches Verteilungsmuster der Thromboangiitis obliterans. In : Heidrich H ed. Thromboangiitis obliterans Morbus Winiwarter-Buerger. Stuttgart : Georg Thieme, 1988, pp 31-6.
8. Pirnat L Simič Lj. Epidemiologie und geographisches Verteilungsmuster der Endangiitis obliterans. In : (II-7), pp36-8.
9. Som AL. Thrombo-angiitis obliterans. Ind J Surg 1941 ; 14 : 249-60.
10. Basu AK, The problem of obliterative arterial diseases in India. Ind J Surg 1966 ; 28 : 375-7.
11. Vaidya MP, Goyal GS, Tripathi FM. Peripheral obliterative arterial disease—a study of

incidence, symptomatology, methods of diagnosis and management. Q J Surg Sci 1967; 3: 259-71.
12. Kradjian R, Bowles LT, Edwards WS. Peripheral arterial disease in Ceylon. Surgery 1971; 69: 523-5.
13. Nigam R, Narayanan PS, Sharma SR, Beohar PC, Saha MM. Thromboangiitis obliterans and arteriosclerosis obliterans as causes of limb ischemia in Delhi. Ind J Surg 1980; 42: 9-15.
14. Booshanam VM. Role of sympathectomy in Buerger's disease, read before 7th Congress of the Asian Surgical Association in Penang, February 1989.
15. Whyte GD. Thrombo-angiitis obliterans. China Med J 1917; 31: 371-8.
16. Ludlow AI. Four cases of thrombo-angiitis obliterans. China Med J 1920; 34: 18-22.
17. Ludlow AI. Thrombo-angiitis: a review and report of the disease in Koreans. China Med J 1931; 45: 487-514.
18. McKusick VA, Harris WS. The Buerger syndrome in the Orient. Bull Johns Hoskins Hosp 1961; 109: 241-91.
19. Hill GL, Moeliono J, Tumewu F, Brataamadja D, Tohardi A. The Buerger syndrome in Java: a description of the clinical syndrome and some aspects of its aetiology. Br J Surg 1973; 60: 606-13.
20. Noble TP. Thrombo-angiitis obliterans in Siam. Lancet 1931; 220: 288-91.
21. Tashiro T. Epidemiology of Buerger's disease. In: Ishikawa K ed. Annual Report of the Buerger's Disease Research Committee of the Ministry of Health and Welfare of Japan. 1976, pp 3-17(in Japanese).
22. Matsubara J, Sasaki R, Shionoya S. Epidemiology of Buerger's disease by case-control study. In: Aoki K ed. Annual Report of the Epidemiology of Intractable Diseases Research Committee of the Ministry of Health and Welfare of Japan, 1984, pp 363-5 (in Japanese).
23. Nishikimi N, Shionoya S, Mizuno S, Sasaki R, Aoki K. Result of national epidemiological study of Buerger's disease. J Jpn Coll Angiol 1987; 27: 1125-30 (in Japanese).
24. Gaylis H. Thromboangiitis obliterans in a female. Angiology 1957; 8: 259-65.
25. Buerger L.(I-48).
26. Horton BT, Brown GE. Thrombo-angiitis obliterans among women. Arch Intern Med 1932; 50: 884-907.
27. LeFevre FA, Burns J. Thromboangiitis obliterans in women. Cleveland Clin Q 1944; 11: 49-52.
28. Silbert S. Further experience with thromboangiitis obliterans in women. Am Heart J 1948; 36: 757-71.
29. Koyano K. A clinical study of one hundred and twenty cases of thromboangiitis obliterans among the Japanese. Acta Scholae Med Univ Imp Kioto 1921; 4: 489-99.
30. Karatsu E. A study of spontaneous gangrene. J Jpn Surg Soc 1935; 36: 1389-463 (in Japanese).
31. Kumamoto M. A statistical study of Buerger's disease. Jitchiikatorinsho 1940; 17: 560-83 (in Japanese).
32. Nakamura Y. Seventy-three cases of spontaneous gangrene. Grenzgebiet 1940; 14: 535-58 (in Japanese).
33. Sato T. A study of spontaneous gangrene. J Jpn Surg Soc 1941; 42: 577-600 (in Japanese).
34. Kawada Y. A statistical study of spontaneous gangrene. Geka 1954; 16: 415-21 (in Japanese).

REFERENCES

35. Urakubo F, Shinyama K. A statistical study of spontaneous gangrene. Geka 1954 ; 16 : 422-5.
36. Shichino S, Sakakibara K. The statistical studies of spontaneous gangrene. J Jpn Surg Soc 1955 ; 56 : 433-55 (in Japanese).
37. Cutler EL. Thromboangiitis obliterans affecting women: report of a case and review of the literature. Angiology 1959 ; 10 : 91-8.
38. Morris-Johnes W, Jones CDP. Buerger's disease in women : a report of a case and a review of the literature. Angiology 1973 ; 24 : 675-90.
39. Mills JL, Taylor LM, Porter JM. Buerger's disease in the modern era. Am J Surg. 1987 ; 154 : 123-54.
40. Booshanam M.V. Cyril R. Lower limb ischemia in women. Ind J Surg 1984 ; 46 : 572-80.
41. Leu HJ. Thromboangiitis obliterans Buerger : Pathologisch-anatomische Analyse von 53 Fällen. Schweiz med Wschr 1985 ; 115 : 1080-6.
42. Ohta T, Yamada I, Matsubara J, Shionoya S, Ban I. Chronic arterial occlusive disease of the lower extremity in the young female. J Jpn Coll Angiol 1985 ; 25 : 119-25 (in Japanese).
43. Leavitt RY, Bressler P, Fauci AS. Buerger's disease in a young woman. Am J Med 1986 ; 80 : 1003-5.
44. Tseng WP, Chen MY, Sung JL, Chen JS. A clinical study of blackfoot disease in Taiwan, an endemic peripheral vascular disease. Mem Coll Med Nat Taiwan Univ 1961 ; 7 : 1-18.
45. Tseng WP. Prognosis of blackfoot disease : a 10-year follow-up study. J Formosam Med Ass 1970 ; 69 : 1-21.
46. Wu HY, Chen KP, Tseng WP, Hsu CL. Epidemiologic studies on blackfoot disease. Mem Coll Med Nat Taiwan Univ 1961 ; 7 : 33-50.
47. Yu HS, Sheu HM, Ko SS, Chiang LC, Chien CH, Lin SM, Tserng BR, Chen CS. Studies on blackfoot disease and chronic arsenism in southern Taiwan: with special reference to skin lesions and fluorescent sustances. J Dermatol. 1984 ; 11 : 361-70.

Chapter III
ETIOLOGY

While the cause of Buerger's disease is not yet known, many etiologic factors have been suggested for years.

Cold injury

Winiwarter[1] thought much of the influence of cold injury on an outbreak of the disease, from reviewing the case history of the patient who underwent the leg amputation.

From the fact that a very large proportion of cases of Buerger's disease had a history of frostbite, it was said that frostbite might be not an indifferent episode in predisposing the patient to vascular complications.[2] Cold climate has a deleterious effect on patients with the disease, and the manifestations of the disease tend to be worse during the winter months. The farmers' hard farm work with naked feet and hands in the cold waters for many hours explains why farmers ranked first in the occupations of patients with Buerger's disease, and the decreased ratio of laborers including farmers might be due to the present improvement in labor environment, though the farming population has decreased in Japan. Although this tells a great deal about an important role of cold and traumatic injury in the development of the disease, its etiologic relationship to Buerger's disease is probably secondary, in view of the geographic distribution of the patients with the disease. It is another thing that the patients with Buerger's disease should always prevent themselves from cold and traumatic injury.

It has been suggested that the disease affected chiefly laborers in the lower socioeconomic classes in the Southeast Asia,[3] but our own experience[4] fails to substantiate a greater prevalence of the disease in one occupation or socioeconomic class than in another in Japan at the present time.

Infection

Incipient researchers got it into their head that syphilis might be the cause of the disease, in view of clinical and pathohistologic findings.[5,6] Although the syphilis-theory was not substantiated, Buerger's conviction that disease was an infectins disease in which a specific type of organism was at work urged him to a gruesome experiment on a human body.[7]

Thereafter, infection has been still regarded with suspicion of being the causative agent of Buerger's disease for a long time. In 1936 Allen and Lauderdale[8] reported a shocking case of accidental transmission of Buerger's disease from man to man: a spicule of bone from the patient's amputated toe accidentally pierced the flesh of the palmar surface of the third finger of the surgeon's right hand, and ischemic symptoms appeared in the third, fourth, and fifth fingers of his right hand one month later. They asked a surgeon to be careful about the operation of the extremities of patients with Buerger's disease lest he likewise contract the disease. In 1923 Rabinowitz[9] isolated a specific organism from the blood of the local affected portion and from the general blood stream in patients with Buerger's disease: the lesions produced by in the ear and feet of a rabbit by the bacillus were similar to those in patients with the disease. However, his finding obtained no people's approval.

Syphilis,[5,6] typhus,[10] streptococcus,[11] dermatomycoses,[3,12,13] rickettsia[14] and HB virus[15] have been proposed as etiological agents without general acceptance, as they were not able to explain the entire syndrome. Dermatophytosis is present in many patients with Buerger's disease, but it has been always looked upon merely as a complication which must be treated to avoid ulceration and gangrene. In seeking a possible relationship between dermatophytosis and Buerger's disease, one need not necessarily have the concept that the fungi are the sole cause of the vascular disease. It may be that fungi, being concentrated in the blood-vessels of the extremities, act on these vessels in such a manner that other agents such as tobacco or streptococci may bring on an inflammatory reaction. Another possibility is that fungi may precipitate or intensify an inflammatory reaction in blood vessels previously acted upon by other agents such as tobacco or bacteria.[13]

There were some reports[16,17] on experimental angiitis due to intraluminal or periarterial injection of chemical substances and/or bacteria, but it might be questionable to come to a conclusion regarding to the etiology of the disease, only based on a morphological resemblance of the lesions between thromboangiitis obliterans and experimental angiitis. Although ischemic ulceration frequently occurs associated with dermatophytosis in the interdigital region in patients with Buerger's disease, it does not seem to be reasonable to accept an etiological relationship between fungi and the disease. The same may be said of bacteria, rickettsias and virus.

Ergotism

Ergot, which exists as a toxic contaminant of flour, has been known to produce organic vascular changes, thrombosis and ultimately gangrene. In the present state of things that rye bread is no universal diet in the world, ergotism became the theory of the past.[18]

Hyperadrenalinemia

Based on a hypothesis[19,20] of adreno-sympathetic overactivity and histological evidence of atrophy of the zona glomerulosa with hyperplasia of the zona fasciculata in patients with Buerger's disease, adrenalectomy or adrenomedullectomy, combined with sympathectomy had been attempted to correct the hormonal imbalance.[21,22]

In 1963 Iwase[23] noticed an increased urinary excretion of both adrenaline and noradrenaline in addition to dopa and 3-methoxy-4-hydroxy manderic acid (V M A) in patients with Buerger's disease and arteriosclerosis obliterans, and observed a decreased urinary excretion of adrenaline after adrenomedullectomy. In 1989 Ono[24] also reported urinary levels of adrenaline and noradrenaline were significantly higher in patients with Buerger's disease than in those with arteriosclerosis obliterans and controls.

According to histological examination of the removed adrenal glands in 58 patients with true or pseudo- Buerger's disease by Kunlin et al.[25] in 1973, there was no difference in the incidence of structural changes or of signs of hyperadrenalism between the patients and those whose disease evolved toward atheromatosis. As adrenalectomy did not significantly influence the clinical course of the patients,[25,26] adreno-sympathetic overactivity does not seem to be an etiologic factor of Buerger's disease, though sympathetic activity may participate in manifestation of the vasospastic symptoms in patients with the disease.

Metabolic abnormalities

Thorn test: A slower rate of decrease in the eosinophile count was noticed in 40 patients with the disease compared with patients with Raynaud's disease or venous thrombosis.[27]

17 OHCS and 17 KS excretion: Although urinary 17 OHCS and 17 KS was within normal limits in 25 patients with Buerger's disease, adrenal gonadal fraction ratio of 17 KS was higher than 2.0, namely, a decrease in adrenal component (fraction III+VI+VII) and an increase in gonadal component (fraction IV+V) in 9 of 15 patients.[27] There was a tendency that the longer the duration of the disease became, the more the fraction ratio increased. Such an adrenal cortical disfunction might be related with the course and duration of the disease. Stress due to intractable pain and longstanding abuse of analgesics might have an unfavorable influence on the adrenal cortical function.

Estrogen excretion: Estrogen excretion level in urine of 20 patients with Buerger's disease was from 9.0 to 7.7.0 r (average: 34.98 r), which was much higher than that of healthy males[28]. The increased level of estrogen might be a manifestation of a kind of defense mechanism against vasoactive factors.

Histamine: Blood histamine level in 17 patients with the disease was from 0.0065 to 0.0115 mg/l, while that was from 0.002 to 0.006 mg/l in controls.[29] It was speculated that the destruction of platelets in the process of gradual development of the thombus would be responsible for the high level of blood histamine, and the presence of peripheral necrotic changes would be related with the increased level of blood histamine.

Fat metabolism: In 35 male patients with Buerger's disease, the serum cholesterol showed a higher level than that of controls, but there was no difference in the cholesterol-ester ratio between the two groups[30]. In 23 patients with the disease, the serum levels of total phospholipids, cephalin, lecithin and sphingomyelin were 90 to 272 mg/dl (mean: 204 mg/dl), 62 to 151 mg/dl (mean: 87.3 mg/dl), 50 to 149 mg/dl (mean: 94.9 mg/dl) and 0 to 55 mg/dl (mean: 21.6 mg/dl): in healthy subjects the mean values were 154 mg/dl, 54 mg/dl, 76 mg/dl and 24 mg/dl, respectively. Although total phopholipids, cephalin and lecithin were higher in the patients than in the controls, the level of syphingomyelin was reversed.[31] It was unknown whether a change in fat metabolism could be related with the pathologic physiology in Buerger's disease.

Protein metabolism: In 18 patients with Buerger's disease, there was a reduction in albumin and an increase in globulin, especially in r-globulin fraction: the changes in plasma protein fraction were normalized after the administration of predonisolone. There was significantly less prolongation of coagulation time after the administration of heparin in patients with the disease than in patients with Raynaud's disease[32]: the result coincided with deTakats' one[33]. It was speculated that an unknown change in protein metabolism in patients with Buerger's disease might cause the abnormal reaction against heparin, resulting such less prolongation of coagulation time.

Electrolytes: The serum levels of sodium, potassium and calcium were within normal limits in patients with Buerger's disease.[32]

The above described abnormalities in hormone, fat, and protein metabolism in patients with Buerger's disease do not seem to be changes of etiologic significance in the disease, though these metabolic changes may be concerned in development of various morbid states of the disease.

Changes in the blood

While a primary alteration of the vessel wall cannot be excluded as factor in the thrombosi in patients with Buerger's disease, the impression one gained from the study of the vessels in all stages of the lesions was that the site of the acute primary alteration might be in the thrombus itself[34,35,36] rather than in the vessel wall, though Buerger also laid more emphasis on thrombosis than on changes of the vessel wall at first.

A number of hematologic investigations have been carried out in patients with Buerger's disease, and the results were compared with those obtained in patients with arteriosclerosis obliterans and healthy subjects. Craven and Cotton[37] indicated that the patients with Buerger's disease had significantly higher concentrations of heparin-precipitable fractions of fibrinogen (HPF) in their plasma and there was a highly significant increase in the ration of this fraction to fibrinogen and their HPF was positively correlated to a highly significant degree with both fibrinogen and erythrocyte sedimentation rate (ESR), which was similar to the pattern observed in healthy subjects: in the arteriosclerotic group, there was no correlation between HPF and ESR, and HPF and fibrinogen. Furthermore, whereas the euglobulin lysis times were influenced by the serum triglyceride level in the arteriosclerotic group, this correlation was completely lacking in patients with the disease. However, there are no conclusive evidences that the changes in the blood favoring hypercoagulability occur in patients with Buerger's disease and the laboratory findings are helpful to the diagnosis of the disease.

At the first examination in our series, the number of erythrocytes, hemoglobulin, hematocrit, antithrombin III, plasminogen, fibrinogen, α_2-macroglobulin, α_1-antitrypsin, and ADP-induced platelet aggregation were measured in 67 patients with Buerger's disease, but a systemic hypercoagulable state was not proven. As coagulation factor and fibrinolytic activity are unstable, repeated hematological examinations are necessary to investigate a possible correlation between hypercoagulability and progression of the disease. By repeated measurements of antithrombin III, plasminogen, fibrinogen, α_2-macroglobulin, and α_1-antitrypsin, an intimate relationship of remission and relapse of the disease to the changes in thrombogenic factors was observed[38]: a decrease in the first two factors or an increase in the latter three factors is considered as favorable to thrombus formation. Although these results encouraged us to pursue further hematological investigation into the pathogenesis of this distressing condition, it is very far from here that the concept of angiitis leading to thrombosis could be replaced by a view that the process is primarily thrombotic.

Allergy

An idea that Buerger's disease is caused by hypersensitiviness of an allergic type is time-honored, as an allergic reaction has been considered to have a part in the causative relationship of tobacco[39] or fungi[12] to Buerger's disease. Because of the low prevalence of the patients with the disease among numerous smokers or innumerable persons with dermatomycoses, it is no wonder that a hypersensitivity to such factors might exist in patients with the disease. However, on the contrary, another studies[40,41] considered the skin reaction as due to some of the many nonspecific reactions from chemical irritation.

In 1959 Takahashi[42] prepared an extract of 98 per cent denicotinized tobacco and the results he obtained were as follows: Skin reaction to the denicotinized tobacco extract was positive in 65.9% of 41 patients with Buerger's disease, in 37.5% of 8 patients with arteriosclerosis obliterans, in 3.8% of 26 patients with Raynaud's disease, and in 14% of 79 healthy subjects; the reaction was regarded as positive when the skin wheal was reddened and more than 10 mm in diameter 30 minutes after the intradermal injection of 0.1 ml of 5% saline solution of a 98% denicotinized tobacco extract. When the subjects of the investigation were limited to smokers, the test was positive in 65.9% of 41 patients with Buerger's disease, in 35.1% of 37 patients with other peripheral vascular disease, in 14.4% of 167 patients without peripheral vascular disease, and in 25.0% of 32 healthy persons.

With the serum obtained from the patients who were positive to the denicotinized tobacco extract, Prausnitz-Kuster test was positive in 33% of 15 patient with Buerger's disease and in 16.7% of 12 smokers with other disease or of health. Skin reaction to intradermal injection of 0.1 ml of a nicotine saline solution of the strength of 1/5,000 was positive in 17.2% of 29 patients with Buerger's disease, in 14.3% of 7 patients with arteriosclerosis obliterans, in 0% of 15 patients with Raynaud's disease, and in 9.5% of 21 patients with venous thrombosis. When the subjects of the investigation were limited to smokers, the test was positive in 17.2% of 29 patients with Buerger's disease, in 12.1% of 33 with other vascular diseases, in 6.9% of 87 patients without peripheral vascular diseases, and in 15.4% of 13 healthy persons. The patients with Buerger's disease showed more hypersensitive skin reaction to the denicotinized tobacco extract compared with the patients with other diseases or healthy smokers.

We have no definite view of an atopic condition of the sentization of the vascular system to tobacco or reagins for tobacco on passive transfer tests, and the explanation seems to be inconclusive unless we understand the concept of "allergy" in a broad sense.

Autoimmune mechanism

With advance of studies on autoimmune disease, various hypotheses suggesting the contribution of autoimmune mechanism in the pathogenesis of Buerger's disease have been postulated. Evidence of an immunopathogeneis for the disease included an increase in complement factor C 4,[43] antielastin,[44] and anticollagen antibody and cellular sensitivity to human type I or type III collagen[45,46] in patients with Buerger's disease, compared to patients with arteriosclerosis obliterans.

Because Smolen et al.[47] detected circulating antibodies to heat-denatured human collagen (ACA) in seven (35%) and a significant lymphocyte stimulation after culture with collagen in seven (35%) out of 20 patients with Buerger's disease and there was a significant correlation between the occurrence of HLA B 8 and the occurrence of ACA, it was concluded that autoimmune mechanism might be involved in the pathogenesis of the disease, or that the observed immune reactivity to collagen might be an epiphenomenon due to the chronicity of the disease, as most of the patients with ACA or lymphocyte transformation to collagen belonged to the group of patients with severe and often long-standing disease history.

Gulati and his colleagues[48] observed organ specific autoantibodies (IgM, IgG, IgA) and C 3 component in the diseased vessels of patients with Buerger's disease in addition to non-organ specific antibody (ANA) and antibodies, antiarterial, in their sera, and then they[49] reported that the immunoglobulins in the circulating immune complexes in the patients were predominantly of mixed type and the immune complexes were biologically active. Furthermore Gulati's research team[50] indicated that the patients with the disease showed specific inhibition of migration of leukocytes against arterial as well as tobacco antigens in comparison to the controls, and they concluded that these observations strenghtend the concept of involvement of tobacco smoking in causing angiitis in Buerger's disease by maneuvering the immune homeostasis. In 1989 Roncon et al.[51] also confirmed the presence of circulating immune complexes in patients with the disease.

These results may suggest the possibility of differentiating between Buerger's disease and arteriosclerosis obliterans by autoimmunologic means. However, determining whether these findings are primary or secondary phenomena due to the vascular lesions remains a difficult problem, and the significance of these immunologic findings remains to be resolved.

Smoking

While the cause of Buerger's disease is not yet known, smoking is very closely related with exacerbations and remissions of the disease. In general, if the patient absolutely abandons smoking, the natural history will invariably be benign, but if smoking continues, any treatment will ultimately prove futile and the course will progressively worsen.

In 1904 Erb[52] stated that smoking was an important contributing cause of this condition. Lilienthal[53] noted this relationship in 1914, and Meyer[54] expressed the conviction that the disease was due to the use of tobacco in 1920. Meyer considered the term "thromboangiitis" as only one of the features of the disease, like intermittent claudication, gangrene, etc., not the disease itself: the disease proper might be of the blood, not of the blood vessels, because the disease could be caused by the absorbed tobacco-smoke poisons circulating with the blood and in the lymph. The vasoconstricting effects of smoking on the peripheral vessels was demonstrated in man by Bruce et al.,[55] using the volume changes in the hand and arm. In 1932 Maddoch and Coller[56] noted a lowering of the surface temperature and an increase in pulse rate and blood pressure after tobacco smoking in young healthy smokers: these changes were most marked in the tips of fingers and toes, lasting as long as one-half hour, usually of greater duration in the toes.

Barker[57] confirmed the above observations in normal subjects, patients with Buerger's disease and patients with vasospastic disturbances: this effect seemed to depend on individual hypersensitiviness and not on the amount of tobacco habitually used. Wright and Moffat[58] observed slowing and even stoppage of the blood flow in the capillaries of the nail fold during the process of smoking, in addition to a marked drop in surface temperature at the tips of the fingers and toes: the length of time a subject had been a smoker and the number of cigarette habitually smoked daily had no determinable effect on the degree of the temperature drop. While these studies explained why smoking was definitely aggravating any condition when the circulation was normal or impaired, they did not prove that smoking was the original causative factor of Buerger's disease.

In 1933 Harkavy[39] studied skin reactions following intracutaneous injection with 0.01 ml of the tobacco extract in 87 patients with Buerger's disease, 36 with coronary disease and 262 controls: positive skin reactions were found in 87%, 36% and 16%, respectively. From these observation, he concluded that tobacco sensitiveness might play an important role in the pathogenesis of Buerger's disease and the patients might belong to the category of allergic individuals. His paper on tobacco sensitiveness, read at a State Meeting of the Academy, gave the audience a shock, and the discussants expressed their surprise in the following manner: I came here somewhat frightened at what might be said against my kindly friend, tobacco, or he intended unnecessarily to take some of the joy out of life.

In 1934 Sulzberger[59] lent support to Harkavy's work and attributed the failures of purely toxicologic experiments with nicotine to the attempts performed without employing the method of sensitizing the test objects or experimental animals. It was well known that all attempts experimentally to reproduce and study the harmful effects of tobacco, which were often so evident clinically in smokers, had failed. Sulzberger reported that 78% of the patients with Buerger's disease had positive reactions of the skin to the denicotinized extracts of tobacco: 36% of the smokers without the disease and 16% of the nonsmokers gave positive reactions. That part of the tobacco which elicited the skin reaction of hypersensitivity was coctostablile and thermostabile and was not destroyed by ultraviolet rays or x-rays; it was not nicotine. However, the persons afflicted with Buerger's disease were not atopic, and there were no regularly demonstrated reagins in their serums. He regarded these results as highly suggestive that sensitization of the vascular system to tobacco might play a causal or contributory role in many cases of Buerger's disease.

In 1959 Itakura[60] observed thickening of the adventitia with fibrinoid distension of the connective tissue, thickening of the media with vacuolization and degeneration of the muscle cells and loss of the elastic fibres mainly in small and medium-sized arteries in rats after a 3 to 4-month intravenous or intraperitoneal injection with nicotine free extracts of tobacco: pretreatment with DOCA, concomitant adrenaline or exposure to cold enhanced the changes. In 1960 Oono[61] noticed a kind of non-suppurative inflammation of all layers of the visceral and limb arteries in mice subjected to forced smoking for 8 months: similar lesions were seen in some accompanying veins.

It is also clear that millions of men and women smoke incessantly without developing this disease. Why is it that a practice which so many indulge with impunity is so harmful to a few? In 1945 Silbert[62] concluded that Buerger's disease was caused by smoking in individuals constitutionally sensitive to tobacco, on the basis of a 10-20 year follow-up study of 100 patients with Buerger's disease, who all stopped smoking at the beginning of treatment and in all of them the disease had remained completely arrested following the initial period of treatment. Silbert thought that certainly a constitutional factor, a special sensitivity of the blood vessels to the effects of tobacco, must also be present: only those who have such a constitutional factor will develop Buerger's disease from smoking. He attributed the objection that instances of Buerger's disease had been seen in nonsmokers to confuse peripheral vascular disease due to the disease with that due to presenile arteriosclerosis, an entirely different disease.

Judging from that millions of smokers without developing ischemia of the extremities, it is no wonder to think of a special sensitivity of the body to the effects of tobacco, though a simple view of tobacco hypersensitivity was denied. What is a constitutional factor which develops Buerger's disease from smoking?

Ohtawa et al.[63] first noted an increase in the incidence of HLA-A 9, BW 10, and a Japanese specific antigen (J-1-1) together with an absence of HLA-A 12 in Japanese patients with Buerger's disease in 1974. HLA-typing study was followed by McLoughlin et al.[64], and several Japanese researchers[65-68], in which a high frequency of Bw 22.2 (J-1-1), A 9 or B 5 and a low frequency of B 12 were recognized as a rule, but the results varied in the other antigens.

In 1986 Numano[69] reported significant high frequencies of Aw 24, Bw 40, Bw 54, Cw1, and DR 2 antigens and a low frequency of DR 9 and DRw 52 in HLA analysis in patients with Buerger's disease compared with those in normal Japanese individuals. As the haplotype Aw 24-Bw 54-Cwl-DR 4 is known to be common among Japanese, a significant high frequency of haplotype Bw 54-DR 2 found in cases of Buerger's disease, instead of that of Bw 54-DR 4, may suggest a possible cross-linkage occurrence in chromosome 6, which could prove to be an important causative phenomenon in the pathophysiology of Buerger's disease. Although controversy continues regarding characteristic association of HLA-antigens in Buerger's disease, it has been speculated that there may be a gene in mankind controlling susceptibility to the disease, linked to the presence or absence of some HLA-antigens.[70]

On the other hand, a major contribution towards a better understanding of relationship of Buerger's disease to smoking was made. In 1941 Theis and Freeland[71] observed that tobacco smoking was usually accompanied by a greater reduction in the oxygenation of the arterial blood in patients with Buerger's disease than in normal individuals, and they suggested that failure of physiologic adjustments to compensate for the lowered oxygen tension in the tissues and internal organs might be an etiologic factor in Buerger's disease. In 1964 Astrup[72] observed that the oxygen association curve of a patient with Buerger's disease showed a shift to the left at low tension, that is to say, the hemoglobin was less ready to part with its oxygen under the condition of the peripheral tissues : this phenomenon was confirmed in heavy cigarette smokers by other workers and was deemed to be due to the absorption of carbon monoxide[73]. In 1965 Ashby et al.[74] reported that platelet stickness increased significantly in healthy volunteers when they smoked two cigarettes in quick succession. Astrup et al.[75] investigating possible reasons for damage to blood vessels by smoking found that the greatest rate of cholesterol accumulation in the aortic tissues was in rabbits fed on cholesterol and exposed to carbon monoxide.

Hess and Frost[76] electromicroscopically noticed deposition of thrombocytes, erythrocytes, fibrin, unidentified cells and desquamation of endothelial cells on the intima of the aorta and the carotid artery of the rabbit forced to inhale tobacco smoke. In 1973, it was found by Wald et al.[77] in the age group 30-69 years that a patient with a carboxyhemoglobin level of 5 per cent or more was 21 times as likely to be affected by occlusive arterial disease as another person of the same age and sex with a carbon monoxide level less than 3 per cent, notwithstanding similar smoking history and current smoking habits.

In 1988 Mukaiyama et al.[78] studied the acute effects of smoking three cigarettes over 15 min on coagulation-fibrinolysis, plasma levels of prostaglandins, catecholamines and serotonin and the number of circulating endothelial cells : 1) prothrombin time, plasma levels of fibrinogen and fibrinopeptide A, and fibrinopeptide A/fibrinopeptide B 15-42 ration were significantly higher in smokers before smoking, compared with non-smokers ; 2) APTT, α_2-PI activity and plasma level of factor VIII related antigen were significantly elevated in smokers 10 min after smoking; 3) plasma level of TXB_2 was significantly higher and 6-keto-$PGF_1\alpha$/TXB_2 ratio was significantly lower in smokers compared with non-smokers, and plasma 6-keto-$PGF_1\alpha$ level showed a tendency to decrease in smokers, though no definite changes in plasma TXB_2 level was seen after smoking (Fig. III-1); 4) plasma level of dopamine decreased significantly and that of serotonin significantly increased in smokers after smoking; and 5) the number of circulating endothelial cells significantly increased after smoking, in proportion to blood level of COHb, in smokers after smoking (Fig. III-2). From these results, it is suggested that smoking might induce a prethrombotic state due to hypercoagulability, reduced fibrinolytic activity and the damaged vessel wall denuded of endothelium. Judging from above-mentioned observations smoking might facilitate the thrombus formation, from the both sides of blood and vessel wall.

A subject of environmental tobacco smoke and passive smoking has recently attracted public attention. Passive smoking refers to the involuntary exposure of nonsmokers to the combination of tobacco combustion products released by the burning cigarette (sidestream) with smoke components exhaled by the active smoker (mainstream). Mainstream smoke is the complex aerosol mixture inhaled by the smoker, filtered in the lungs, and exhaled. Sidestream smoke is the aerosol emitted directly into the surrounding air from the lit end of a smoldering tobacco product. Qualitatively, the two types of smoke share similar components, including

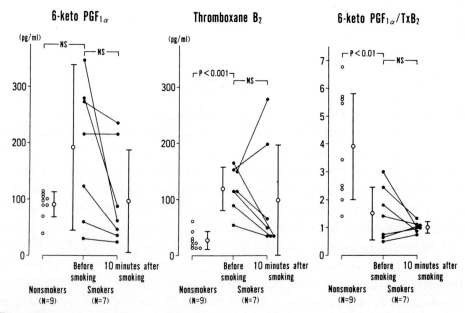

Figure III-1. 6-keto-$PGF1\alpha$ and $TXB2$ in nonsmokers and smokers before and after smoking. (From Mukaiyama H, et al. J Jap Coll Angiol 1988;28:331-8.)

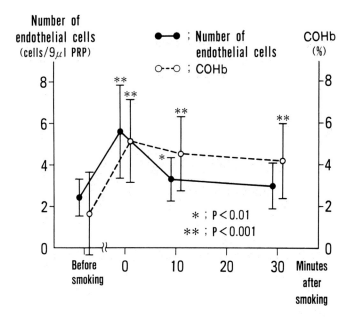

Figure III-2. Changes in number of endothelial cells and COHb in the blood by smoking (From Mukaiyama H, et al. J Jap Coll Angiol 1988; 28 : 331-8.)

oxides of nitrogen, nicotine, carbon monoxide, and various carcinogens and cocarcinogens. However, undiluted sidestream smoke has a higher pH, smaller particles, and higher concentrations of carbon monoxide, as well as many toxic and carcinogenic components that are found in mainstream smoke, including ammonia, volatile nitrosamines, certain products of nicotine decomposition, and aromatic amines. Although an estimated 85 percent of the smoke generated in an average room during cigarette smoking is composed of sidestream smoke, passive smokers are exposed to a smaller amount of smoke and a lower concentration of chemicals that have known adverse health effects than are active smokers. The quantification of a nonsmoker's exposure to environmental tobacco smoke is affected by such factors as the type of cigarette, smoking rate, room size, ventilation rates, duration of exposure, and other factors.[79]

Considerable work is being undertaken at present to identify sensitive markers with which to measure tobacco-smoke exposure in nonsmokers. The absorption markers most studied to date include carbon monoxide, thiocyanate, and cotinine. Carbon monoxide and thiocyanate are nonspecific markers of tobacco smoke exposure because they have other environmental sources, but nicotine and its major metabolite, cotinine, are specific for tobacco smoke.[80] Nicotine and cotinine have received the most attention, with cotinine becoming increasingly accepted as a short-term marker in epidemiologic studies because of its relatively long half-time (20 hours, as compared with 2 hours for nicotine), lack of susceptibility to fluctuations during smoke exposure, and capacity for noninvasive ascertainment in urine and saliva. There is a strong correlation including a dose-response relation, between urinary cotinine levels and self-reported exposure to other people's tobacco smoke,[81] including passive smoking on airline flights.[82,83] Saliva cotinine concentrations in nonsmoking schoolchildren were strongly related to the smoking habits of their parents: when neither parent smoked the mean concentration was 0.44 ng/ml, rising to 3.38 ng/ml when both parents were cigarette smokers, and mothers' smoking had a stronger influence than did fathers'[84]. Another study[85] indicated that the prevalence of a detectable salivary level of cotinine was about 35% of children whose parents did not smoke, and emphasized the need to consider exposures outsides of the home.

The mean urinary cotinine level in the smokers was 8.57 ± 0.39 µg per milligram of creatinine — significantly higher than the level in the nonsmokers (0.68 ± 0.07): urinary creatinine was also measured, and urinary cotinine excretion is expressed as micrograms per milligram of creatinine to avoid the influence of urine volume.[86] When smokers were separated according to the number of cigarettes smoked daily, the urinary cotinine values increased with increasing consumption. The urinary cotinine levels of nonsmokers who lived with smokers or worked with smokers were increased, in proportion to the degree of the exposure to the tobacco smoke. For example, nonsmokers who lived with smokers of more than 40 cigarettes per day excreted a significantly higher amount of cotinine ($1.56 + 0.57$ µg per mg of creatinine), and their cotinine levels were nearly identical to those of smokers of less than 3 cigarettes per day.[86]

Sinzinger and Kefalides[87] measured platelet sensitivity to the antiaggregatory prostaglandins (E_1, I_2, D_2) before, during, and after passive smoking in an enclosed room: the test subjects were exposed to the smoke for 15 min. Passive smoking reduced platelet sensitivity to the antiaggregatory PGs, being more severe in nonsmokers than in smokers. These epidemiological and clinical studies demonstrated that passive smoking occurred in the home, the workplaces, and the community, and called our attention to the health effects of involuntary smoking.

It remains an open question whether non-smokers will develop Buerger's disease. Someones insist that they have not seen one in non-smokers, but others state that instances of this disease have been seen in nonsmokers. The difficulty of explaining this discrepancy of opinion might be due to lack of objective evidence for real non-smokers.

Lie described a case[88] of Buerger's disease who had never smoked but had chewed tobacco for approximately 20 years, and he also reported an unusual case[89] of the disease affecting the upper extremities in a man who allegedly had discontinued smoking fifteen years earlier. Complete clinical remission in Buerger's disease during abstinence from tobacco[90] is an established fact. If nonsmokers are attacked by the disease or the disease recurs after cessation of cigarette smoking in reality, however, smoking might clear itself a false charge.

On the basis of the results that the mean urinary cotinine level in smokers was 596 ng/mg Cr, 12.4 ng/mg Cr in nonsmokers exposing to the tobacco smoke of smokers, and 6.1 ng/mg Cr in nonsmokers unexposed to the tabacco smoke (Fig. III-3, and 4), Matsushita et al.[91] regarded ones with more than 50 ng/mg Cr of urinary cotinine level as smokers; those with between 10 and 50 ng/mg Cr as passive smokers, and those with less than 10 ng/mg Cr as nonsmokers without passive smoking.

Many factors probably participate in the etiology of Buerger's disease, but it is indisputable that smoking holds the key to the solution of the question. Judging from the degree of the involuntary smoking estimated by measurement of a sensitive marker of tabacco smoke, cotinine, the health effects of the passive smoking should not be underrated. If the influence of the involuntary smoking on occurrence of Buerger's disease in nonsmokers and on recurrence of the disease after cessation of active smoking could be explicated, it would break the deadlock in studying the etiology of the disease, though a high priority for future studies is more reliable

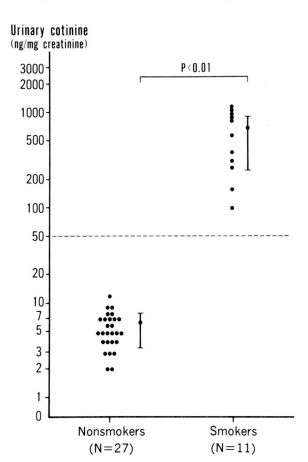

Figure III-3. Urinary cotinine excretion in nonsmokers and smokers.

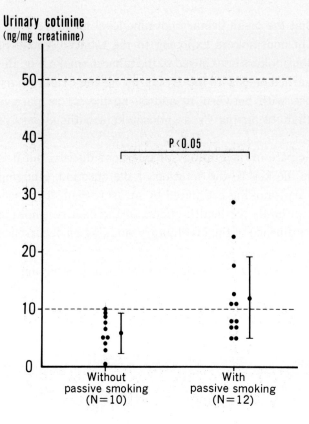

Figure III-4. Effect of passive smoking on urinary cotinine excretion in nonsmokers.

measurement of exposure to tobacco smoke in the environment, including sources other than household exposure.

REFERENCES

1. Winiwarter F.(I-7).
2. Mallory TB. Case records of the Massachusetts General Hospital. NEJ of M 1936 ; 214 : 882-4.
3. Hill GL et al.(II-19).
4. Nishikimi N et al.(II-23).
5. Haga E.(I-17).
6. Buerger L(I-34).
7. Buerger L(I-54).
8. Allen EV, Lauderdale M. Accidental transmission of thrombo-angiitis obliterans from man to man. Proc Staff Meet Mayo Clin 1936 ; 11 : 641-4.
9. Rabinowitz HM. Infectious origin of thrombo-angiitis obliterans : Experiments on the infectious origin of thromboangiitis obliterans and the isolation of a specific organism from the blood strem. Surg Gynecol Obstet 1923 ; 37 : 353-60.

10. Goodman C. Thrombo-angiitis and rickettsia-etiologic relationship. J Mt Sinai Hosp 1941; 7: 391-404.
11. Horton BT, Dorsey AHE. Experimental thrombo-angiitis obliterans: bacteriologic and pathologic studies. Arch Path Lab Med 1932; 13: 910-25.
12. Thompson KW. The relationship of the dermatomycoses to certain peripheral vascular infections. Internat Clin 1941; 2: 156-70.
13. Naide M. The causative relationship of dermatophytosis to thrombo-angiitis obliterans. Am J Med Sci 1941; 202: 822-31.
14. Bartolo M, Rulli F, Raffi S. Buerger's disease: is it a rickettsiosis? Angiology 1980; 31: 660-5.
15. Roncon A, Lecour H, Ribeiro T, Isolette A, Amélia R. The prevalence of hepatitis B makers in endarteritis obliterans in young men. Adv Vasc Surg. In: de Oliveira F ed. Proc III Internat Meeting Vasc Surg 1983; 95-115.
16. Schmidt-Weyland P. Experimentelle Untersuchungen zur Erzeugung von Gangrän und ihre Beziehungen zur Thrombo-angiitis obliterans. Klin Wschr 1932; 2: 2148-51.
17. Winternitz MC, LeCompte PM. Experimental infectious angiitis. Am J Pathol 1940; 16: 1-12.
18. Kaunitz J. Chronic endemic ergotism: its relation to thrombo-angiitis obliterans. Arch Surg 1932; 25: 1135-51.
19. Oppel WA. Die Raynaudsche Krankheit als Hyperadrenalinaemia. Arch klin Chir 1928; 149: 301-30.
20. Orban F. New trends in the treatment of thromboangeiosis (Buerger's disease) Ann Roy Coll Surg Engl 1961; 28: 69-100.
21. Durante L. Adrenal medullectomy in symdromes caused by hypersecretion of the adrenal medulla and in many conditions of the mesenchyma: results of 605 unilateral and bilateral intervention. JAMA 1954; 156: 646.
22. Kamiya K, Takao T, Hachisuka K, Narita H, Iwase M, Shionoya S, Suzuki M, Nakamura K. Adrenomedullectomy for arterial occlusive diseases. Geka 1963; 25: 1469-74 (in Japanese).
23. Iwase M. Urinary excretion of free catecholamine and 3-methoxy-4-hydroxy mandelic acid in patients with peripheral vascular disease and their levels following adrenomeduulectomy. J Nagoya Med Ass 1963; 86: 108-41(in Japanese).
24. Ono K. Sympathetic activity in patients with Buerger's disease—evaluation based on urinary excreted catecholamines—J Jap Coll Angiol 1989; 29: 381-6 (in Japanese).
25. Kunlin J, Lengua F, Testart J, Pajot A. Thromboangiosis or thromboangiitis treated by adrenalectomy and sympathectomy from 1942 to 1962: a follow-up study of 110 cases. J Cardiovasc Surg 1973; 14: 21-7.
26. Van der Stricht J. Goldstein M, Flamand JP, Belenger J. Evolution and prognosis of thromboangeitis obliterans. J Cardiovasc Surg 1973; 14: 9-16.
27. Sugihara E. Adrenocortical function in Buerger's disease: especially on urinary 17 OHCS, the amount of 17 KS excreted and its fractions. J Nagoya Med Ass 1959; 78: 1026-44 (in Japanese).
28. Kamiya K, Narita K, Okamoto H. Urinary excretion of estrogen in peripheral vascular diseases. Naibunpitotaisha 1958; 1: 130-6 (in Japanese).
29. Nakanishi E. Clinical and experimental studies on the relation between histamine content of blood and peripheral vascular diseases. J Nagoya Med Ass 1959; 78: 1103-17 (in Japanese).

30. Sakurai T. Studies on the metabolism of blood cholesterin in diseases of the peripheral blood vessels, especially in thrombophlebitis. J Nagoya Med Ass 1959 ; 77 : 1963-88 (in Japanese).
31. Yoshida F. Phospholipid metabolism in peripheral vascular disease, especially in thrombophlebitis. J Nagoya Med Ass 1959 ; 79 : 1471-98 (in Japanese).
32. Kamiya K. Buerger's disease. Vasc Dis 1964 ; 1 : 186-202.
33. de Takats G. Heparin tolerance : a test of the clotting mechanism. Surg Gynecol Obstet 1943 ; 77 : 31-9.
34. McKusick VA et al. (I-71).
35. Kinare SG, Kher YR, Sen PK. Pattern of occlusive peripheral vascular disease in India. Angiology 1976 ; 27 : 165-80.
36. Williams G. Recent view on Buerger's disease. J clin Path 1969 ; 22 : 573-8.
37. Craven JL, Cotton RC. Some hematologic differences between thromboangiitis obliterans and atherosclerosis. Angiology 1968 ; 19 : 450-9.
38. Shionoya S, Ban I. Prognostic estimation of Buerger's disease by score method. In : (II-21), pp 203-7 (in Japanese).
39. Harkavy J. Tobacco sensitiveness in thromboangiitis obliterans, migrating phlebitis and coronary artery disease. Bull New York Acad Med 1933 ; 9 : 318-28.
40. Trasoff A, Blumstein G, Marks M. The immunologic aspect of tobacco in thromboangiitis obliterans and coronary artery disease. J Allergy 1936 ; 7 : 250-3.
41. Westcott FH, Wright IS. Tobacco allergy and thromboangiitis obliterans. J Allergy 1938 ; 9 : 555-64.
42. Takahashi M. On skin tests with nicotine free extracts of tobacco in diseases of the peripheral vessels. J Nagoya Med Ass 1959 ; 78 : 30-59 (in Japanese).
43. Bollinger A, Hollmann B, Schneider E, Fontana A. Thromboangiitis obliterans : Diagnose und Therapie im Licht neuer immunologischer Befunde. Schweiz med Wschr 1979 ; 109 : 537-43.
44. Horsch AK, Horsch S, Mörl H. Beitrag zur Diagnose der Thromboangiitis obliterans (Morbus v. Winiwarter-Buerger) durch den Nachweis von Anti-Elastinantikörpern. VASA 1985 ; 14 : 5-9.
45. Trentham D, Dynesius RA, Rocklin RE, David JR. Cellular sensitivity to collagen in rheumatoid arthritis. N Engl J Med 1978 ; 299 : 327-32.
46. Adar R, Papa MZ, Halpern Z, Mozes M, Shoshan S, Sofer B, Zinger H, Dayan M, Mozes E. Cellular sensitivity to collagen in thromboangiitis obliterans. N Engl J Med 1983 ; 308 : 1113-6.
47. Smolen JS, Youngchaiyud U, Weidinger P, Kojer M, Endler AT, Mayr WR, Menzel EJ. Autoimmunological aspects of thromboangiitis obliterans (Buerger's disease). Clin Immunol Immunopathol 1978 ; 11 : 168-77.
48. Gulati SM, Madhra K, Thusoo TK, Nair SK, Saha K. Autoantibodies in thromboangiitis obliterans (Buerger's disease). Angiology 1982 ; 33 : 642-50.
49. Gulati SM, Saha K, Kant L, Thusoo TK, Prakash A. Significance of circulatory immune complexes in thromboangiitis obliterans (Buerger's disease). Angiology 1984 ; 35 : 276-81.
50. Sharma V, Agarwal V, Saha K, Gulati SM. In vitro study of cell mediated immunity against tobacco in patients with thrombo-angiitis obliterans (T.A.O.). Vasc Med 1985 ; 3 : 35-9.
51. Roncon A, Delgado L, Correia P, Torrinha JF, Serrao D, Braga A. Circulating immune complexes in Buerger's disease. J Cardiovasc Surg 1989 ; 30 : 821-5.

52. Erb W. Ueber Dysbasis angiosclerotica ("intermittierendes Hinken"). Münch med Eschr 1904; 51: 905-8.
53. Lilienthal H. Thrombo-angiitis obliterans: multiple ligation of varicose veins of the leg. Ann Surg 1914; 59: 796-9.
54. Meyer W. A further contribution to the etiology of thromboangiitis obliterans. Med Rec 1920; 97: 425-30.
55. Bruce JW, Miller JR, Hooker DR. The effect of smoking upon blood pressure and upon the volume of the hand. Am J Physiol 1909; 24: 104-16.
56. Maddock WG, Coller FA. Peripheral vaso-constriction by tobacco demonstrated by skin temperature changes. Proc Soc Exp Biol Med 1932; 29: 487-8.
57. Barker NW. Vasoconstrictor effects of tobacco smoking. Proc Staff Meet Mayo Clin 1933; 8: 284-7.
58. Wright IS, Moffat D. The effects of tobacco on the peripheral vascular system: further studies. JAMA 1934; 103: 318-23.
59. Sulzberger MB. Recent immunologic studies in hypersensitivity to tobacco. JAMA 1934; 102: 11-7.
60. Itakura M. Inflammation of blood vessels by nicotine free extracts of tobacco. J Nagoya Med Ass 1959; 80: 755-67 (in Japanese).
61. Oono H. Experimental studies on the effects of tobacco on the vascular system: histological and histochemical investigations. J Nagoya Med Ass 1960; 81: 826-45 (in Japanese).
62. Silbert S. Etiology of thromboangiitis obliterans. JAMA 1945; 129: 5-9.
63. Ohtawa T, Juji T, Kawano N, Mishima Y, Tohyama H, Ishikawa K. HL-A antigens in thromboangiitis obliterans. JAMA 1974; 230: 1128.
64. McLoughlin GA, Helsby CR, Evans CC, Chapman DM. Association of HLA-A9 and HLA-B5 with Buerger's disease. Br Med J 1976; 2: 1165-6.
65. Tanabe T, Yasuda K, Yokota A, Sugie S, Wakisaka A, Yakura H, Itakura K. HLA in patients with Buerger's disease. In: (II-21), pp 86-7 (in Japanese).
66. Mishima Y, Ohtawa T, Kawano N, Juji T, Tohyama H. HLA antigens in Buerger's disease. In: (11-21), pp 88-91 (in Japanese).
67. Takahashi M, Ozaki M, Nagano T, Sugisaki H, Tsuji T, Watakuji M, Sasaki M. Immunologic studies of Buerger's disease. In: (II-21), pp 92-5 (in Japanese).
68. Shionoya S, Matsubara J. HLA-typing in Buerger's disease. In: (II-21), pp 96-7 (in Japanese).
69. Numano F, Sasazuki T, Koyama T, Shimokado K, Takeda Y, Nishimura Y, Mutoh M. HLA in Buerger's disease. Expl clin Immunogenet 1986; 3: 195-200.
70. Ohtawa T. HLA antigens in arterial occlusive diseases in Japan. Jap J Surg 1976; 6: 1-8.
71. Theis FV, Freeland MR. Smoking and thrombo-angiitis obliterans. Ann Surg 1941; 113: 411-23.
72. Astrup P. An abnormality in the oxygen-dissociation curve of blood from patients with Buerger's disease and patients with non-specific myocarditis. Lancet 1964; 2: 1152-4.
73. Birnstingl M, Cole P, Hawkins L. Variations in oxyhaemoglobin dissociation with age, smoking, and Buerger's disease. Br J Surg 1967; 54: 615-9.
74. Ashby P, Dalby AM, Millar JHD. Smoking and platelet stickiness. Lancet 1965; 2: 158-9.
75. Astrup P, Kjeldsen K, Wanstrup J. Enhancing influence of carbon monoxide on the development of atheromatosis in cholesterol-fed rabbits. J Atheroscler Res. 1967; 7: 343-54.

76. Hess H, Frost H. Rauchen und arterielle Verschlußkrankheiten. Fortschr Med 1968 ; 86 : 841-3.
77. Wald N, Howard S, Smith PG, Kjeldsen K. Association between atherosclerotic diseases and carboxyhaemoglobin levels in tobacco smokers. Br Med J 1973 ; 1 : 761-5.
78. Mukaiyama H, Matsumoto T, Shionoya S, Asai M. Effects of cigarette smoking on platelet MAO activity, coagulation-fibrinolysis, plasma levels of prostaglandins, catecholamines and serotonin, and circulating endothelial cell counts. J Jap Coll Angiol 1988 ; 28 : 331-8 (in Japanese).
79. Fielding JE, Phenow KJ. Health effects of involuntary smoking. N Engl J Med 1988 ; 319 : 1452-60.
80. Benowitz NL, Kuyt F, Jacob P III, Jones RT, Osman AL. Cotinine disposition and effects. Clin Pharmacol Ther 1983 ; 34 : 604-11.
81. Wald NJ, Boreham J, Bailey A, Ritchie C, Haddow JE, Knight G. Urinary cotinine as marker of breathing other people's tobacco smoke. Lancet 1984 ; 1 : 230-1.
82. Foliart D, Benowitz NL, Becker CE. Passive absorption of nicotine in airline flight attendants. N Engl J Med 1983 ; 308 : 1105.
83. Mattson ME, Boyd G, Byar D, Brown C, Callahan JF, Corle D, Cullen JW, Greenblatt J, Haley NJ, Hammond SK, Lewtas J, Reeves W. Passive smoking on commercial airline flights. JAMA 1989 ; 261 : 867-72.
84. Jarvis MJ, Russell MAH, Feyerabend C, Eiser JR, Morgan M, Gammage P, Gray EM. Passive exposure to tobacco smoke : saliva cotinine concentration in a representative population sample of non-smoking schoolchildren. Br Med J 1985 ; 291 : 927-9.
85. Coultas DB, Howard CA, Peake GT, Skipper BJ, Samet JM. Salivary cotinine levels and involuntary tobacco smoke exposure in children and adults in New Mexico. Am Rew Respir Dis 1987 ; 136 : 305-9.
86. Matsukura S, Taminato T, Kitano N, Seino Y, Hamada H, Uchihashi M, Nakajima H, Hirata Y. Effects of environmental tobacco smoke on urinary cotinine excretion in nonsmokers : evidence for passive smoking. N Engl J Med 1984 ; 311 : 828-32.
87. Sinzinger H, Kefalides A. Passive smoking severely decreases platelet sensitivity to antiaggregatory prostaglandins. Lancet 1982 ; 2 : 392-3.
88. Lie JT. Thromboangiitis obliterans (Buerger's disease) and smokeless tobacco. Arthritis and Rheumatism 1988 ; 31 : 812-3.
89. Lie JT. Thromboangiitis obliterans (Buerger's disease) in an elderly man after cessation of cigarette smoking—a case report. Angiology 1987 ; 38 : 864-6.
90. Gifford RW, Hines EA. Complete clinical remission in thromboangiitis obliterans during abstinence from tobacco : report of case. Proc Staff Meet Mayo Clin 1951 ; 26 : 241-5.
91. Matsushita M, Shionoya S, Matsumoto T. An investigation of active and passive smoking in female patients with Buerger's disease. In : Mishima Y, ed. Annual Report of the Research Committee on Systemic Vascular Disorder of the Ministry of Health and Welfare of Japan, 1990, pp 77-79 (in Japanese).

CHAPTER IV
PATHOLOGY

Buerger's disease is an inflammatory occlusive disease primarily involving small and medium-sized arteries and veins of the extremity. Arguments concerning the status of Buerger's disease as a distinct entity center on the specificity of the acute lesion.[1,2,3] Understanding of the pathologic arterial changes in Buerger's disease has been handicapped by the relative paucity of anatomic material available for study, particularly from acute stage. However, in superficial arteries, such as the radial or the posterior tibial artery, an acute lesion is not uncommomly recognized, for the skin over the artery reddens and subsequently darkens or blackens.[4] To many, this interesting appearance implies a marked periarterial inflammation. Removed at a time when the area is painful and tender and the pulse is reduced or absent, the specimens shows the characteristics of the acute lesion, as described below.

Acute stage

Macroscopically, the occluded artery appears to be tense or swollen and the periarterial tissue edematous, but no suppurative pus or exudate is seen. Mobilizing the affected artery from the surrounding tissue is not so difficult. The occluded segment is definitely indurated due to occluding thrombus but not brittle. The lumen is obstructed with fresh thrombus, and the degree of the adhesion of the thrombus to the inner surface of the vessel wall is various.

  Microscopically, a focal inflammation, consisting of multinucleated giant cells, epithelioid cells, and leukocytes, in the form of microabscess, is frequently observed, like Buerger described[1] (Fig. IV-1,2,3 and 4). Careful examination of serial sections not infrequently reveals phagocytic giant cells in the cellular thrombus: the giant cells exist mainly in the periphery of the thrombus. Intimal cells proliferate slightly, and the giant cell foci and the proliferated intimal cells seem to be near related. The internal elastic membrane remains essentially intact, though it is sometimes partially destroyed. Inflammatory cells, mainly lymphocytes and fibroblasts, infiltrate throughout the media and adventitia, but no necrotizing lesions are found in the media.[5] Unlike in the thrombus, no microabscess is seen in the media and adventitia.

  The granulomatous reaction with giant cells lends a characteristic apperance to

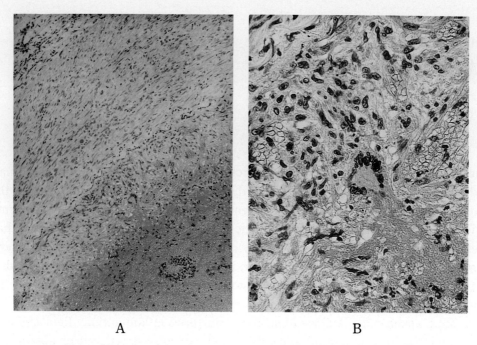

Figure IV-1. Photomicrographs of acute lesion in the brachial artery of a 34-year-old man with Buerger's disease. A : Left upper corner is the media and adventitia, and right lower corner is the lumen. There are a giant cell and collection of leukocytes in the periphery of the organizing thrombus.(Hematoxylin and eosin stain; original magnification ×125.) (From Shionoya S, et al. Surgery 1974 ; 75 : 695-700.) B : Enlargement of a giant cell contiguous to agglomerated fibrins.(Hematoxylin and eosin stain;original magnification ×400.)

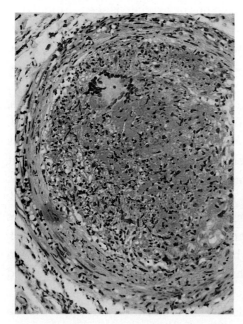

Figure IV-2. Photomicrograph of acute lesion in a small muscular branch artery in the left leg of a 41-year-old man with Buerger's disease. There is a remarkable inflammatory cell infiltration in the vessel wall and the thrombus, in which a multinucleate giant cell is seen. (Hematoxylin and eosin stain;original magnification ×200.) (From Shionoya S. Pathologia et Microbiologia 1975 ; 43 : 163-6.)

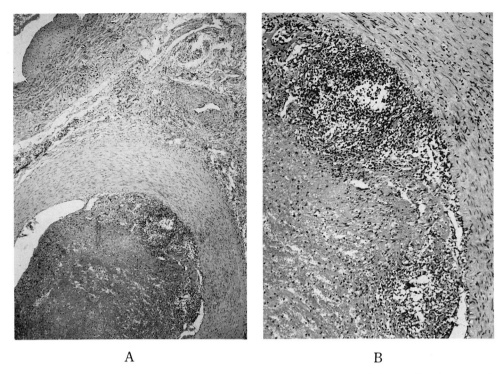

A B

Figure IV-3. Photomicrographs of acute lesion in a branch artery of the popliteal artery of a 41-year-old man with Buerger's disease. A : Microabscesses with giant cells are seen in the periphery of the thrombus, and the accompanying vein (left upper corner) shows a localized intimal thickening and a moderate inflammatory cell infiltration throught the vessel wall. (Hematoxylin and eosin stain ; original magnification ×100.) B : Enlargement of the microabscesses with giant cells. (Hematoxylin and eosin stain ; original magnification ×200.) (From Shionoya S. World J Surg 1983 ; 7 : 544-51.)

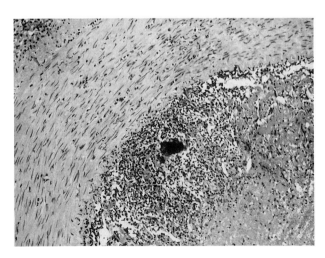

Figure IV-4. Photomicrograph of acute lesion in a branch artery of the popliteal artery of a 41-year-old man with Buerger's disease. Microabscess with multinucleate giant cells is located in the periphery of the thrombus. There is an inflammatory cell infiltration throughout the vessel wall. (Hematoxylin and eosin stain ; original magnification ×200.)

the thrombotic lesion of Buerger's disease at the acute stage[2,3,4]; it is characteristic in that this picture is never seen in thrombi associated with arteriosclerosis obliterans or simple thrombosis. Two conditions are necessary for the presence of phagocytic giant cells in a thrombus: 1) the existence of slightly soluble materials, such as fibrin; and 2) local mesenchymal cell activation.[6] As the giant cells are near related fibrin in the thrombus, the multinucleated giant cells might be formed to phagocytose the slightly soluble fibrins. In Buerger's disease, there seems no fibrinolytic activation equivalent to an increase in fibrinogen.[7]

In the vascular lesion of Buerger's disease, three types of multinucleated giant cells are recognized: 1) in the thrombus; 2) around the internal elastic membrane, and 3) in the media. The giant cells around the internal elastic membrane are elasticophatic in nature for the fragments of the internal elastic membrane, and are not specific for Buerger's disease because the elasticophagic giant cells are more frequently seen in giant cell arteriitis and Takayasu arteriitis than in Buerger's disease (Fig. IV-5). In the media, a probably myogenic giant cell is rarely noticed in the granulation tissue following destructive muscle lesions in the media: this type of giant cell is rather exceptional[8](Fig. IV-6). Among the three types of giant cell, that in the periphery of the thrombus is most characteristic of the disease. Although it is difficult to define a period of time of the acute stage, these typical pathohistologic findings might be observed within a few months after the onset of the thrombotic occlusion.

Determining where the initial vascular lesion occurs in the disease remains an unsolved problem. An initial damage in the endothelium before a thrombus formation might be based on a mere conjecture. Considering that an etiologic agent which provokes the primary lesion in the vessel wall is also effective in calling forth the coagulation of the blood, as Buerger[1] said, the actual condition of "an initial

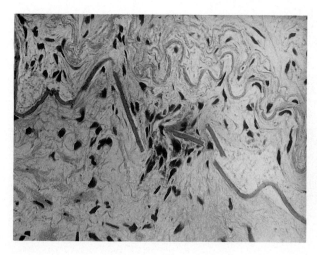

Figrure IV-5. Photomicrograph of a elasticophgic giant cell contiguous to a fragment of the internal elastic lamina in the popliteal artery of a 38-year-old man with Buerger's disease. (Hematoxylin and eosin stain; original magnification ×400.)

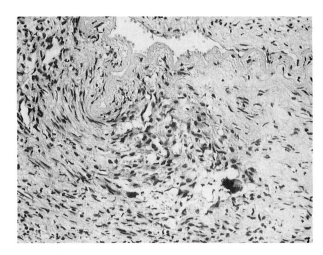

Figure IV-6. Photomicrograph of a probably myogenic giant cell adjacent to disintegrated muscle cells in the media of the superficial femoral artery of a 43-year-old man with Buerger's disease. (Hematoxylin and eosin stain; original magnification ×200.) (From Shionoya S. Pathologia et Microbiologia 1975; 43: 163-6.)

vascular lesion" might be a mere guesswork. Whether the initial vascular lesion of Buerger's disease is primarily thrombotic or primarily inflammatory has never been satisfactorily settled and probably never will[3], in the strict sense of the word.

The initial lesion of Buerger's disease or arteriosclerosis might be triggered by an interaction between the blood and the intima. In the former, however, the lumen is promptly occluded with thrombus without remodeling of the artery wall; in the latter, there is a remarkable alteration of the vessel wall due to a defect in removal of plasma constituents from the vessel, or an increase in insudation of plasma constituents, i.e., a disturbance of perfusion in the vessel wall.[9]

Intermediate stage

The inflammatory reaction throughout the vessel reduces intensity, and the thrombus becomes organized with formation of new vessels. In the thrombus, the microabscess usually disappears, but the giant cells sometimes persist (Fig. IV-7). Persistence of giant cells might be dependent on the local vascularity, namely, vascularization, in the same way as in the course of giant cells in tuberculous or syphilitic lesions.[10]

Chronic stage

Macroscopically, the occluded artery appears to be contracted and indurated. The artery and accompanying veins may be bound into a rather firm cord so that they can be separated only with difficulty.

Microscopically, the advanced lesion is characterized by a marked recanalization of the thrombus, a fibrous thickening of the intima and increased fibrous tissue

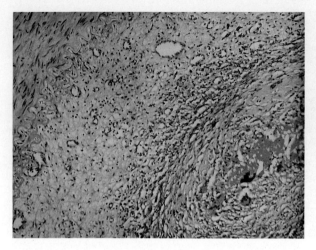

Figure IV-7. Photomicrograph of intermediate lesion in the femoral artery of a 27-year-old man with Buerger's disease. Right lower corner is the lumen, and giant cells remain near the fibrin nets in the well-organized thrombus. Left upper corner is the media and adventitia, and new vessels are formed in the media. (Hematoxylin and eosin stain; original magnification × 125.)

in the media and adventitia. While the internal elastic membrane is partially destroyed or fragmented, the general architecture of the vessel wall is well preserved (Fig. IV-8). Although blood pigments and remnants of the inflammatory reaction remain in the thrombus, they gradually disappear, and the vascular lesions proceed to healed stage. The thrombus and the vessel wall are well recanalized.

Characteristic of the metamorphosis of the obstructive clot at the acute stage is the absence of elastic tissue, and also the absence of the excessive reduplication of the internal elastic layer so characteristic of arteriosclerotic processes. As the canalizing vessels become older, however, new formed ealstic tissue disposes itself about them in concentric layers, and a centrally or eccentrically placed recanalized channel that crowds the organized clot into the crescentic mass on the lateral might be mistaken for endarteritis obliterans[1]. As the large recanalizing lumina suggest

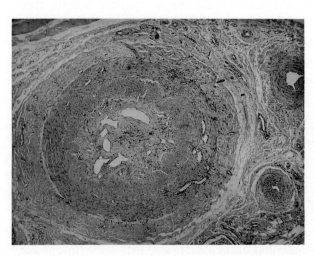

Figure IV-8. Photomicrograph of chronic lesion in the radial artery of a 54-year-old man with Buerger's disease (onset at the age of 44 years). The thrombus and the vessel wall are well recanalized, and general architecture of the vessel wall is preserved. (Hematoxylin and eosin stain;original magnification ×50.) (From Shionoya S. World J Surg 1983 ; 7 : 544-51.)

endarteritis obliterans rather than thromboangiitis obliterans, no wonder then that these lesions should so long have been misinterpreted.

Site of the initial lesion

Where does an incipient lesion of Buerger's disease originate in? As above described, it is impossible to define morphologically a lesion as the initial pathologic feature, because the initial stage of damage of the endothelium or thrombus formation might be similar, notwithstanding etiological factors for circulatory disturbances are diverse.

It is agreed that the initial lesion begins in the peripheral small vessels. Buerger[1] said that it probably might not originate in the capillaries or smallest arterioles, but begin in branches of moderate size. Although he showed no convincing evidence for his idea, it seems to be true that the initial obstructive lesion does not originate in the capillary vessels under the epidermis of the skin, judging from that a localized skin necrosis is not an initial symptom in Buerger's disease. Drawing an inference from angiograms obtained in symptomatic and asymptomatic affected limbs of patients with Buerger's disease, the disease seems to commence in the digital, metatarsal, tarsal, calcaneal, arcuate, and arcus plantaris arteries or their branches in the lower extremity: it begins in the digital, metatarsal and palmar arch arteries or their branches in the upper extremity. As the process may pass unnoticed until the occlusive lesions involve the crural arteries in the majority of the affected lower extremity, no anatomical material for study is available at the initial stage. Even at the time when the occlusive lesions reach the forearm arteries, ischemic symptoms of the fingers are infrequently recognized.

Besides the small vessels of the most peripheral region of the extremities, the disease might originate in the branch arteries in the proximal area, namely, intramuscular arteries or small branches of the iliofemoropopliteal segment, independent of the lesions in the toe and foot vessels. Some patients with the patent popliteal and posterior tibial arteries have claudication in the calf, which must be attributed to obstruction of the muscular branches of the main vessels,[11] though biopsy of the calf muscle was of no advantage to the histologic investigation of the disease.[5] The branches of the iliac arteries and the intramuscular vessels in the calf and thigh might be protected more favorably from traumatic injury, compared with the superficial vessels.

Interpretation of pathologic findings

As gross pathology of Buerger's disease, Buerger[1] emphasized three findings: 1) thrombotic occlusion; 2) periarteritis; and 3) arteriosclerosis.

Arteriosclerotic thickening of the vessel wall is never pronounced in those rare instances in which the patient has suffered from the disease for many years and has reached the latter part of the fourth decade: a very slight degree of whitening or thickening of the intima is noted here and there in the patent portions of the vessels as a rule, and small atheromatous patches are present in a very few cases. It deserves more attention that he thought the two diseases might be associated, based on the fact of the coexistence of thromboangiitic and arterieoscleoric lesions in the affected arteries with Buerger's disease. It is a natural consequence that he was interested in the periaretritis as an evidence that justifies his "inflammation" theory.

Microscopically, the granulomatous reaction with giant cells lends a characteristic appearance to the thrombotic lesion of the disease. Buerger[1] laid stress on "purulent foci," foci of leukocytes, in the occluding thrombus: the existence of the miliary abscess favored the assumtion that some specific agent was responsible for the disease. The perulent foci were regarded as precursor of giant cell foci, and such aggregation of leukocytes was considered to owe its existence to immigration of cells by way of the media. According to him,[2] angioblasts proliferate at the periphery of purulent foci, and as the leukocytes disintegrate and the toxic products are absorbed, the atypical distorted angioblasts—now looking like typical epithelioid cells—together with giant cells, gradually replace the leukocytes from periphery toward the center, a picture resulting that closely resembles miliary tubercles: angioblasts approach a purulent focus to organize the thrombus, but some angioblasts become impotent and distorted, as it were, at the periphery of purulent focus, and unable to enter the leukocytic area at all, others pass in for a short distance, or proliferate in loco into a giant cell. In a word, the giant cells are regarded as abortive attempts on the part of the angioblasts to produce new vessels.[2]

However, we will not take up the histogenesis of the giant cell further, but, in any case, existence of foreign bodies which a phagocytosis is indispensable to and a mesenchymal cell activation in loco are necessary for the occurrence of the giant cells, phagocytic in nature. Solubility of fibrin in the thrombus depends on an intrathrombotic fibrinolytic activity, and the fibrin might become a slightly soluble foreign body-like material in case of a decreased local fibrinolytic activity. Ooneda[12] revealed a fibrinlike material in a giant cell in the thrombus in the femoral artery of a patient with Buerger's disease. While the affected vessels with Buerger's disease are provided with these prerequite conditions, no giant cell foci could be formed in the occluding thrombus due to arteriosclerosis obliterans or simple arterial thrombosis, probably because of lack of either of the two factors.

In short, the lesions in Buerger's disease are changeable in chronological order; from an acute inflammatory lesion with fresh thrombosis, via the stage of organization, to a chronic lesion without typical granulomatous giant cell reaction in the thrombus. But it took only a very short time for the process of organization of the thrombus to metamorphose these purulent area, and that is why many of biopsies were disappointing.

Skip lesion

In the arteriograms of patients with Buerger's disease, the arteries proximal to the occlusions appear to be smooth and normal as a rule. However, the stenosis, dilatation or irregularity of the main patent artery, principally of the femoropopliteal segment, is sometimes recognized; this lesion corresponds to the intimal thickening described as arteriosclerotic lesion.

This skip lesion is considered an early stage in the proximal progression of the inflammatory process and presages occlusion of the large vessel. The preexisting lesion in the femoropopliteal segment favors occurrence of the thrombotic occlusion, namely, skip progression. What is that pathogenesis of the skip lesion?

Takao and his colleagues[13] found skip occlusion in 26 of 137 limbs with Buerger's disease: the site of the skip lesion was the femoral artery in 12 cases and the popliteal artery in 14. Biopsy[14] of the 18 skip lesions showed the typical histologic feature as Buerger's disease, including giant cells, round cell infiltration, proliferation of new vessels and partial destruction of the elastic membrane, and the artery contiguous to the prominant inflammatory focus was occluded with simple thrombosis. Based on the finding that the occlusion of the main arteries at early stage of the disease was recognized around the ankle and the wrist joint, they attributed the cause of the skip lesion to the repeated traumatic injury near the hip-and the knee joint and Hunter's canal.

The same agent that elicits the vascular inflammation in the distal small vessels may provoke a parietal thrombus in the medium-sized or large artery, which results in various intimal changes as a result of the inflammatory lesions of the vessel, instead of the occluding thrombus[15]. If the thromboangiitis process recurs at the precursory lesion, the lumen will be occluded with a thrombus (Fig. IV-9 and 10). Elucidation of the pathogenesis of the skip lesion in the main artery is a topic for further discussion.

There are two patterns of progression of the arterial occlusion in Buerger's disease: continuous progression and skip one[16]. At the early stage, the lesions are distinctly focal or segmental, and apparently normal segments of vessels are situated between diseased segments. When the patent segment among the diseased arteies becomes affected, the finished feature is a diffused occlusive lesion. It is difficult to find the origin of a fire from the ruins of a fire.

In case of the skip occlusion in the popliteal artery, serial section showed an older process in its branch artery, though the popliteal artery was occluded with a

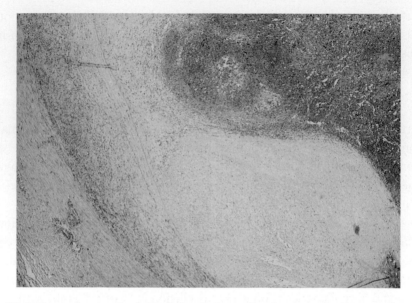

Figure IV-9. Photomicrograph of skip lesion in the popliteal artery of a 41-year-old man with Buerger's disease. Right upper corner is the lumen, and microabscesses with giant cells in the periphery of the fresh thrombus formed on the thickened intima (skip lesion). Left lower corner is the media and adventitia which are infiltrated with inflammatory cells. (Hematoxylin and eosin stain; original magnification ×95.)

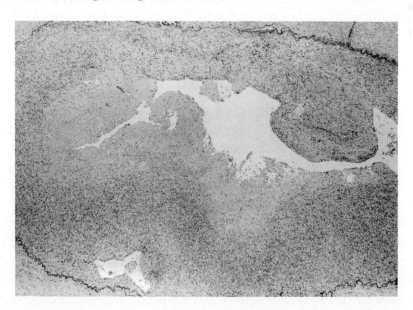

Figure IV-10. Photomicrograph of skip lesion in the popliteal artery of a 29-year-old man with Buerger's disease. The lumen is occluded with fresh thrombus on the thickened intima (skip lesion). (Elastic van Gieson stain; original magnification ×40.) (From Shionoya S, et al. Heidrich H. ed. Thromboangiitis obliterans Morbus Winiwarter-Buerger. Georg Thieme, 1988, pp 42-5.)

fresh thrombus: the more distally the branch was examined, the more the lesion was older. Judging from the finding, the skip lesion in the popliteal artery might be caused by ascending progression of the occlusive process in the branch artery (Fig. IV-11 and 12). In the sural artery, a branch vessel of the popliteal artery, the skip lesion is also observed (Fig. IV-13).

In an advanced case with Buerger's disease, segmental occlusions were seen in the inferior gluteal artery and the obturator artery, in addition to obstruction of the superficial and deep femoral arteries, and the branch artery of the obturator artery showed the healed stage of thromboangiitis obliterans (Fig. IV-14). Therefore, the disease might occur in the branch vessels of the iliac artery, and the skip lesion of the pelvic main arteries might owe its cause to such an ascending progression of the process in the branch vessels, as the disease originates in the toe and foot vessels and it then ascends in the leg.

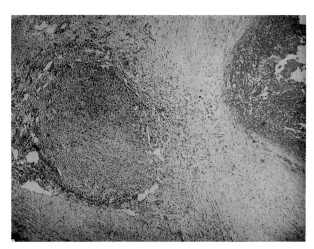

Figure IV-11. Photomicrograph of new and old lesions in the popliteal artery (on the right) and its branch artery (on the left) of a 34-year-old man with Buerger's disease. The former is occluded with fresh thrombus, and the latter is obstructed with organizing thrombus. The branch artery shows more advanced lesion than the main artery (Hematoxylin and eosin stain; original magnification ×50.) (From Shionoya S. et al. Surgery 1974; 75: 695-700.)

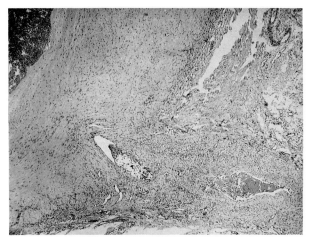

Figure IV-12. Photomicrograph of new and old lesions in the popliteal artery (on the left upper corner) and its branch artery (on the right lower corner) of a 41-year-old man with Buerger's disease. The former is occluded with fresh thrombus, and the latter is obstructed with organizing thrombus containing a giant cell. (Hematoxylin and eosin stain; original magnification ×50.) (From Shionoya S. VASA 1978; 7: 253-7.)

IV PATHOLOGY

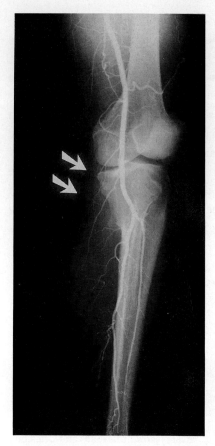

Figure IV-13. Femoral arteriogram of a 49-year-old man with Buerger's disease. The sural aretry is segmentally occluded (arrows). (From Shionoya S. VASA 1978 ; 7 : 253-7.)

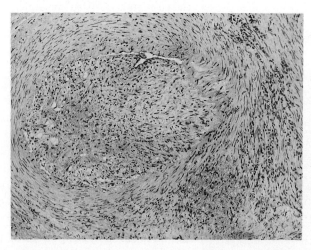

Figure IV-14. Photomicrograph of a branch artery of the obturatory artery of a 30-year-old man with Buerger's disease. The lumen is occluded with organizing thrombus. Inflammatory cell infiltration and hemorrhage are seen in the media. (Hematoxylin and eosin stain;original magnification ×100.) (From Shionoya S. et al. J Cardiovasc Surg 1978 ; 19 : 69-76.)

Lesions outside the extremities

Buerger[17] observed what he termed the acute lesion of the disease in the territories other than the vessels of the extremities, namely, in the spermatic artery, in the veins of the spermatic cord; and old lesions in one of the branches of the gastric artery in a case of ulcer of the stomach. Because no macroscopic or microscopic feature about the lesions was demonstrated in his paper, we do not know what it really was. While Buerger himself reported three autopsy cases with the disease, whose death causes were coronary artery disease or thrombosis of the aorta and its main braches, only marked lesions of atherosclerosis and thrombosis were revealed and there was no evidence of the identical lesion with thromboangiitis obliterans in the vessels examined.

In 1932 Jäger[18] reported four autopsy cases with Buerger's disease, and he concluded that the disease was not localized in the arteries of the extremities, but involved the generalized arterial system. According to him, the pathology of the disease might rest on a specific reaction of the intima to various damages; the reaction in the large arteries was similar to recurrent thromboendocarditis; the medium-sized arteries showed fibrin thrombosis with organization including giant cell; and in the small arteries the feature was similar to periarteritis nodosa. He thought the disease bore a close parallel to rheumatic vascular damage and periarteritis nodosa.

Since then, there are a number of reports of "generalized" Buerger's disease, namely, of involvement of the cerebral,[19-21] coronary,[22,23] visceral[24,25] and large elastic arteries.[26,27] In 1940 Hausner and Allen[28] estimated the incidence of disease of the coronary arteries in Buerger's disease at 5.6 per cent in Mayo series; in 1952 Lippmann[29] estimated the overall incidence of cerebrovascular complications in the disease in the literatures at less than 0.5 per cent. In 1976 Ooneda and Shinkai[30] reported a case of generalized Buerger's disease among about 130,000 autopsy cases from 1966 to 1971 in Japan.

In 1957 Asang and Mittelmeier[31] reported 75 autopsy cases with generalized Buerger's disease, in München-Schwabing Hospital, from 1948 through 1955. The incidence of the lesion in the organs was as follows: 96% in heart, 90% in aorta, 86% in kidney, 65% in lower extremity, 64% in spleen, 56% in intestine, 38% in liver, 32% in cerebrum, 21% in stomach and duodenum, 15% in pancreas, and 15% in lung.

The death causes were due to intestine (infaction or ileus) in 28%; kidney (uremia, hypertension or cerebral bleeding) in 22%; heart (coronary thrombosis, myocardial degeneration) in 18%; cerebrum (infarction) in 13%; pancreas (necrosis or apoplexy) in 6%; lung (right ventricle failure) in 6%, and aorta (thrombosis of rupture) in 6%. Their clinical features were completely different from those in our series, and they insisted that the name "thromboangiitis obliterans" should be discarded and "endangiitis obliterans" should be adopted, because thrombus formation was a secondary phenomenon and proliferation of the intima might play an important role in the pathogensis. According to them, proliferation of the intimal (subendothelial) cells be regarded as inflammation of the intima, a tissue lacking in capillary : they considered proliferation of the intimal mesenchymal cells as an inflammatory granulation tissue without capillary. Apart from the question of approving a only productive cellular reaction from the beginning to the end of an inflammation, their definition of the vascular inflammation seems to have no authority, because the intimal cells proliferate under various hemodynamic changes, in addition to exogenous or endogenous stress.[32]

The majority of the occlusive lesions outside of the extremities were interpreted as arteriosclerotic in nature. The question arises as to whether the arteriosclerosis of the visceral arteries is a coincidental occurrence in no way related to Buerger's disease, whether the sclerotic lesion of the visceral arteries is merely a different stage (end stage) of thromboangiitis obliterans, or whether the visceral artery sclerosis develops as an entirely different entity on the basis of Buerger's disease.

It is obvious that in acute and chronic stages characteristic differences exist between Buerger's disease and arteriosclerosis. The region of the organized thrombus in the former is almost completely devoid of elastic tissue, wheares elastic lamellas are found in arteriosclerotic thickening of the intima : the reduplication of the internal elastic membrane is also characteristic of the latter disease. However, as Buerger[1] mentioned, where the lesion of thromboangiitis obliterans was of long duration, secondary thickening of the intima and proliferation of elastic fibres around the recanalized vessels took place : changes which in their earlier stages were specific for the disease became less and less characteristic, and only fibrosis and hyalinization remained. These lesions apparently formed the basis of arteriosclerosis. Therefore, it is quite possible that true arteriosclerosis developed secondary on the primarily diseased vessel with Buerger's disease, as arteriosclerotic lesions develop secondarily on a primary syphilitic arteritis. In other words, a primary inflammatory lesion of the artery may be at least one factor in the causation of arteriosclerosis.

Doerr[33] classified modes of progression of arteriosclerosis into four types : 1) physio-sclerosis ; 2) marked incorporation of fibrin-components and microthrombi ; 3) atherosclerosis due to impaired perfusion of blood-components and fat-phanecrosis ; and 4) monoclonal cellular plaques. The former three types belong to "benign" one, and the "benign" type of arteriosclerosis is characterized by longitudinal edema at the intima-media-junction in the aorta up to 30 cm of length, wheares the last type is attached to "malignant" one, and it shows focal-circumscribed plaque which may be subject to secondary changes : the "malignant" type is characterized by disseminated intimal proliferation, edema rich in proteoglycan, and necrosis.

According to him,[34] arteriosclerosis does not begin focally, but the most common mode of arteriosclerosis is generalized with extensive edema within the deep intimal layers, contrary to a general concept of arteriosclerosis. The second type has been described under the name "inflammatory arteriosclerosis" in the German-speaking world, and has been sometimes confused with "endarteritis obliterans." While the first, second, and third types are caused by a disturbance of plasma perfusion, the fourth one is connected with cellular proliferation: the second and fourth types depend on the basis of an inflammatory mechanism for their origin, from the phenomenologic standpoint of view. The fourth type is mainly recognized in the coronary artery, and it may occur in the second or third decade of life. One of the most important causes of the sudden death in the younger generation is attributed to this type (presenile arteriosclerosis; arteriitis stenosans coronariae or coronary Buerger's disease[35]): hypoxia might bring the cellular proliferation of the intima to edematous necrosis of the tissue.

Reviewing the reports on Buerger's disease of the coronary artery, the patients afflicted with the disease of the peripheral vessels occasionally revealed cardiac symptoms and died mostly from acute cardiac failure. The pathology of the occlusive lesion of the coronary artery was deemed to belong to the fourth type of mode of progression of arteriosclerosis by Doerr. Arteriosclerosis is not a nosologic entity. It is a complex of morphological fingdings, which is the result of various constitutional changes and exogeneous disturbances.[34] The idenitfication of the early stages of arteriosclerosis is the key for the understanding of its morphogenesis. Arteriosclerosis is not only the response of the arterial wall to a series of changes in general metabolism and certainly not simply a response to changes in the vessel-wall-metabolism. From this point of view, there are different patterns of arteriosclerosis with different initial changes, and it is no wonder that arteriosclerotic lesions associated with ageing manifest themselves in the visceral vessels in patients who suffered from Buerger's disease in their younger days.

Venous involvement

Although attention has been riveted to venous involvement in Buerger's disease for a long time,[36] the site and extent of the occlusive lesions and the incidence of involvement in the venous system remains unknown. While the accompanying veins are frequently afflicted with the inflammatory process and adhered to the arteries, a full detail of the morbid state is not given yet. There are few venographic studies[37] available, because the venous involvement brings about no practically noticeable disturbance of venous return as a rule. Revascularization of the ischemic limbs with the disease was tried through the venous route by arteriovenous anastomosis at the beginning of this century. Buerger aroused attention to the patency of the superficial and deep veins of the lower extremity in case of arteriovenous anastomosis as a cure for the ischemic limb, because he found obliteration of the deep veins in seven of 19 amputated limbs with the disease.[38]

It is generally said that the pathohistologic feature of the affected deep veins is identical with that of the arteries. However, very few studies went into details of the problem for the above described reason. Thrombophlebitis migrans is a recurring migratory phlebitis that usually affects segments of superficial peripheral veins, more frequently in the leg and foot than in the upper extremity. Buerger[36] emphasized the association of migrating thrombophlebitis with the disease, and he concluded that we were dealing with one and the same disease, because of sufficient resemblance between the histopathology of the lesion of the deep and that of the superficial vessels. Although the thrombophlebitis migrans is a representative feature of inflammatory character of Buerger's disease, the incidence of the migrating phlebitis was not 100 per cent.

At acute stage, the media, adventitia and perivascular tissue of the vein are infiltrated with inflammatory cells and the lumen of the vessel is completely filled with red clot, in the periphery of which larger or smaller foci of leukocytes (purulent foci) begin to form and giant cell foci also develop[36]. However, even in the case of migrating phlebitis associated with Buerger's disease, it is not an easy matter to produce material in the proper stage of the disease. It is seldom that the patient will consult us at the very onset of the phlebitis, and that is why many of biopsies were disappointing, yielding lesions already in the stage of healing and connective tissue organization. In the pathohistologic study on materials harvested from 7 patients with recurring superficial thrombophlebitis (Buerger's disease in 4, idiopathic in 3), no difference was noticed in histologic features between patients with disease and patients without arterial occlusion.[39]

Although Buerger emphasized the association of thrombophlebitis migrans and thromboangiitis obliterans and the necessity of examining patients who have thrombophlebitis migrans for existent evidence of arterial disease and of watching for future development of arterial lesions, there were many reports on cases of superficial thrombophlebitis migrans without evidence of arterial disease. In 1905 Briggs[40] stated that there was a disease which had to be classified as "idiopathic recurrent thrombophlebitis," and the condition was primarily phlebosclerosis resulting from an anatomic constitutional fault. Subsequently a number of such cases have been reported[41-45] as instances of "phlebitis migrans" or "thrombophlebitis migrans," which is called saltans[46] also, but it has never had a clearcut definition.

While these cases of idiopathic thrombophlebitis were divided into two groups according to whether there were multiple episodes (recurrent) or only one, it is possible that some of the patients who had a single episode of thrombophlebitis will have recurrences in the future, and it is recognized that the interval between episodes in some cases of the recurrent type is rather long.[47] In 1936 Barker[47] reviewed 79 cases with idiopathic or primary thrombophlebitis in his series: recurrent in 40 cases, and single in 39. The former involved chiefly small and midium-sized veins and occurred most commonly among young and middle-aged males; the latter affected medium-sized and large veins and occurred as a single episode without particular preponderance as to age or sex. Recurrent idiopathic thrombophlebitis was histopathologically similar to thromboangiitis obliterans. Judging from the clinical course, the latter type occurred as deep vein thrombosis without evident etiologic factors as operation, trauma or infection. In 1949 Gerber and Mendlowitz[48] reported six autopsy cases of visceral thrombophlebitis migrans: venous thrombosis was seen in the central nervous system, lung, heart, liver, spleen, kidney, adrenal gland, or intestine. Considering the fatal clinical course, the thrombophlebitis of this type should be named as malignant thrombophlebitis. As no evidence of arterial involvement was found in all the cases, these patients seemed to belong to another category and have no relation to Buerger's disease.

Taking some cases of Buerger's disease who died of thrombosis of the mesenteric vessels into consideration, however, visceral thrombophlebitis might deserve attention: Baehr and Klemperer[49] reported recurrent portal and splenic vein thrombosis with death due to mesenteric vein thrombosis in a male with a long history of Buerger's disease. Sakaguchi and his colleagues[50] found no significant difference in blood coagulation, fibrinolytic activity, immunological reaction and complements between patients of Buerger's disease with phlebitis migrans and those without phlebitis migrans. Generally speaking, in migratory thrombophlebitis associated with Buerger's disease, the vein involvement is usually peripheral and superficial; the visceral veins are spared.

Nerve lesions

Although the most important manifestation of Buerger's disease is a constant and distressing pain, Buerger thought the nerve lesions were secondary, apparently dependent upon the fibrotic perivascular changes: considerable connective tissue proliferation around the nerve bundles, thickening of the perineurium, and even atrophy of nerve fibers wherever the periarteritis was marked and where the nerves were intimately connected with the vessels.[1]

In a histopathologic study of the peripheral nerves (the anterior and posterior tibia nerves and the popliteal nerve) in a series of 20 amputated limbs with Buerger's disease, Barker[51] found various combinations of wallerian degeneration, fibrosis, edema, atrophy, lymphocytic infiltration, inflammation and thrombosis of the vasa vasorum in all but one case. He attributed the invalidity of surgical section of the peripheral nerve trunks to the progression of wallerian degeneration proximal to the level of surgical section of the nerves. These significant changes in the nerves are a result of severe ischemia and pain due to ischemic neuritis will not be immediately relieved after restoration of arterial flow.

On the other hand, Hillenbrand[52] made the first report on the alterations of the terminations of the vegetative nervous system in the vessel wall in patients with Buerger's disease: vacuolization, lumping, and proliferation of Schwann's cells were seen at the advanced stage of the disease. He thought these slight changes might indicate a stimulative condition of the termination of the vegetative nervous system and central impulses and the alterations of the termination should have a particular significance. In 1958 Hachisuka[53] found degeneration of plasmodial strands, probably the terminations of the vegetative nervous system in the altered vessel wall not only of the occluded segment but of the patent one, in the materials obtained from patients with Buerger's disease: the degeneration of plasmodial strands was considered as promoted degeneration of the vascular wall, though it was difficult to decide whether such degeneration was primary or secondary. Early degeneration of plasmodial strands might indicate a state of stimulation of the terminations of the vegetative nervous system, and participate in the pathogenesis of Raynaud's phenomenon. Further, regenerated nerve fibers were recognized in the organized thrombus.[53] Although determining whether the regenerated nerve fibers were vegetative or somatic remained a difficult problem, they might be one of the causes of the continued stimulation as stated in Leriche's hypothesis— "the spasm of collateral vessels is caused by the stimulation of the occluded blood vessel.[53]"

Aneurysm formation

Although the thromboangiitic lesion is originally occlusive or stenotic one, rare cases with aneurysmal dilatation of the vessel wall probably due to Buerger's disease have been reported.

In 1973 Takao and his colleagues[54] reported two cases of aneurysm due to Buerger's disease: one occurred in the popliteal artery and the other in the ulnar artery. In 1975 Sakaguchi[55] reported two cases of the disease in whom aneurysm appeared in the follow-up period: one in the anterior tibial artery and the other in the popliteal artery. The aneurysm of the anterior tibial artery was about 2 cm in diameter and ruptured: intimal thickening and organized thrombus were seen but no histologic feature characteristic of the disease was recognized. The aneurysm of the third segment of the popliteal artery became occluded during a 2-year-long follow-up period, and no biopsy was performed. In 1978 Uchida et al.[56] angiographically recognized aneurysmal dilatation of the bilateral common carotid arteries and the brachiocephalic trunck in a 33-year-old man with the disease. In 1979 Giler and et al.[57] reported a case of aneurysm of the radial artery in a patients with a long history of Buerger's disease: the aneurysm was occluded with thrombus shortly after angiography and no pathologic examination was carried out.

As the skip lesion of the popliteal artery shows frequently an aneurysmal dilatation, the diagnosis of aneurysm requires circumspection. Considering the inflammatory process with no necrotizing damage of the media at the acute stage and the preservation of the general architecture of the vessel wall at the chronic stage of Buerger's disease, destruction of the media enough to cause an aneurysmal dilatation might rarely occur. An aneurysm of the deep femoral artery was found in a patient with a long history of Buerger's disease in our series (Fig. IV-15).

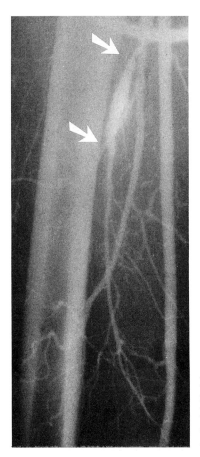

Figure IV-15. Right femoral arteriogram of a 46-year-old man with Buerger's disease. The proximal part of the lateral circumflex femoral artery shows an aneurysmal appearance (arrows). The infrapopliteal arteries are occluded.

A peculiar form of the lesion

In 1985 Ferguson and Starkebaum[58] reported an interesting case of Buerger's disease associated with idiopathic hypereosinophilia. A 47-year-old male smoker with chronic eosiophilia developed progressive ischemia in his extremities, and pathologic examination of vessels in the amputated digits revealed changes of Buerger's disease. Focal segments of some arteries, however, revealed marked eosiophilic infiltration of the thrombus and vessel wall. Furthermore, the patient developed a totally occluded temporal artery, which on biopsy specimen showed marked eosinophilic infiltration of the thrombus and vessel wall. In contrast to most patients with the hypereosinophilic syndorme, however, this patients had no evidence of endomyocardial thrombosis or fibrosis. In view of the recent evidence that eosinophil granule proteins are toxic to endothelial cells, and the strong association of Buerger's disease with cigarette smoking, the authors speculated that in some patients, long-term smoking incited an allergic reaction with hypereosinophilia that could be a mechanism for chronic vascular injury.

Based on the study of three smokers of thromboangiitis obliterans with eosinophilia of the temporal arteries, Lie and Michet[59] suggested that Buerger's disease could be found in an improbable segment of the vascular tree, such as the superficial temporal artery and the cytotoxic properties of the eosinophil major basic protein might be potentially relevant in the pathogenesis of vascular injury in Buerger's disease, though it might be circumscribed within narrow bounds.

Characteristic of pathologic findings

Buerger said[60] that the lesions in thromboangiitis obliterans were in chronological order : 1) an acute inflammatory lesion with occlusive thrombosis, the formation of miliary giant cell foci ; 2) the stage of organization or healing, with the disappearance of the miliary giant cell foci, the organization and canalization of the clot, the disappearance of the inflammatory products ; and 3) the development of fibrotic tissue in the adventitia that bound together the artery, vein and nerves. The pathology of Buerger's disease is not static but floating, and pathologic diagnosis of Buerger's disease should be made on the basis of the clinical data and course. In other words, the diagnosis of Buerger's disease is a historical one.

Determining what an initial change in the vessel wall in Buerger's disease is remains an unsolved problem. In 1985 Leu[61] found electronmicroscopically small and focal necroses, polynuclear leukocytes, lymphocytes, macrophages, and invasion of capillaries, fibroblasts and activated myocytes in the focal necrotic region in the intima and media, especially in the media, of the arteries and veins harvested by biopsy or amputation due to Buerger's disease. From the findings, he thought a primarily inflammatory process might exist in the vessel wall in Buerger's disease. Buerger[62] exquisitely said that thromboangiitis obliterans was a pathological but not a clinical entity in the formal sense. The clinical course in toto rather than over a short period of its existence, often furnishes adequate data for diagnosis.

REFERENCES

1. Buerger L.(I-34).
2. Buerger L.(I-41).
3. Lie JT.(I-80).
4. Shionoya S. Pathologie der Thromboangiitis obliterans. VASA 1978 ; 7 : 253-7.
5. Leu HJ, Brunner U. Zur pathologisch-anatomischen Abgrenzung der Thromboangiitis obliterans von der Arteriosklerose. Dtsch med Wschr 1973 ; 98 : 158-61.
6. Shionoya S, Tsunekawa T, Kamiya K. Elastolysis and giant cell reaction against disintegrated elastic fibres. Nature 1965 ; 207 : 311-2.
7. Shionoya S, Ban I.(III-38).
8. Shionoya S. Pathology of Buerger's disease. Pathol Microbiol 1975 ; 43 : 163-6.
9. Doerr W. Perfusionstheorie der Arteriosklerose. Stuttgart : Georg Thieme, 1963, pp 4-68.
10. Rau L. Über Vokommen, Bedeutung und Entstehung der Riesenzellen in normalen und pathologischen Zuständen. Ergebn Path Anat 1932 ; 26 : 229-352.
11. Kinmonth JB. Thrombo-angiitis obliterans : results of sympathectomy and prognosis. Lancet 1948 ; 255 : 717-9.
12. Ooneda G. Buerger's disease : pathology of the extremity vessels. Byoritorinsho 1983 ; 1 : 1167-76 (in Japanese).
13. Takao T, Nakai T, Ooiwa S, Naiki K, Kato R, Fukuta I, Nagata Y, Yano T, Terasawa T. Skip lesions of Buerger's disease. In : Shiokawa Y, ed. Annual Report of Vascular Lesions of Collagen Disease Research Committee of the Ministry of Health and Welfare of Japan, 1978, pp 183-9 (in Japanese).
14. Takao T, Nakai T, Naiki K, Kato R, Fukuta I, Nagata Y, Yano T, Kazui H, Kobayashi M, Terasawa T, Ito H. Histopathological study on skip lesion of Buerger's disease. In : Shiokawa Y, ed. Annual Report of the Vascular Lesions of Collagen Disease Research Committee of the Ministry of Health and Welfare of Japan, 1979, pp 365-72 (in Japanese).
15. Shionoya S. (I-79).
16. Shionoya S, Matsubara L, Kamiya K. Fortschreiten des Verschlussprozesses bei Thromboangiitis obliterans. VASA 1977 ; 6 : 249-54.
17. Buerger L. (I-48).
18. Jäger E. Zur pathologischen Anatomie der Thromboangiitis obliterans bei juveniler Extremitätengangrän. Virchows Arch path Anat 1932 ; 284 : 526-622.
19. Lindenberg R, Spatz H. Über die Thromboendarteriitis obliterans der Hirngefäße (Cerebrale Form der v. Winiwarter-Buergerschen Krankheit). Virchows Arch path Anat 1939 ; 305 : 531-57.

20. Antoni N. Buerger's disease, thrombo-angiitis obliterans, in the brain: report of three (four) cases. Acta Med Scand 1941; 108: 502-28.
21. Scheinker IM. Cerebral thromboangiitis obliterans: histogenesis of early lesions. Arch Neurol Psychiat. 1944; 52: 27-37.
22. Allen EV, Willius FA. Disease of the coronary arteries associated with thrombo-angiitis obliterans of the extremities. Ann Intern Med 1929; 3: 35-9.
23. Saphir O. Thromboangiitis obliterans of the coronary arteries and its relation to arteriosclerosis. Am Heart J 1936; 12: 521-35.
24. Cohen SS, Barron ME, Thrombo-angiitis obliterans with special reference to its abdominal manifestations. N Engl J Med 1936; 214: 1275-9.
25. Wolf EA, Sumner DS, Strandness DE. Disease of the mesenteric circulation in patients with thromboangiitis obliterans. Vasc Surg 1972; 6: 218-23.
26. Julitz R. Die klinischen Ausdrucksformen der Endarteriitis obliterans und ihre Differentialdiagnose. Z f d ges Inn Med 1953; 8: 343-61.
27. Gilkes R, Dow J. Aortic involvement in Buerger's disease. Br J Radiol 1973; 46: 110-4.
28. Hausner E, Allen EV. Generalized arterial involevement in thrombo-angiitis obliterans including report of a case of thrombo-angiitis obliterans of a pulmonary artery. Proc Staff Meet Mayo Clin 1940; 15: 7-13.
29. Lippmann HI. Cerebrovascular thrombosis in patients with Buerger's disease. Circulation 1952; 5: 680-92.
30. Ooneda G, Shinkai H. A pathological study of Buerger's disease with special reference to generalized Buerger's disease. In: Shiokawa Y, ed. Annual Report of the Vascular Lesions of Collagen Disease Research Committee of the Ministry of Health and Welfare of Japan, 1977, pp 45-50.
31. Asang E, Mittelmeier. Die systematisierte Endangiitis obliterans (Zugleich ein Beitrag zur Pathogenese der Arteriosklerose). Arch Kreisl 1957; 26: 143-217.
32. Zollinger HU. Adaptive Intimafibrose der Arterien. Virchows Arch path Anat 1967; 342: 154-64.
33. Doerr W. Gangarten der Atteriosscklerose. Heidelberg: Springer, 1964.
34. Doerr W. Arteriosclerosis without end. Virchows Arch A Path Anat Histol 1978; 380: 91-106.
35. Albertini A. Studien zur Aetiologie der Arteriosklerose. 2. Teil: Koronarsklerose: Die Bedeutung entzündundlicher Erkrankungen der Koronarterien, (im besondere der "Arteriitis stenosans coronariae") für die Pathogenese der Koronarsklerose. Schweiz Z Path 1938; 1: 163-87.
36. Buerger L. (I-37).
37. Chopra BS, Zakariah T, Sodhi JS, Khanna SK, Wahi PL. Thromboangiitis obliterans: a clinical study with special emphasis on venous involvement. Angiology 1976; 27: 126-32.
38. Buerger L. (I-38).
39. Tabuchi S. A histological study on recurring superficial thrombophlebitis. J Nagoya Med Ass 1959; 80: 672-82 (in Japanese).
40. Briggs JB, Recurring phlebitis of obscure origin. Johns Hopkins Hops Bull 1905; 16: 228-33.
41. Lipschitz M. Zur Frage der Thrombophlebitis migrans. Dtsch med Wschr 1929; 55: 744-6.
42. Kletz N. Thrombo-phlebitis migrans. Lancet 1932; 223: 938-9.
43. Keibl E, Köberle. Ueber Thrombophlebitis migrans Wien klin Wschr 1939; 52: 648-50.

44. Swirsky MY, Cassano C. Thrombophlebitis migrans. J Lab Clin Med 1943 ; 28 : 1812-6.
45. Lefemine AA, Warren R. Thrombophlebitis migrans. Angiology 1957 ; 8 : 266-71.
46. Bollinger A, Leu HJ. Thrombophlebitis saltans. Dtsch med Wschr 1974 ; 99 : 1433-6.
47. Barker NW. Primary idiopathic thrombophlebitis. Arch Intern Med 1936 ; 58 : 147-59.
48. Gerber IE, Mendlowitz MM. Visceral thrombophlebitis migrans. Ann Inern Med 1949 ; 30 : 560-79.
49. Baehr G, Klemperer P. Thrombosis of the portal and of the hepatic veins. Med Clin North Am 1930 ; 14 : 391-410.
50. Sakaguchi S, Nakamura S, Koyano K, Kamiya T, Muro H, Shirasawa H, Takada A, Takada T, Kanamaru M. Significance of thrombophlebitis migrans in Buerger's disease. In : Fukuda Y, ed. Annual Report of the Vascular Lesions of Collagen Disease Research Committee of the Ministry of Health and Welfare of Japan, 1980, pp 319-25 (in Japanese).
51. Barker NW. Lesions of peripheral nerves in thromboangiitis obliterans. Arch Intern Med 1938 ; 62 : 271-84.
52. Hillenbrand HJ. Die feinsten Endausbreitungen des vegetativen Nervensystems in den Gefäßwänden bei Kranken mit Endangiitis obliterans und ihre klinische Bedeutung. Langenbecks Arch Dtsch Z Chir 1956 ; 283 : 291-315.
53. Hachisuka K. Histopathological studies on the nerve fibers in the vascular wall in thromboangiitis obliterans. Nagoya J Med Sci 1958 ; 21 : 190-204.
54. Takao T, Kato K, Kusano M, Nagashima T, Fujioka S, Yano T, Ishigaki H. Peripheral arterial anearysms. Ketsuekitomyakkan 1973 ; 4 : 1087-96 (in Japanese).
55. Sakaguchi S. Two cases of Buerger's disease with peripheral arterial aneurysm. In : Ishikawa K, ed. Annual report of the Buerger's Disease Research Committee of the Ministry of Health and Welfare of Japan, 1975, pp 95-8 (in Japanese).
56. Uchida H, Teramoto S, Yasuhara M, Mano M, Furutani S, Ohtsuka A, Matsui T, Sanoo K. Buerger's disease and perihperal arterial aneurysm. Geka 1978 ; 40 : 904-7 (in Japanese).
57. Giler Sh, Zelikovski A, Goren G, Urca I. Aneurysm of the radial artery in a patient with Buerger's disease. VASA 1979 ; 8 : 147-9.
58. Ferguson GT, Starkebaum G. : Thromboangiitis obliterans associated with idiopathic hypereosinophilia. Arch Intern Med 1985 ; 145 : 1726-8.
59. Lie JT, Michet CJ. Thromboangiitis obliterans with eosinophilia (Buerger's disease) of the temporal arteries. Hum Pathol 1988 ; 19 : 598-602.
60. Buerger L.(I-45).
61. Leu HJ.(II-41).
62. Buerger L.(I-55).

CHAPTER V
PATHOPHYSIOLOGY

The most characteristic feature of peripheral arterial occlusive disease is a stagnation of arterial circulation in the most peripheral region of the extremity as a rule, independently of the site of arterial occlusion. "Dependent rubor," abnormally red skin color of the digits, is a representative feature of the peripheral arterial stagnation in patients with Buerger's disease. Persistence of the impaired peripheral circulation causes a breakdown of the microvascular system and the tissue gets into a critical ischemia.

Critical limb ischemia

Critical limb ischemia is ischemia which endangers the limb or part of a limb and the pathophysiology of critical limb ischemia in humans remains to be established.

The microcirculation comprises the arterioles, venules and capillaries, and microvascular flow regulating system (MFRS) and microvascular defence system (MDS) are supposed to participate in maintaing microvascular circulation. The MFRS regulates and distributes blood flow in the normal microcirculation, and it is characterized by normal vasomotion, with regular, periodic perfusion of capillary networks: microcirculatory flow is influenced by endothelium-derived relaxing factor (EDRF) and one or more endothelium-derived constricting factors (EDCF). The MDS consists of an appropriate interaction of the platelets, leucocytes and endothelium as a defensive reaction to injury and infection[1].

In critical limb ischemia there is breakdown of the MFRS, principally due to the decrease in the arterial perfusion pressure, with maldistribution of blood flow in the microcirculation, especially the nutritive skin capillaries. There may be constriction of precapillary arterioles and the balance between EDRF and EDCF shifting in favor of the latter. In addition, activated platelets and leucocytes release vasoconstrictor substances, e.g., leukotrienes, TXA_2 and 5-HT. In critical limb ischemia there is also inappropriate activation of the MDS, with activation of leucocytes and platelets, and damage to the endothlium. This is always associated with local hypoxia and metabolic changes. In addition, there is release of growth factors by the endothelium, macrophages and platelets which stimulate proliferation of vascular smooth muscle. Endothelial swelling, platelet plugging, leucocyte plugging and tissue edema occur in this inflammatory reaction.[1] As a multiple and widespread occlusion of the peripheral arteries is the essential feature of Buerger's disease, the affected limb is liable to get into critical limb ischemia due to breakdown of the MFRS and MDS. While it is controversial whether all arterioles in the critically ischemic area are already maximally dilated, information elucidating the pathophysiology of critical limb ischemia not only has prognostic value but may also place in perspective the role of surgical or conservative treatment in the disease. Therefore, the pathophysiology of Buerger's disease should be reviewed from the standpoint of blood flow velocity, vasospasm, vasomotion and hemorheology, with an insight into the microcirculation: it is indispensable to understanding of various pathologic manifestations due to the disease.

Blood flow velocity

Ischemic symptoms in Buerger's disease manifest themselves most evidently in the distal region of the extremity and trophic lesions occur exclusively in the finger or the toe.

Although measurement of regional blood flow, at rest and during exercise, is a goal of pathophysiologic investigation in peripheral arterial occlusive disease, there is currently no ideal nonivasive diagnostic method that permits a quantitative assessment of regional blood flow through any given vessel at any instant without disturbing the flow itself, especially in the limb with trophic lesion. Furthermore resting blood flow does not discriminate between normal and ischemic limbs, and the maximum blood flow during exercise or reactive hyperremia is useful in distinguishing the limbs with arterial insufficiency from normal ones.[2]

There are two methods of obtaining quantitative arterial flow velocity measurements in the extremity: Doppler flowmeter[3,4] and radioisotopic tracer technique.[5,6] The former[3,4] is restricted for such main arteries as the femoral, posterior tibial, or dorsalis pedis arteries, and resting mean flow velocity is not a reliable index of arterial insufficiency because of peripheral vasomotor adjustment which tends to maintain mean flow even in the presence of arterial obstruction.[7]

The radioisotopic tracer method has been applied to measure flow velocity by calculating the difference of arrival time of the radioactive bolus between two target points. By means of a tracer technique with ^{99m}Tc-pertechnetate, flow velocity at various levels of the artery in normal subjects was reported as follows: 16.8cm/sec in the aorta, 8cm/sec in the iliac artery, 6cm/sec in the femoral artery, and 5.2cm/sec in the crural artery.[5] By means of a tracer technique with ^{99m}Tc-pertechnetate, provided with seven zonal regions of interest, 6.7 mm in width, placed at equal spaces of 20.1 mm, from the toe tip to the midfoot at a right angle to the long axis of the foot, arterial flow velocity in the foot during reactive hyperemia

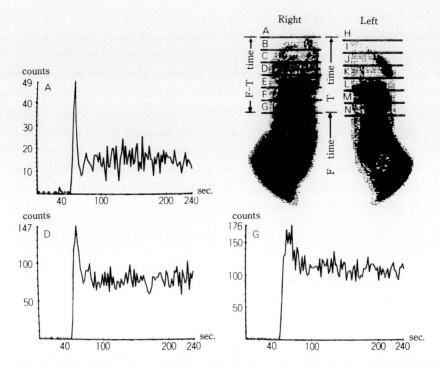

Figure V-1. Regions of interest in the foot and time activity curves of a normal subject. A thick horizontal line indicates a zonal ROI, 6.7 mm in width. The curve of any ROI shows an activity peak. G and N, the most proximal ROI; A and H, the most distal ROI. F time, transit time at G or N; T time, transit time at A or H; F-T time, difference between F time and T time, namely, isotope transit time from the midfoot to the toe tip, mean flow velocity, 16.0 cm/ F-T time. (From Shionoya S, et al. Surgery 1981; 90: 10-9.)

was measured[8](Fig. V-1 and 2). The mean velocity in the foot was 6.8±1.9cm/sec in 16 normal limbs, 1.6±1.1cm/sec in 27 limbs with distal TAO (Buerger's disease of infrapopliteal occlusion type), 0.9±0.7cm/sec in 30 limbs with proximal TAO (Buerger's disease of supra-and infrapopliteal occlusion type), and 1.0±0.8cm/sec in 25 limbs with ASO (arteriosclerosis obliterans): the difference in the velocity between normal and each ischemic limbs was significant ($p<0.001$).

By the following formula;

the lower limit of velocity = normal mean velocity $-2.5 \times$ standard deviation of velocity

the lower limit of the normal value of the velocity in the foot was calculated as 2.0 cm/sec. By this criteria, 20 of 27 limbs with distal TAO (74%), 27 of 30 limbs with proximal TAO (90%) and 21 of 25 limbs with ASO (84%) showed abnormal levels of the velocity respectively.

Comparing the velocity with toe blood pressure index (TPI) in 43 limbs with ischemic ulceration (11 limbs with distal TAO; 20, proximal TAO; and 12, ASO),

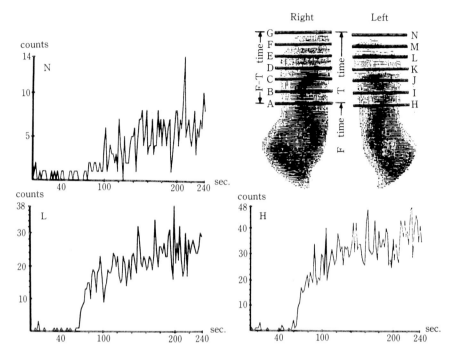

Figure V-2. Regions of interest in the foot and time activity curves of a patient with Buerger's disease. The curve of any ROI shows no activity peak, but isotope transit time at each ROI is measurable. (From Shionoya S. In: Shionoya S, Ohara I, Sakaguchi S, eds. Noninvasive diagnostic techniques in peripheral vascular disease. Nagaishoten, 1983, pp 235-53.)

the velocity was abnormal in all but one limb with distal TAO, mostly below 1.0cm/sec, and TPI was pathological in all the limbs. From these results, ischemic ulceration might be ready to occur when the velocity in the foot reduces below 1.0 cm/sec and TPI decreases below 0.3 in ischemic limbs.

After successful arterial reconstruction in 9 limbs with proximal TAO, ulceration healed favorably in 5 limbs and intermittent claudication disappeared in 4 limbs. While the velocity returned to normal in all the cases after surgery, TPI remained pathological in all but 1 and ankle blood pressure returned to normal in 6 of the 9 limbs. After lumbar sympathectomy in 16 limbs (14 limbs with TAO; 2; ASO), ankle and toe blood pressure remained unchanged postoperatively, but the velocity significantly increased after surgery ($p < 0.05$). In 13 limbs with ischemic ulceration, ulcers healed favorably in four limbs with postoperative normalization of the velocity, but healing of the lesion was delayed in the other nine limbs without recovery of it. In view of reduction or unchangeability of the toe blood pressure after lumbar sympathectomy or by sympathetic nerve block, postoperative clinical course correlated better with flow velocity in the foot than with distal blood pressure.

The most distinctive difference in the hemodynamics in the foot between normal subjects and patients with peripheral arterial occlusive disease was a remarkable reduced flow velocity and a noticeable decreased toe blood pressure: ankle blood pressure is not indicative of ischemia in patients with Buerger's disease in whom the peripheral arteries below the ankle are most severely occluded. When the velocity in the foot was normalized after arterial reconstruction or lumbar sympathectomy, however, ulceration healed favorably and the ischemic limb was salvaged in spite of an incomplete recovery of the toe blood pressure. The pathophysiology of the impaired peripheral arterial circulation in Buerger's disease is reflected better in the flow velocity than in the distal blood pressure, and an improvement of the decreased flow velocity is a goal of surgical or conservative treatment in Buerger's disease.

The dependent rubor, a peculiar blush of the toes and forepart of the foot in Buerger's disease, indicates vasodilatation and repletion in the subpapillary plexes of the skin, namely, stagnation of arterial circulation in the microcirculatory system. As such a stagnant and atonic status in the microvascular system is beyond sympathetic vasomotor regulation, the rubor often persists after arterial reconstruction and/or sympathetic denervation.

Vasospasm

Vasospasm implies a reversible constriction of the vascular tree. The term "arteriospastic" might be more accurate, but it would exclude the possibility of venous spasm contributing to the presentation in some of vasospastic phenomenon.

Apart from the question of the role of vasospasm in the pathogenesis of Buerger's disease, the vasospastic mechanism participates in the pathophysiology of the disease and decorates its clinical features. The vasospastic phenomena in Buerger's disease can be divided into two categories: 1) Raynaud's phenomenon, namely, an episode of constriction of the precapillary arterioles and small arteries of the extremities; and 2) an increase in vasoconstrictor tone of the more proximal arteries and veins.

The former, secondary Raynaud's phenomenon, is characterized by episodic changes in color of the fingers or toes: pallor, cyanosis, and rubor. Raynaud's attacks are often precipitated by cold, and elucidation of pathophysiology of cold sensitivity is indispensable to understand Raynaud's phenomenon. Several different mechanisms may be involved in the pathogenesis of Raynaud's phenomenon: increased vasoconstrictor tone, vascular abnormality (local fault), blood pressure, viscosity of blood, and immunologic factors[9]. These factors might be more or less related with the secondary Raynaud's phenomenon in Buerger's disease, respectively. Nielsen and his colleagues[10] studied responses to local cooling of the digital arteries in different groups of arterial obstructive diseases on the upper extremity, i.e., Buerger's disease in 15 patients, Raynaud's disease (primary Raynaud's phenomenon) in 7, subclavian stenoses in 5, and normals in 15: the response to finger cooling registered as a decrease in finger systolic blood pressure indicated an increase of digital arterial tone. In all three patient groups, digital arterial tone increased more than in normals during finger cooling. Patients with Raynaud's disease showed a pathological increase in arterial tone at 23.5℃ with closure of the digital arteries at a mean temperature of 18.5℃. The temperature eliciting these phenomena in patients with Buerger's disease was about 7℃ lower (16.5 and 11.0℃), respectively. Accordingly, cold sensitivity and Raynaud's phenomenona in the two groups may have a different pathophysiological mechanism, namely, a pathological arterial tone in Raynaud's disease vs. a normal arterial tone in obliterative diseases acting on a narrow vessels.

Based on the analysis of cold sensitivity of the fingers in patients with Buerger's disease, arteriosclerosis obliterans, primary Raynaud's phenomenon or secondary Raynaud's phenomenon due to collagen disease, Hirai[11] concluded that impaired arterial circulation due to occlusions in the digital arteries or more proximal arteries was a necessary precondition for cold sensitivity in the arterial occlusion group, and an increased sympathetic response to cold was of less importance as an etiologic factor: a patient with cold sensitivity of the hand and normal digital blood pressure should not be considered to have arterial occlusive disease as the underlying cause of cold sensitivity. Because of hypotension in the acral region due to arterial occlusive lesions in patients with Buerger's disease, the diseased digital vessels will close by a normal increase in vascular tone acting on an abnormal vessel (local fault).

By sticking a microelectrode into the tibial nerve of patients with Buerger's disease, Yamamoto et al.[12] found a decreased basal activity of muscle sympathetic nerve activity, innervating the gastrocnemius and the soleus, but an increased response of muscle sympathetic nerve activity to local cold stimulus, compared to healthy subjects. In operative procedures, especially arterial reconstructive surgery in patients with Buerger's disease, a marked vasospasm of the arteries and veins is frequently encountered: the mobilized crural artery or saphenous vein so constricts evidently that the distal anastomosis with the artery or the employment of vein graft is considered as unsuccessful, in spite of preventing measures. From "corrugated" or "accordion-like" appearance of the leg arteries and markedly delayed visualization of the distal arteries by angiography in patients with the disease, it is reasonable to assume that the arteries or veins of the extremities develop vasospastic phenomena.

Vasomotion

It was agreed that peripheral circulation might act independently of the rest of the circulatory system, and some ascribed this to the individual contractility of the capillaries[13] and others ascribed it to the reactions of the terminal arterioles.[14]

By means of constriction of terminal arterioles and precapillary sphincters, the capillary blood flow is subject to continuous variation and the rhythmical change in diameter of these microcirculatory units is called "vasomotion.[15]" A significant feature of vasomotion is its relative independence of the blood flow, and the vasomotion is pronouncedly affected by local conditions in the tissue. Although the nervous factor participates in vasomotion,[15] rhythmical active vasomotion is still present after sympathetic denervation.[16] Rhythmical variations in human skin blood flow were studied with Doppler flowmetry, and the frequencies of the oscillations on the forehead, forearm, upper arm and dorsal foot were 8.6±0.7 cycles/min[17] (Fig. V-3).

The rhythmic activity might be an inherent property of smooth muscle cells rather than the response of vascular muscle to rhythmical demands from the vasomotor center, from humoral influences or physical conditions, and it is likely to be dependent on the local metabolism, electrolyte balance and temperature. In severe ischemic limbs, cutaneous forefoot vasomotion was not detected when the ankle blood pressure was less than approximately 80 mmHg, and the vasomotion was restored 24 hours post angioplasty when the ankle blood pressure was increased to about 80mmHg or greater.[18] Because vasomotion is thought to reflect arteriolar autoregulation as a means limiting microvascular perfusion, its absence

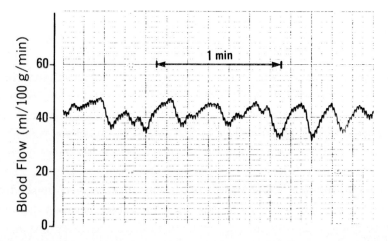

Figure V-3. Recording of blood flow value in the finger skin of a 30-year-old healthy subject by He-Ne Laser Doppler flowmeter. (ALF 2100, Advance Co.) Rhythmical variation in blood flow (vasomotion) is seen.

would be expected under ischemic conditions requiring maximal vasodilatation.

As the degree of ischemia is extremely severe in the acral region in Buerger's disease, cutaneous toe vasomotion is unable to be detected with Doppler flowmetry in the majority of patients with the disease[16](Fig. V-4). Dependent rubor in the toes and forefoot symbolizes the disappearance of vasomotion in the diseased foot, and persistence of the rubor even after arterial reconstruction or lumbar sympathectomy indicates the irreversible damage of the micocirculatory units due to severe and prolonged ischemia in Buerger's disease. Rubor means the dilated subpapillary vessels filled to repletion, and the regional blood flow that is normal in volume may be quite abnormal in pulsatile characteristics—a phenomenon worthy of detailed investigation in apparently ischemic feet.[19]

No rhythmical variation in blood flow in the microcirculatory bed implies the lack of the functional autonomy of the peripheral vascular system, the responsiveness of which is readily affected by local tissue conditions. In time of low functional demand the blood flow is largely limited to the bypass channels (preferential thoroughfare channels) with the majority of the precapillary sphincters closed. Periodic opening and closing of different sphincters irrigates different parts of the capillary net. With increasing functional demand, the nutritive blood flow to the tissues may increase greatly following the opening of many sphincters. Abnormal vasomotion produces maldistribution of blood flow with some capillaries not perfused or underperfused, and the outbreak of a necrotic lesion is imminent. As the skin is short of local blood flow autoregulation compared with the brain, kidney or muscle, the skin deprived of vasomotion is ready to be in the face of ruin. Discriminating measurement of blood flow through the true capillaries and the arteriovenous anastomoses in the finger with laser Doppler flowmetry and venous occlusion plethysmography is a topic for further discussion.[20]

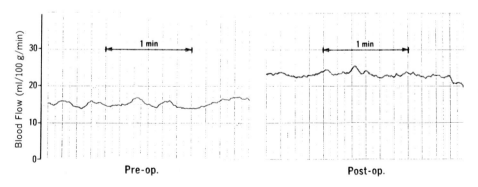

Figure V-4. Recordings of blood flow value in the toe skin of a 46-year-old man with Buerger's disease before and after femorotibial bypass grafting and concomitant lumbar sympathectomy by He-Ne Laser Doopler flowmeter. (ALF 2100, Advance Co.) The blood flow value can be seen to increase, but vasomotion remains unchanged after operation.

Hypercoagulable state

In 1948 Hagedorn and Barker[21] demonstrated heparin tolerance in vivo by measuring the prolongation of the whole blood clotting time produced after the intravenous injection of standard doses of heparin : there was a high incidence of "non-reactors" and "hyporeactors" both in patients with Buerger's disease and ASO as compared with healthy controls. The term "hypercoagulable state" is generally used to denote any condition in which the normal balance between clotting and anticlotting mechanisms becomes altered in such a way that the patient is predisposed to thrombus formation. However, determining whether hypercoagulable state exists in Buerger's disease remains an unsolved question, though some new sensitive assays to detect hypercoagulability were recently developed. Properly speaking, hypercoagulable (prethrombotic) state belongs to local problem, and a thorough analysis of the pathophysiology of local field is a prerequiste for the study.

In 1989 Sato[22] reported the hematological characteristics in 20 patients with Buerger's disease (TAO), compared with those obtained in 85 patients with peripheral occlusive vascular disease or aortic aneurysm and 18 healthy subjects. β-thromboglobulin (β-TG) was significantly elevated in all the patients than in the controls. The levels of fibrinopeptide A (FPA), fibrinopeptide B β_{15-42} (FPB$_{15-42}$) and D-dimer signficantly increased in arteriosclerosis obliterans (ASO), aneurysms (AA), acute arterial occlusion (AAO), and deep vein thrombosis (DVT) compared with TAO and controls. Therefore, while ASO, AA, AAO and DVT groups exhibited platelet activation, hypercoagulability and increased fibrinolysis, TAO showed only platelet hyperactivity. These results may be dependent on difference in the amount of thrombi formed at the diseased regions. As D-dimer is a reliable indicator for detecting the degree of thrombolysis, patients with ASO, aneurysms, AAO, and DVT, especially the latter three groups, seemed to abound with unorganized thrombi. Protein C level in controls, TAO, ASO, AA, AAO and DVT was 111.5 ± 23.4 ng/ml, 125.3 ± 15.4, 106.8 ± 21.0, 99.1 ± 19.6, 98.5 ± 26.8, and 113.7 ± 33.1, respectively, and the level in ASO, AA, AAO was significantly lower than in TAO. Antithrombin III (ATIII) in AA, AAO and DVT was significantly decreased than that in TAO: the decrease of ATIII in AA, AAO and DVT might be caused by consumption of ATIII due to hypercoagulability. Tissue plasminogen activator (t-PA) in controls, TAO, ASO, AA, AAO and DVT was 2.4 ± 1.1, 2.7 ± 1.3, 2.8 ± 1.2, 3.1 ± 1.5, 4.6 ± 1.7 and 5.8 ± 5.5 ng/ml, respectively; it was significantly higher in AAO and DVT. α_2-plasmin inhibitor (α_2-PI) in ASO and AA was significantly decreased than that in TAO: the decreased α_2-PI level in ASO and AA might be caused by consumption of α_2-PI due to activated fibrinolysis. There was no difference in α_1-antitrypsin and α_2-macroglobulin between TAO, ASO and AA.

Judging from the results, there was no difference in fibrinolytic activity between TAO and controls, though an increased level of β-TG suggested platelet hyperactivity in TAO. The cause of no marked increase in D-dimer in TAO migth be attributed to a relatively small amount of thrombus which is ready to be soon organized and resistant to fibrinolysis, contrary to the thrombus in ASO, AAO, and AA.

Based on the investigative results of coagulation factors, fibrinolysis, and platelet function in patients with atherosclerotic vascular lesions, Breddin[23] concluded that the following tests or factors seemed promising candidates to be tested as possible indicators of a prethrombotic state and as possible predictors in future prospective studies: spontaneous aggregation (platelet aggreagtion test—PAT III), antigen to von Willebrand factors, and fibrinogen, perphaps also Factor VII. Saito et al.[24] found that the levels of β-TG and FPA were inversely correlated with Tl/2 of platelets and fibrinogen in patients with thrombotic tendency such as diabetes mellitus, malignancy and stroke. The progress in biochemistry, molecular biology and pathophysiology of the prethrombotic state, might find a clue to the solution of the question as to the hypercoagulable state in Buerger's disease.

Blood viscosity

Although viscosity is independent of shear rate in a Newtonian fluid, blood, which is a suspension of red cells and other particulate matter in a solution containing large asymmetric protein molecules (e.g., fibrinogen), has distinctly anomalous viscous properties.

In 1912 Maeshima[25] clinically measured the blood viscosity by Hess' viscometer and defined the normal limits as 3.8 to 4.8 for males and 3.4 to 4.1 for females. In the next year, Koga[26] detected an increase in the blood viscosity in patients with Bueger's disease, and found reduction of the blood viscosity by infusion of saline or Ringer's solution, in keeping with improvement in ischemic symptoms. In 1930 Silbert et al.[27] found an average reduction of 21 per cent in blood volume by the dye method in 69 of 87 patients with Buerger's disease, and they suggested that a concentration of the blood is usually present in the disease. In 1939 Theis and Freeland[28] noticed increased viscosity of the blood, rapid sedimentation of the cells, rapid coagulation, greatly increased alkalinity, low or normal cell counts and arterial oxygen saturation and a low carbon dioxide content of the blood in 7 cases of acute Buerger's disease. As these conditions were not present in 21 clinically improved or recovered patients with the disease, they concluded that a disturbance in the utilization of oxygen might be one of the conditions in the complex physiology of the blood and tissue metabolism which were responsible for the acute symptoms of Buerger's disesae.

The blood is a non-Newtonian fluid and its viscosity depends not only the flow velocity but also the dimention of the conducting vessel. The blood viscosity greatly varies when the velocity is changed within the range of low flow rate, while it does not much vary at high flow rate. Therefore, a low shear measurement is suitable for the hemodynamic study of blood rheology. Using a new viscometer,[29] in 1967 Iino[30] measured the blood viscosity at very low shear rate (0.05/sec to 250/sec) without anticoagulant drugs in 5 healthy subjects, 21 patients with arterial disease (Buerger's disease in 10, aneurysm in 4, ASO in 2, aortitis syndrome in 1, thrombosis in 1, embolism in 1 and renovascular hypertension 1), 11 patients with venous disease (thrombosis in 8, varicose veins in 2, and superior vena cava syndrome in 1) and 2 patients with arteriovenous fistula. The results showed a tendency toward elevation of the blood viscosity in the patients with vascular disease, especially it was most remarkable in patients with venous thrombosis. In patients with Buerger's disease, no significant elevation of the blood viscosity was recognized.

The most important factor affecting viscosity is hematocrit, and viscosity increases according to hematocrit. Except for such peculiar morbid states as polycythemia or hyperfibrinogenemia, however, the viscosity of the systemic blood is not deemed to correspond to the viscosity in the acral region where blood is passed through microcirculatory vessels. Since the microvasculature and the venous system are in series with the arterial system, the rheology of flow in these "relative low shear" areas is an important determiner of arterial inflow. In spite of the confusion regarding the non-Newtonian behavior of blood, red cell aggregation, and anomalous viscosity of blood in vivo, it is an established fact that a reduction in viscosity of blood may improve the microvascular circulation. Therefore, methods for lowering blood viscosity have a rational basis in the treatment of peripheral arterial occlusive disease.

Muscle circulation

Intermittent claudication is a characteristic symptom in obliterating arterial disease of the legs, and it is generally agreed that this symptom is caused by inadequate blood flow in the muscles of the legs during walking.[31] In Buerger's disease, intermittent claudication occurs most commonly in the sole of the foot at early stage, and the foot claudication, which is less accurately called instep claudication, is a typical symptom in the infrapopliteal arterial occlusion. The basic and clinical researches on msucle circulation have been promoted by Lassen and his school,[32,33] and the muscle ischemia in Buerger's disease has been vigorously investigated by Hirai.

Plantar muscle

In 1976 Hirai[34] measured muscle blood flow in the flexor hallucis brevis muscle by Xe-133 clearance technique, in 20 limbs of 10 healthy subjects and 55 limbs of 41 patients with occlusive arterial disease of the lower extermity: all the patients showed no necrotic lesion or rest pain (Fig. V-5). All the limbs were divided into three groups according to the site of arterial occlusion and pain: 1) no claudication group in 25 limbs whose occlusions were located in the infrapopliteal and/or foot arteries without claudication; 2) foot claudication group in 17 limbs whose occlusions were localized in the infrapopliteal and/ or foot arteries with foot claudication; and 3) calf claudication group in 13 limbs whose occlusions were extended to the suprapopliteal arteries with calf claudication. In normal group, the mean of resting muscle blood flow was 2.8 ± 1.3 ml/100g/min, and there was no significant difference in resting blood flow among the four groups including normal one. After ischemic exercise on tiptoe for two minutes, maximal blood flow after the exercise and duration of reactive hyperemia were significantly lower and prolonged in the foot or calf claudication group, compared with the normal and no claudication groups (Fig. V-6).

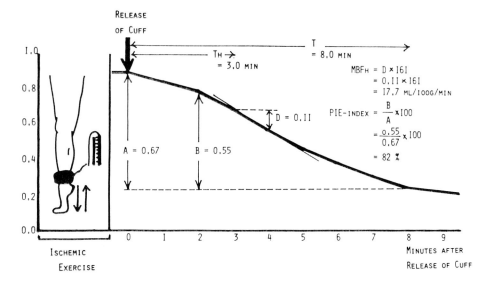

Figure V-5. Xe-133 clearance curve from the flexor hallucis brevis of a patient with intermittent claudication of the foot. The curve shows maximal blood flow after the ischemic exercise (MBFH). The time from the release of the cuff to the commencement of MBFH (TH) is 3.0 min and the total duration of reactive hyperemia (T) is 8.0 min. The remaining hyperemia (PIE-index) is that percentage of the total fall of the clearance curve which occurs 2 min after the release of the cuff. Longitudinal axis means Log 10 (CPS/N): CPS, counts per second; N, initial CPS/10 and ranges from 200 to 500. (From Hirai M. Jap Circul J 1976; 40: 313-7.)

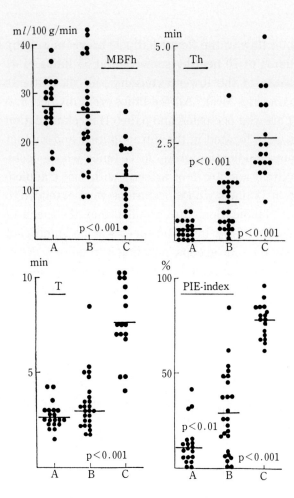

Figure V-6. The means and values of MBFH, TH, T, and PIE-index during reactive hyperemia in healthy subjects and patients with arterial occlusive disease. A: healthy group. B: no claudication group. C: foot claudication group. (From Hirai M. Igakunoayumi 1975; 95: 654-5.)

On the other hand, one hundred and two limbs of 84 patients with occlusive arterial disease of the lower extremity were divided into three groups according to arteriographic findings: 1) 24 limbs with occlusion of the anterior tibial, dorsalis pedis and/or peroneal arteries, but no involvement of the posterior tibial or plantar arteries; 2) 30 limbs with occlusion of the posterior tibial artery and visualization of the plantar artery through collaterals; and 3) 48 limbs with occlusion of the plantar arteries with or without occlusion of the posterior tibial artery. In group 1, no limbs had foot claudication; in group 2, 13 of 30 limbs complained of the pain in the foot during walking, and in group 3, 21 of 48 limbs were foot claudicators.

From the clearance curves of cases with foot claudication that showed the reduction in maximal blood flow with predominant delay in onset and markedly prolonged duration of hyperemia, the underlying pathologic mechanism of foot claudication might be an ischemia in the plantar muscle during walking. From the results that patients with occlusion of the anterior tibial, dorsalis pedis and/or peroneal arteries without involvement of the posterior tibial or plantar arteries did not complain of foot claudication, it might be an indispensable condition for the occurrence of foot clandication that the posterior tibial and/or plantar arteries are involved. The anterior tibial, dorsalis pedis or peroneal artery may be useful as collaterals in case of occlusion of the posterior tibial artery. Whether foot claudication will develop in case of occlusion of the posterior tibial and/or plantar arteries might rest on the degree of compensatory function of the collaterals and/or damage of the nutrient arteries in the plantar muscles.

Anterior tibial muscle

From Xe-133 clearance curves in the anterior tibial muscle four parameters were calculated[35]:
1. MBFe: maximal blood flow during exercise
2. MBFh: maximal blood flow after exercise
3. T-time: duration of the postexercise hyperemic reaction measured in minutes and extending from the cessation of the exercise until the curve reaches its pre-exercise level.
4. R-index: percentage of the remaining part of the hyperemia that occurs one minute after the cessation of the exercise to the total hypermia during and after the exercise.

Hirai[35] defined the following as normal values:
1. MBFe $\geq$ 12.0 ml/100g/min
2. T-time $<$ 2.6 min
3. R-index $<$ 22.0%
4. When MBFe is less than 24.0 ml/100g/min:
T-time $<$ 1.8 min, R-index $<$ 10.0% and MBFe$\geq$MBFh.

While the cases with complete occlusion or severe stenosis at the origin of the anterior tibial artery showed abnormal clearance curves, they complained of no pain in the muscle during walking, though the anterior tibial artery is the sole feeding artery to the muscle: the anterior tibial muscle does not seem to contribute a large share to walking, compared with the gastrocnemius muscle.[36] In patients with Buerger's disease, abnormal clearance curves were obtained in case of patency of the anterior tibial artery, and it might indicate that occlusive lesions of the muscular branches resulted in insufficiency of the nutiritive circulation in the muscle. Viewed at the initial lesions of Buerger's disease in the muscular branch arteries, this finding is worth notice.

Gastrocnemius muscle

Normal clearance curve of the gastrocnemius muscle was defined as follows[36]:
1. MBFe $\geq$ 12.0ml/100g/min
2. R-index $<$ 38.0%
3. T-time $<$ 3.1 min.

Judging from that abnormal clearance curves were recognized in case of occlusion of the sural arteries or the posterior tibial artery at its origin respectively, the gastrocnemius muscle receives blood supply from the sural arteries as well as the posterior tibial artery. Occlusion of the sural arteries at their origin or the posterior tibial artery at its origin or bifurcation, produced abnormal clearance in the gastrocnemius muscle, but the degree of the circulatory insufficiecny was mild and the patients usually did not suffer from calf claudication. Only in patients with Buerger's disease who had occlusion of the posterior tibial and sural arteries, marked abnormal clearance curves of the gastrocnemius muscle were seen and they complained of usual calf claudication, notwithstanding no occlusive lesions were observed in the arteries proximal to the popliteal bifurcation: the muscular nutritive arteries must have been severely affected in addition to occlusion of the posterior tibial and sural arteries in theses cases.

Soleus muscle

The normal limits of clearance curves of the soleus mescle were defined as follows[37]:
1. $MBFe \geq 12.0 ml/100g/min$
2. T-time < 2.7 min
3. R-index $< 28.0\%$.

As the circulation to the soleus muscle is derived from at least five separate main arteries, which enter the structure at various points in its longtudinal axis,[38,39] it may well be that the collateral circulation to the soleus muscle will be established in the fact of a complete block of one or even several of the main channels.[39] Although Jackson[40] described soleus claudication causes discomfort in the back and inner sides of the calf, and hypoxia of the gastrocnemius provokes an ache behind the knee, distal one third of the posterior thigh, and back of the calf, this report remains to be confirmed.

A patient with Buerger's disease in whom the anteior tibial and the peroneal artery were occluded but the posterior tibial and suprapopliteal arteries were patent complained of pain at the lateral side of the lower leg during walking. From the abnormal clearance curve of only the soleus muscle in spite of the normal clearance curves of the anterior tibial and gastrocnemius muscles, his intermittent claudication seemed to be due to circulatory insufficiency of the soleus muscle.[37]

Red muscle (soleus muscle) seems to be controlled by motoneurons that are characterized by a relatively small fiber diameter and a predominantly tonic pattern of activity as compared with the phasic motoneurons controlling white muscle (gastrocnemius muscle): red muscle fibers are specialized to produce sustained contractions and are involved in the maintenance of body posture; the relative slowness of their single twitch makes them especially suited for this type of function[41]. Red muscle is supplied by a more dense capillary network than white muscle, and its resting blood supply is higher that of white muscle: this is the case with its maximal blood flow capacity as well.

Maximal vasoconstrictor fiber activity increased blood flow resistance for the soleus muscle only 150%, at most, compared with 500-600% for the gastrocnemius muscle: the soleus blood flow always increased relatively less than that of the gastrocnemius for a given increase of stimulation rate.[41] Therefore, the gastrocnemius muscle may play the principal role in the pathogenesis of calf claudication due to occlusion of the poplieal artery or higher. In Buerger's disease with occlusion of the infrapopliteal arteries, however, claudication due to hypoxia of the soleus muscle is worth due consideration. From the standpoint of pathophysiology, the X-133 clearance curves in the anterior tibial, soleus, and gastrocnemius muscles respectively are indispensable to understanding the hypoxia of these muscles due to occlusive lesions of the muscular branch arteries in patients with Buerger's disease.

Distribution of perfusion

As long as obstruction is limited to one or two major arteries, compesatory dilatation of collateral arteries and the peripheral vascular bed will maintain an adequate blood supply at rest. However, when the hydraulic capacity of the collateral bed is exceeded during exercise, a relative ischemia develops in the muscle, resulting in intermittent claudication. In the presence of three or more levels of obstruction or when the obstruction is located far distally, as in the digital vessels, the dilatation of collateral channels and the peripheral vascular bed is no longer able to compensate for the increased resistance even at rest and ischemic symptoms such as rest pain, ulceration, and gangrene develop.

The term "ischemic ulceration" has been used to denote a skin lesion with tissue loss related to arterial disease, rather than using the term as a description of the perfusion state of the lesion. There is no doubt that arteriography is essential for a detailed anatomical evaluation of peripheral vascular disease. However, this information is incomplete unless it is supplemented by knowledge of the actual status of tissue perfusion. Assessment of perfusion distribution in the extremity during resting state and during stress has provided insights into the physiologic effect of documented intraraterial disease, objective evidence of diffuse small vessel disease, and prognostication of the healing ability of ischemic ulcers.[42]

A tracer technique with ^{99m}Tc-pertechnetate, a diffusible substance, measures both arterial and capillary blood activity as well as the diffusion interface for the injected tracer.[43,44] As it has been noted that intravenous thallium-201 distributed in cardiac muscle in proportion to blood flow,[45] and in skeletal muscle its distribution reflected the fractional distribution of cardiac output and was related to regional blood flow,[46] thallium-201 peripheral perfusion scan is most suitable to evaluate blood perfusion on the acral region.[47] In contrast to particulate tracers[48] which are physically intrapped during the first passage of the tracers through the organ, the ionic thallium-201 is in constant metabolic flux.

It would be very useful clinically to be able to evaluate extremity perfusion during the rest and stress states and identify differences in perfusion between the two states[42]. Inherent in healing process is the ability to develop an inflammatory response and hyperemia that are necessary requirements for this revitalization process.[49] An objective, reliable prognostic criterion for determining the healing potential of an ischemic ulcer is needed to prevent unnecessarily prolonged hospitalization or premature surgery.

In 1985 Ohta[50] classified forty-two ischemic ulcers in the foot into four types according to the presence and degree of the inherent inflammatory response of the ulcer in both the initial and delayed distributions after simultaneously intravenous injection of 2mCi of thallium-201 with releasing of the cuff pressure, 50 mmHg above the brachial systolic pressure, applied above the ankle (Fig. V-7).

Type I : a prominent localized increase of thallium accumulation (a hot spot) in the postocclusive initial distribution, and a decreased accumulation in the delayed (3 hours later) distribution, i.e., redistribution.

Type II : a hot spot in the initial distribution, and an increased accumulation in

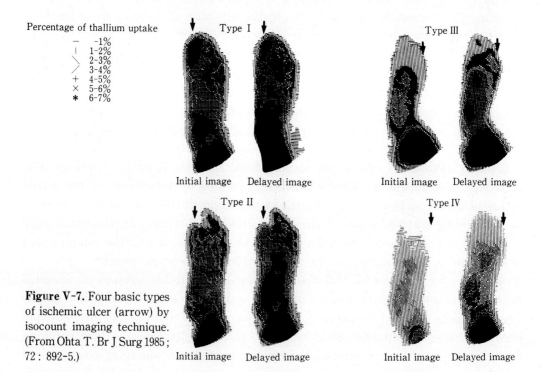

Figure V-7. Four basic types of ischemic ulcer (arrow) by isocount imaging technique. (From Ohta T. Br J Surg 1985; 72 : 892-5.)

the redistribution.

Type III: no hot spot in the initial distribution, but one demontsrated in the redistiribution.

Type IV: no hot spot at all in either distribution.

One of 21 patients with Buerger's disease suffering from ischemic ulceration in his series belonged to type I; 10, to type II; 9, to type III; and 1, to type IV. An ulcer of type I was healed by pharmacotherapy. Of 10 ulcers of type II, 6 were healed with pharmacotherapy, and 4 were healed with lumbar sympathectomy. Of 9 ulcers of type III, 2 were cured with pharmacotherapy, and 7 were cured with lumbar sympathectomy. An ulcer of type IV was cured with arterial reconstruction.

Judgin from the results, ulceration of type I and II has a good healing potential and will heal in response to conservative treatment: ulcers of type III require surgical treatment to prevent protracted hospitalization, though they have fair healing potential. As ulcers of type IV have no spontaneous healing potential, surgical treatment should be recommended. Out of the 21 ulcers, 11 had good healing potential and 9 had fair healing potential. Ischemic ulceration in Buerger's disease has better spontaneous healing potential than generally expected.

REFERENCES

1. Dormandy J. European consensus document on critical limb ischaemia. Berlin: Springer, 1989.
2. Sumner CS, Strandness DE Jr. The relationship between calf blood flow and ankle blood pressure in patients with intermittent claudication. Surgery 1969; 65: 763-71.
3. Bernstein EF, Murphy AE, Shea MA, Housman LB. Experimental and clinical experience with transcutaueous Doppler ultrasonic flowmeters. Arch Surg 1970; 101: 21-5.
4. Fronek A, Coel M, Bernstein EF. Quantitative ultrasonographic studies of lower extremity flow velocities in health and disease. Circulation 1976; 53: 957-60.
5. Müller US. Veränderungen der peripheren arteriellen Hämodynamik. Bern: Hans Huber, 1979, pp 42-6, 84-94.
6. Shionoya S, Hirai M, Kawai S, Ohta T, Seko T. Hemodynamic study of ischemic limb by velocity measurement in foot. Surgery 1981; 90: 10-9.
7. Fronek A, Johansen KH, Dilley RB, Bernstein EF. Noninvasive physiologic tests in the diagnosis and characterization of peripheral arterial occlusive disease. Am J Surg 1973; 126: 205-14.
8. Shionoya S. Blood flow velocity In: Shionoya S, Ohara I, Sakaguchi S, eds. Noninvasive diagnostic techniques in peripheral vascular disease. Osaka: Nagaishoten, 1983, pp 235-53 (in Japanese).
9. Thulesius O. Pathophysiology of cold sensitivity. VD & T, Barrington Publications, 1981, pp 17-21.
10. Nielsen SL, Nobin BA, Hirai M, Eklöf B. Raynaud's phenomenon in arterial obstructive disease of the hand demonstrated by locally provoked cooling. Scand J Thor Cardiovasc Surg

1978 ; 12 : 105-9.
11. Hirai M. Cold sensitivity of the hand in arterial occlusive disease. Surgery 1979 ; 85 : 140-6.
12. Yamamoto K, Iwase S, Mano T, Shionoya S. Evaluation of muscle sympathetic nerve activity by microneurography in patients with Buerger's disease compared to healthy subjects. Proceedings of the 10th Annual Meeting of Japanese Society of Noninvasive Diagnostics on the Vessel, 1990, pp 35-6 (in Japanese).
13. Bensley RR, Vimtrup BJ. On the nature of the rouget cells of capillaries. Anat Rec 1928 ; 39 : 37-55.
14. Nesterow AJ. Über Contractilität der Blutcapillaren beim Menschen. Pflügers Arch Physiol 1925 ; 209 : 465-75.
15. Chambers R, Zweifach BW. Topography and function of the mesenteric capillary circulation. Am J Anat 1944 ; 75 : 173-205.
16. Io A, Kuroyanagi Y, Taguchi M, Nishikimi N, Mukaiyama H, Sakurai T, Yano T, Shionoya S. Changes in skin blood flow after sympathectomy. In : Proceedings of the 9th Meeting of Japanese Society of Noninvasive Diagnostics on the Vessel, 1989, pp 9-10 (in Japanese).
17. Salerud EG, Tenland T, Nilsson G, Öberg P Å. Rhythmical variations in human skin blood flow. Int J Microcirc : Clin Exp 1983 ; 2 : 91-102.
18. Moneta GL, Schneider E, Jager K, Brulisauer M, Thuring-Vollenweider U, Bollinger A. Vasomotion and Laser Doppler flux before and after transluminal angioplasty for limb salvage. In : Tsuchiya M, Asano M, Mishima Y, Oda M, eds. Microcirculation—an update, vol.1. Amsterdam : Elsevier Science, 1987, pp 370-3.
19. McEwan AJ, Stalker CG, Ledingham I McA. Foot skin ischaemia in atherosclerotic peripheral vascular disease. Br Med J 1970 ; 3 : 612-5.
20. Nagasaka T, Hirata K, Nunomura T. Contribution of arteriovenous anastomoses to vasoconstriction induced by local heating of the human finger. Jap J Physiol 1987 ; 37 : 425-33.
21. Hagedorn AB, Barker NW. Response of persons with and without intravascular thrombosis to a heparin tolerance test. Am Heart J 1948 ; 35 : 603-10.
22. Sato H. Studies on coagulation and fibrinolysis in peripheral vascular diseases and thrombolytic therapy. J Jap Coll Angiol 1989 ; 29 : 1183-90 (in Japanese).
23. Breddin K. Detection of prethrombotic states in patients with atherosclerotic lesions. Seminars Thromb Hemost 1986 ; 12 : 110-23.
24. Saito H. Pathogenesis and pathophysiology of prethrombotic states. Annual report of the Research on Cardiovascular Diseases by National Cardiovascular Center, 1987, pp 550-62 (in Japanese).
25. Mayesima J. Klinische und experimentelle Untersuchungen über die Viskosität des Blutes. Mitteil Grenzgebieten Med Chir 1912 ; 24 : 413-43.
26. Koga G. Zur Therapie der Spontangangrän an den Extremitäten. Dtsch Z Chir 1913 ; 121 : 371-82.
27. Silbert S, Kornzweig AL, Friedlander M. Thrombo-angiitis obliterans (Buerger) IV : reduction of blood volume. Arch Intern Med 1930 ; 45 : 948-57.
28. Theis EV, Freeland MR. The blood in thrombo-angiitis obliterans. Arch Surg 1939 ; 38 : 191-205.
29. Yamaguchi T. Rheological studies on peripheral circulation—especially on the blood viscosity —. J Nagoya Med Ass 1967 ; 90 : 179-99 (in Japanese).

30. Iino S. Experimental and clinical studies on peripheral circulation with rheological considerations: variability of blood viscosity, and the relation with thrombobus formation. J Nagoya Med Ass 1967; 90: 200-23 (in Japanese).
31. Veal JR. The pathological basis for intermittent claudication in arteriosclrosis. Am Heart J 1937; 14: 442-51.
32. Lassen NA, Lindbjerg L, Munck O. Measurement of blood-flow through skeletal muscle by intramuscular injection of Xenon-133. Lancet 1964; 1: 686-9.
33. Alpert J, Garcia del Rió H, Lassen NA. Diagnostic use of radioactive Xenon clearance and a standardized walking test in obliterative arterial disease of the legs. Circulation 1966; 34: 849-55.
34. Hirai M. Intermittent claudication of the foot in view of foot muscle blood flow measured by 133 Xe clearance technique and arteriographic findings. Jap Circul J 1976; 40: 313-7.
35. Hirai M. Muscle blood flow measured by Xe-133 clearance method and peripheral vascular disease. Part 2.: normals and patients with peripheral vascular diseases. Jap Circul J 1974; 38: 661-6.
36. Hirai M, Shionoya S. Considerations on occlusive diseases of the leg arteries and determination of muscle blood flow by Xe-133 clearance method. J Cardiovasc Surg 1975; 16: 35-42.
37. Hirai M, Ban I, Nakata Y, Matsubara J, Shinjo K, Kawai S, Suzuki S, Tsai WH, Shionoya S. Consideration for intermittent claudication in the calf in view of hemodynamics of leg muscles. Ketsuekitomyakkan 1975; 6: 69-75 (in Japanese).
38. Blomfield LB. Intramuscular vascular pattern in man. Proc Royal Soc Med 1945; 38: 617-8.
39. Abramson DI. Circulation in the extremities. New York: Academic Press, 1967, pp 139-60.
40. Jackson BB. Surgery of acquired vascular disorders. Springfield: Charles C Thomas, 1969, p107.
41. Folkow B, Halicka HD. A comparison between "red" and "white" muscle with respect to blood supply, capillary surface area and oxygen uptake during rest and exercise. Microvasc Res 1968; 1: 1-14.
42. Siegel ME, Stewart CA. Thallium-201 peripheral perfusion scans: feasibility of single-dose, single-day, rest and stress study. AJR 1981; 136: 1179-83.
43. Gerritsen HA, Kazem I, Hasman A, Kuypers PJ. A new approach to the evaluation of peripheral vascular disease using the gamma camera. Nucl Med 1974; 112: 115-21.
44. Shionoya S, Hirai M, Ohshima M. Radioisotopic study on healing of ischemic ulcers. VASA 1978; 7: 242-6.
45. Strauss HW, Harrison K, Langan JK, Lebowitz E, Pitt B. Thallium-201 for myocardial imaging: relation of thallium-201 to regional myocardial perfusion. Circulation 1975; 51: 641-5.
46. Strauss HW, Harrison K, Pitt B. Thallium-201: non-invasive determination of the regional distribution of cardiac output. J Nucl Med 1977; 18: 1167-70.
47. Siegel ME, Stewart CA, Kwong P, Sakimura I. 201 TI perfusion study of "ischemic" ulcers of the leg: prognostic ability compared with Doppler ultrasound. Nucl Med 1982; 143: 233-5.
48. Oshima M, Ijima H, Kohda Y, Kuramoto K, Kikuchi Y, Wada M, Akisada M. Peripheral arterial disease diagnosed with high-count-rate radionuclide arteriography. Nucl Med 1984; 152: 161-6.
49. Siegel ME, Giargiana FA Jr, Rhodes BA, Williams GM, Wagner HN Jr. Perfusion of ischemic

ulcers of the extremity : a prognostic indicator of healing. Arch Surg 1975 ; 110 : 265-8.
50. Ohta T. Noninvasive technique using thallium-201 for predicting ischaemic ulcer healing of the foot. Br J Surg 1985 ; 72 : 892-5.

CHAPTER VI
CLINICAL MANIFESTATIONS

According to Buerger[1], patients afflicted with thromboangiitis obliterans do not suffer directly from the disease itself but from the disastrous occlusive thrombosis which signalizes Nature's method of healing a vascular lesion that has long since disappeared, because it is the interference with circulatory conditions of the limbs brought about by the extensive occlusive process that is responsible for most of the clinical manifestations of thromboangiitis obliterans. Supposing it to be true that Buerger's disease is essentially an inflammatory process, involving particularly the deeply situated arteries and veins of the lower and upper extremities at the onset, is there ever any symptom referable to the inflammatory lesion in the vessels per se?

Initial symptom

According to Buerger[2], during the early stage the symptoms may be obscure. The patient may remember nothing whatsoever and come to hospital later with the manifestation referable to the chronic stage of the disease. Non-localizable shooting pains in the calf or foot, attended with difficulty in walking, with possibly tender muscles of the calf, with or without vasomotor symptoms, and with or without absence of the dorsalis pedis and posterior tibial pulses may be the only symptoms. Although Goodman et at.[3] observed "burning sensation in soles" as the initial symptom in 8 of their 79 patients with Buerger's disease, detecting whatever symptom accompanies the initial lesion at the onset of the disease remains an unsolved question.

A patient with Buerger's disease in our series complained of pain along the brachial artery with pulsation, and pulsation of the artery soon after disappeared. Biopsied specimen of the brachial artery obtained one month after the onset of pain showed characteristic histologic features of the acute stage.[4] Besides such a superficial medium-sized artery as the brachial artery, however, it is difficult to identify some symptoms as originating in the deeply located vessels.

In the lower extremity, the disease first affects the digital, metatarsal, tarsal, calcaneal, arcuate, or arcus plantaris arteries or their branches, i.e., independently in multiple places, and the process usually rapidly ascends to the infrapopliteal arteries, except a small number of patients in whom the occlusive lesions are restricted below the ankle. Therefore, it is not surprising that the first clinical symptom the patients noticed is coldness, numbness, skin color changes, indefinite pain, intermittent foot claudication, or trophic lesions, contrary to patients with arteriosclerosis obliterans whose initial symptom is intermittent claudication as a rule. Fontaine's classification,[5] which is useful for the clinical staging of arterial insufficiency due to arteriosclerosis obliterans, is not valuable in gauging the degree of ischemia in Buerger's disease: gangrene or ulceration does not always follow claudication and may precede it.

Coldness

The fingers or toes are cold and damp to the touch. The patients feel their coldness more severely than actual fall in temperature. Although abnormal coldness of the all finger or toes occurs, some digits are often cooler than the others of the same extremity in Buerger's disease, contrary to Raynaud's disease.

The patient complains not infrequently of coldness of the affected unilateral extremity which is felt warmer by palpation because of the past sympathetic denervation than the contralateral extremity. Coldness and cold sensitivity of the extremities follow the patient throughout his life, though coldness of the acral region is no peculiar symptom to the disease.

Paresthesia

Although various types of paresthesia were thought to occur in association with Buerger's disease, a sensation of numbness in the digits, foot or hand is most common and it occurs mainly after exercise or walking.

Whether various types of sensory disturbances are related with ischemic neuropathy has never been satisfactorily settled. Numbness in the toes or foot after walking is usually associated with color changes, such as blanching of the toes or foot.[6]

Skin color changes

The skin color changes are characteristic of the disease: the affected fingers and toes are abnormally red, particularly with pendency (rubor). Although "rubor" is not a specific color change to Buerger's disease, it is most frequently seen in patients with the disease even at the horizontal position of the extremity(Fig. VI-1).

While the rubor slowly vanishes with elevation of the extremity, the color change reappears and auguments on dependency. The phenomenon of dependent

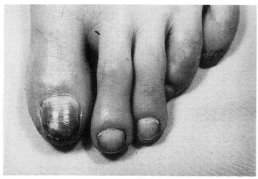

Figure VI-1. Rubor in a patient with Buerger's disease. The toes are abnormally purplish red, particularly on dependency.

rubor can be explained by the presence of numerous dilated capillaries in the skin that contain blood of relatively high oxygen content. Buerger[7] said that whether the delayed rubor indicated belated reflex dilatation or slow chemical response on the part of the capillaries was an open question, and the conclusion was warranted that the finer vessels might be still able to respond and are not wholly inert and paralytic.

Judging from the absence of vasomotion, rhythmical change in blood flow, in the toes with rubor, the microvascular units of the affected limb are atonic and their capacity for interchange of oxygen and other metabolic products becomes impaired. Rare association of typical Raynaud's phenomenon with patients with Buerger's disease and persistence of the rubor after arterial recenrtruction and/or sympathectomy give suggestions as to an extremely atonic state of the microcirculatory vessels, namely, exhaustion of the vasoconstrictor mechanism. The digits of the diseased limbs become abnormally blanched after elevation of the extremities, and on dependency after elevation there may be a delay of more than 20 seconds before the color returns to the skin (venous filling time). In case of acute worsening of occlusive lesions, pallor of the digits or foot manifests itself independently of the position of the afftected extremities with no noticeable effect of posture.

Cyanosis of the skin of the digits occurring in dependent extremities afflicted with chronic arterial insuffciency indicates impairment of circulation for prolonged periods, and this apparently results from dilated minute vessels through which flow inadequate amounts of blood containing excessive quantities of reduced hemoglobin.[8] As regards pathogenesis of cyanosis, venous obstruction, diminution of arterial inflow and impaired vasomotion are enumerated.[7] Diminished arterial perfusion pressure due to occlusive lesions, venous involvement and insufficient vasomotion participate in the occurrence of cyanosis in the digits of patients with Buerger's disease. Cyanosis often involves only certain digits or portion of digits, and persistent intense cyanosis in the localized digit implies that the region has taken in crisis.

Although Raynaud's phenomenon was reported to occur in as many as 57% of the cases of Buerger's disease,[3] typical Raynaud' phenomenon seems to rarely occur in patients with Buerger's disease. However, such color changes as cyanosis and/or pallor solely, instead of the three phases, not infrequently attack the patients. Although the temperature at which the digital arteries begin to close is significantly lower in Buerger's disease than that in Raynaud's disease, the attack is provoked by a normal increase in vascular tone acting on an abnormal vessel under low perfusion pressure in the former.[9]

Edema

Notwithstanding the venous involvement, edema exclusively due to vein obstruction never occurs in patients with the disease as a rule. Edema in the acral region is usually seen in the diseased limb with ulceration or gangrene, because of breakdown of microvascular system, inflammatory reaction and persistent dependency of the affected extremity to relieve pain.

Persistence of such an edema around the necrotic lesion suggests that the local is caught in a vicious circle: by compressing the small vessels the compensatory hyperemia, indispensable to healing of necrotic lesion, is interfered and the microcirculatory disturbance is further deteriolated. In patients with the disease suffering from ulceration or gangrene, continued edema is exceedingly inauspicious.[7]

Intermittent claudication

Pain of intermittent claudication may be an ache, a sense of fatigue, a persistent cramp, or a severe aching, squeezing pain that occurs only after a certain amount of exercise of the affected muscles and that is relieved rather promptly by rest without change of position. The pain does not appear at the start of walking, but gradually manifests itself after some distance of walking, and it fades away in similar manner as the mist clears off while the patient waits for a traffic light. Intermittent claudication originates in insufficient muscle blood flow to maintain the voluntary muscle movements: at rest skeletal muscle blood flow is about 2 ml/100g/min[10]; maximal skeletal muscle blood flow during exercise comes to 50-60 ml/100g/min,[11] by Xe-133 clearance method.

As the arterial occlusive lesions are localized in the infrapopliteal region at early stage of Buerger's disease intermittent claudication occurs most commonly in the arch of the foot. Because the pain is mainly localized in the plantar arch, the term "instep claudication" be abandoned and the term "foot claudication" might be appropriate for the symptom due to occlusion of the arteries distal to the popliteal artery. Considering much more muscle mass of the sole than the instep, unsuitableness of the term "instep claudication" may be understood. As ischemia of the plantar muscles of the foot results in foot claudication,[12] pain in the plantar arch during walking may visit patients with pedal pulsations, though it is a rare occurrence.

Although foot claudication is a characteristic symptom associated with ischemia of the foot due to infrapopliteal arterial occlusion, calf claudication may be experienced if the disease progresses to the suprapopliteal segment, though calf claudication visits patients with infrapopliteal arterial occlusion in case of obstruction of the nutrient arteries in the calf muscles. Looking closely into the patient's past history, a point of time at which the pain during walking changed from the foot to the calf sometimes comes back into his mind: it indicates that the infrapopliteal arterial occlusion has proceeded to the suprapopliteal region. In case of progression of the disease to the iliac region, the site of pain may be in the thigh or lumbar region.

As arterial reconstruction is not infrequently feasible to patients with suprapopliteal arterial occlusion, calf or more proxial claudication can be improved by reconstructive surgery. However, foot claudication usually remains unchanged, because no significant improvement in the foot muscle circulation is available after successful arterial reconstruction of the iliofemoral segment.

Some patients with the disease complains of intermittent claudication in the upper extremity, i.e., fatigueness in the hand or forearm, but the degree is usually not disabling, because of more excellent collateral circulation and less muscle mass subjected to less work, compared with the lower extremity.

Rest pain

The symptom of rest pain is usually described as a severe ache or a numb, disturbing patient's sleep. Skin color is usually purplish-red but occasionally pale, in the same way as in acute arterial occlusion. Ischemic rest pain is pain that occurs in the toes or in the area of the metatarsal heads, occasionally in the foot proximal to the metatarsal heads: it rarely affects fingers or adjacent regions. Ischemic rest pain is sometimes confused with pain of ulceration or gangrene, but they are two different things.

Elevation of the limb above or at the horizontal position aggravates the pain and pendency, to some degree at least, brings relief. Cranley[13] explained the pathogenesis of rest pain as follows: The effective pressure is not sufficient to drive the blood up the gradient of the foot, overcome arteriolar resistance, and reach the capillaries. Furthermore, whatever blood does reach the capillaries of the toes is drained off immediately by gravity through the venous system, because there is no barrier such as is provided by the arterioles between the capillaries and the arteries. According to him, ischemic rest pain is clearly distinguished from ischemic neuritis, as evidenced by the immediate relief obtained after restoration of arterial flow; it seems difficult to imagine a true neuritis clearing so rapidly. Rest pain is characteristically localized to the digits or immediately adjacent areas and often precedes gangrene or ulceration.

Pain of ischemic neuropathy

Pain of ischemic neuritis is various in its manifestation, and it ordinarily does not correspond to any definite distribution of affected nerves[8]. The pain is not localized in the digits and adjacent area, but more widespread in the extremity, contrary to rest pain.

It is usually paroxysmal and is associated with various types of sensory disturbances. The traits characteristic of pain of ischemic neuritis are not readily expressible by words, and the patients state that they are gnawed by the pain and always swayed by misgivings about the coming attack.

Thrombophlebitis migrans

Thrombophlebitis migrans is a characteristic symptom representative of inflammatory feature of Buerger's disease.

The term is derived from a recurring migratory phlebitis that usually affects segments of small and medium-sized superficial nonvaricose veins in the extremities. The lesions develop acutely as red, raised, slightly indurated, and tender cords, several centimeters in length. They are commonly seen of the foot and leg but may occur on the arm: the great and small saphenous veins are infrequently involved. The acute stage of the lesions lasts usually for 2 to 3 weeks; then the redness and tenderness disappear, but the occlusion of the affected vein persists and is palpable as a solid cord, leaving a blackish-brown pigmentation. Although it subsides spontaneously, it tends to recur in another site of the veins at intervals of time varying from months to years (Fig. VI-2).

Thrombophlebitis migrans may occur before the onset of subjective ischemic symptoms of arterial occlusion and after definite manifestation of ischemia in the extremities. The incidence of thrombophlebitis migrans in patients with Buerger's disease is various; 20^{14}-95^{15} per cent. The affection of thrombophlebitis migrans must be depent on the patient's interest and memory about the disease, especially in case of an occurrence before the onset of ischemic symptoms. Buerger[16] emphasized the association of migrating thrombophlebitis with the disease, and regarded it as a bay window through which the real state of the deep vessels might be looked into.

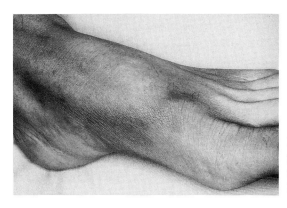

Figure VI-2. Phlebitis migrans in a patient with Buerger's disease. Pigmentation of the skin due to superficial thrombophlebitis of the foot.

Although it remains unsolved whether pathology and course of thrombophlebitis migrans are the same as those of the lesions of the deep arteries and veins, the condition of the disease might be surely regarded to be in activity, as long as migrating thrombophebitis recurs. Ueno and his colleaues[17] reported there was no remarkable difference in the clinical course of the affected limbs between the patients of Buerger's disease with thrombophlebitis migrans and those without thrombophlebitis migrans. "Thrombophlebitis migrans" is a pathognomonic episode characteristic of Buerger's disease (as an angiitis), but its occurrence often escapes the patient's attention.

Gangrene and ulceration

Necrotic lesions, namely, gangrene and ulceration are the most afflicting ischemic symptom in Buerger's disease. These lesions occur most commonly in the digits, mainly around the margins of nails (Fig. VI-3). While the necrotic lesion sometimes occurs without the patient's knowing of its provoking cause (spontaneous gangrene), the necrotic lesion mostly follows mechanical or thermal trauma, including iatrogenic.

A slight trauma to the tissue supplied with impaired blood may provoke necrosis of the tissue, because the severe ischemic tissue is unable to respond to the trauma with reparatory inflammatory reaction. Removal of the nail on the basis of misdiagnosing the necrotic lesion as paronychia around the margins of nails frequently causes an intractable painful ulceration in the nailbed. Pressure on the nail from shoes during walking or careless fall of an object on the foot may be sufficient to cause necrosis of the skin and subcutaneous tissue where the blood supply is impaired. Although the patient's care to protect the extremities from various traumas has its limit, the occurrence of gangrene and ulceartion in Buerger's disease might be depent on his everyday safeguard against trauma to some degree.

Gangrene is usually confined to one digit at first, mainly the tip of the digit, but

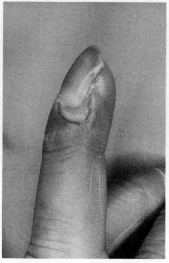

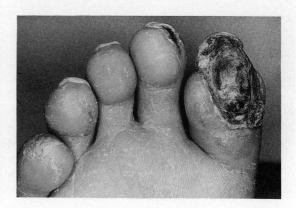

Figure VI-4. Gangrene involving the first toe and the second toe of a patient with Buerger's disease.

Figure VI-3. Ischemic ulceration around the margin of the nail of the second finger of a patient with Buerger's disease.

gangrene may develop on a few digits in course of time, though rare cases with simultaneous involvement of several digits were encountered (Fig. VI-4). After a gangrenous tip has sloughed spontaneously, the gangrenous lesion takes the shape of ulceration. Ulceration may develop in the fold at the base of the flexor surface of the toe or between the toes in association with dermatophytosis, besides on the tips of the digits. External appearance of the base of the ulceration rests on the local blood supply: it is usually yellowish white in case of severe ischemia; it is covered with purulent matter and the margin of the ulcer is swelling if complicated with infection.

Hirai et al.[18] reviewed clinical features of patients with Buerger's disease suffering from gangrene or ulceration in the toes at our hospital: 80 males and one female; the time elapsed from the onset of ischemic symptom to the present investigation was 19 months to 20 years (mean: 7.6 years). One hundred eight limbs of 81 patients were divided by angiographic pattern of occlusive lesion into three types: 1) occlusion of only infrapopliteal arteries in 61 limbs (crural group); 2) occlusion of supra-and infrapopliteal arteries with patent segment of the popliteal artery in 19 limbs (segmental group); and 3) occlusion of supra-and infrapopliteal arteries without interposition of the patent segment in 28 limbs (nonsegmental group). The rate of the patients whose initial symptom was gangrene or ulceration was 21% in crural group, 11% in segmental group, and 25% in nonsegmental group. However, the incidence of the necrotic lesions during whole follow-up period was 56%, 47%

and 89% respectively: the incidence was significantly higher in nonsegmental group ($p<0.01$). The reccurence rate of the necrotic lesions was 16%, 21% and 54% respectively, and it was the highest in nonsegmental group than in the other two groups ($p<0.01$). In crural group, the incidence of gangrene or ulceration in patients who were younger than 40 years old at the onset was 68%; that in patients of older than 40 years was 35%($p<0.01$). No similar tendency was recognized in the other two groups.

The incidence of the necrotic lesions, the recurrence rate and the amptation rate were significantly higher in patients with involvement of the upper limbs and/or thrombophlebitis migrans than in patients with neither of the two. Twenty-seven of the 81 patients were suffered from ischemia in the bilateral legs, and the incidence of the necrotic lesion, the recurrence rate and the amputation rate were significantly higher in the 27 cases with bilateral involvement than in 54 cases with unilateral involvement. There was no significant difference in the rate of recurrence of the necrotic lesions and in the amputation rate between patients whose inital gangrene or ulceration occurred within one year after the onset and patients whose necrotic lesions occurred more than one year after the onset.

The site of the necrotic lesions in 68 limbs was the 1st toe in 38 limbs, 2nd in 25, 3rd in 12, 4th in 14, 5th in 25 and foot in 7: the site of recurred lesions was the 1st toe in 12 limbs, 2nd in 6, 3rd in 4, 4th in 3, and 5th in 6. The most highest incidence of the lesion in the big toe might be attributable to the leading role in walking or exercise, the susceptibility to the external pressure, e.g., shoe sore, and the almost solitary nutrient artery, the first metatarsal artery. In 19 of 46 patients with the necrotic lesions at their first visit to our hospital, definite contributing causes were recognized, such as shoe sore, stumble, fall of an object, removal of the nail or minor surgery. Out of 26 patients with the upper limb involvement, the recurrence rate of the necrotic lesions in the toes and the amputation rate were higher in 15 patients with the necrotic lesion in the finger than in 11 patients without the lesion in the finger (67%, 53% vs. 36%, 18%).

In conclusion, the incidence of gangrene or ulceration in the toes and the recurrence rate of the lesion were significantly higher in patients with nonsegmental occlusion and upper limb involvement and/or thrombophlebitis migrans than in patients of crural or segmental occlusion and with neither of upper limb involvement nor migrating thrombophleitis. In other words, gangrene and ulceration showed a marked trend to recur in patients with three or fourlimb involvement and thrombophlebitis migrans. As a result of secondary infection, the necrotic lesions spread proximally and are associated with intractable pain, and there may be swelling and redness around the margin of gangrenous lesions, abscess formation or cellulitis.

Other trophic changes

Besides gangrene and ulceration, other trophic changes result from chronic ischemia. Nail growth of the toes is so slow that patients with the disease pare the toe nails at long intervals, e.g., once for several months. The nails may become thickened, muddy and deformed or, on rare occasions, thin and papery.

As a result of absorption of the subcutaneous fat and loss of hair, the digits appear shrunken and the skip color seems to be glossy at chronic stage. The muscles of the extremities may become atrophic, due to ischemia and disuse.

Involvement of the upper extremity

Although not only the lower extremity but also the upper extremity is affected with Buerger's disease, scant attention has been given to the upper limb involvement, because of relatively mild ischemic symptoms in the finger, hand and arm.

The incidence of arterial insufficiency in the upper limb in Buerger's disease has been reported to be from 14[19] to 100[20] per cent. The variance in the reported incidence might be attributed to the different diagnostic methods used for confirmation of arterial occlusive lesions in the upper limb, namely, clinical detection of ischemic symptom, noninvasive diagnostic techniques or angiography.

In 34 patients with Buerger's disease who were admitted to the author's institution during the 12 month period from March 1977 to February 1978, the presence of arterial obstruction of the upper limb was investigated by means of brachial arteriography, clinical findings and determination of digital blood pressure[21]. All patients were male and smokers at the onset of symptoms. The initial ischemic symptoms appeared at a mean age of 36 years, with a range of 25 to 48 years. The mean duration from the onset of the symptoms to the time of this investigation was 6.5 years, with a range of 2 months to 23 years. All the patients were otherwise healthy and had no evidence of heart disease, arterial aneurysm, diabetes mellitus or collagen disease: all the patients had normal blood cholesterol levels. Superficial thrombophlebitis had occurred in 20 patients and 17 patients complained of intermittent claudication in the foot. In 31 of the 34 patients (91 per cent) arterial occlusion in at least one upper limb was confirmed. In 27 of these 31 cases arterial obstruction was detected by arteriography; in the remaining 4 cases it was ascertained by the persence of definitive signs of ischemia, such as cyanosis or gangrene, as well as by the absence of wrist pulsations in association with a positive Allen test and a decreased digital blood pressure.

McPherson et al.,[20] who reported an incidence of 100 per cent of the upper limb involvement, considered impaired arterial pulsations in upper extremities with or without ischemic lesions of the fingers as one of indispensable requirements for diagnosis of Buerger's disease. Mozes and his colleagues[15] called 1) migrating phlebitis, 2) vasospastic elements, such as Raynaud's phenomenon, and 3) upper extremity involvement "systemic manifestations" to distinguish them from the local signs and symptoms in the leg that were directly related to arterial insufficiency, namely, claudication, rest pain, gangrene and ulceration. As they made a diagnosis of Buerger's disease when in addition to ischemic manifestation in the leg two or more of the systemic manifestations were present, the incidence of the upper limb involvement in their series was 77%.

In our series, only 6 of the 34 patients were admitted to the hospital, complaining of ischemic symptoms in the upper extremity either associated with lower limb symptoms or not. However, careful interview and physical examination revealed that 22 cases had arterial occlusion in the upper limb. A high incidence of the upper limb involvement with Buerger's disease might be an result of the physician's concern and interest who is well versed in the widespreading distribution of the disease in the upper and lower extremities. However, these findings mean that arterial occlusive lesions in the upper limb do not always bring about observable ischemic symptoms.

Goodman et al.[3] reported that 5 per cent of the patients with Buerger's disease had their initial symptoms in the hand, but involvement of the upper limbs was usually a later finding and should be thought of as a frequent occurrence with progression of the disease. Tanabe et al.[22] found only the upper limb involvement in 8 of 152 patients with Buerger's disease. If no evidence of impairment of arterial blood supply in the lower extremity manifests itself in the 8 cases throughout a long-term follow-up period, it might be necessary to differentiate them from arterial occlusion in the hand and fingers associated with repeated occupational trauma.[23]

Judging from the high incidence of the upper limb involvement in our series, the upper extremities might be almost always affected in severe cases of the disease, though ischemic symptoms in the finger often escapes the patient's attention.

Mental symptoms

It was said that certain personality traits emerged as being characteristic of the patients with Buerger's disease as a whole.[24] The patients were characterized mainly by poorly suppressed hostility, together with guilt over hostile and aggressive impulses; negativism, along with a desire to conform socially; ambition combined with strong unconscious desires for dependency which seemed to be entirely unacceptable at a conscious level.[25]

Buerger gave a living description of the patient with the disease. A haggard look, the staring eyes, the trunk bent with arms clasping and embracing the knee and leg of the affected part, is a striking and well known picture. Or, the foot is held tenaciously, the sole or dorsum rubbed and stroked in fruitless unavailing attempts to mitigate the intensity of the pain. So distressing can the symptoms be, that it is little wonder that intense mental depression is common. The pain, the disability, the threat of gangrene aroused by a knowledge of the fate of fellows in distress, so pervades every thought and action of certain cases as to cause complete demoralization, and in a few instances has led to attempts at suicide.[7] It is for the sake of mitigating the violence of pain to assume a peculiar posture in bed, and the posture makes circumstances inclinable to blood perfusion to the diseased foot.

Although it is not impossible vaguely to delineate familiar looks or features sometimes seen in the patients with disease, it is naturally no personal description of the patients. Almost all the patients with Buerger's disease have a problem with smoking, and it is an established fact that most of the patients won't give up smoking and have to be repeatedly hospitalized. However, it might be not concluded that the patients with the disease have a significantly weaker will to abstain from smoking than general smokers, though it is hard to understand that they smoke again after they sufficiently tasted the bitterness of smoking, namely, intractable painful necrotic lesions.

There were some patients with the disease who continued to smoke until death notwithstanding amputation of bilateral arms and legs.[26] We also experienced two basket cases before the early 1970s. When advised to stop smoking they would often state that they had a "nicotine deficiency"[26] and therefore could not stop. After both arms were amputated they continued to smoke with the help of the family. Abnormal mentality of the basket case who despaired of his future is exceptional, and it is irrational to generalize the abnormal mentality of an extreme example of Buerger's disease.

While the patients with the disease had not infrequently troubles with physicians and nurses regarding smoking and administration of analgesics, their irritation was suppressed within several weeks, and none led to attempts at suicide in our series. Addiction to smoking and weak-mindedness shouldn't be blamed only to the patients with Buerger's disease. Judging from that the patients with the disease did not drink deep as a rule, their smoking habits were not related with alcohol habits. Every man has his own taste. According to our observation of the patients in our series, no peculiar pathological personality was recognized.

Clinical correlations

As the chief traits of Buerger's disease are noticed in its clinical features and course, analyzing of clinical correlations in patients with Buerger's disease who were managed in the author's institution will be helpful to understand profiles of the disease.

Age and sex

From 1977 through 1988, 255 patients with Buerger's disease were treated at the author's institution; 249 were men (98%) and 6 were women (2%). All the patients were smokers.

The age at the onset of symptoms ranged from 19 to 49 years (average, 35.8±7.7 years). The maximum incidence by the age at the onset of the disease was in the fourth decade of life and the fifth, the third and the second decade followed in a decending scale. The time elapsed from the onset to the first examination at the author's hospital was one week to 44 years (average, 5.8±6.7 years). The majority of the patients received the first medical examination at other hospitals than the author's. In spite of changing smoking habits, the incidence in women in Japan is still low. A percentage of smokers in Japanese adult men was 75% in 1978, 68% in 1980 and 65% in 1982; that in Japanese adult women was 13%, 13% and 15% respectively.[27] Although affection of Buerger's disease in real nonsmokers is undeniable, especially in the nonsmokers who are exposed to the tobacco smoke of smokers, its incidence might be very low.

The first clinical manifestations of the disease usually appear between the ages of twenty and fifty years: the youngest case in our series was a man of 19 years at the onset. Laslett et al.[28] described the occurrence of the disease in a female of 17 years who had smoked two packs of cigarettes per day for at least 5 years: the youngest male patient in the Mayo series[29] was seventeen. Buerger's disease may affect men in their 50s, but they might be expected to respond in a different manner to etiologic factors than younger men, because their aged vessels may show arteriosclerotic degenerative changes and have no activity enough to provoke an inflammatory reaction.

Number of limbs involved

Two limbs were affected in 17 per cent of the 255 patients, three in 43 per cent, and four in 40 per cent : involvement was recorded when there was a missing distal pulse other than the dorsalis pedis plus signs of ischemia such as cyanosis, gangrene or ulceration, or angiographic evidence of the occlusive lesions. Thus, 83 per cent of all the cases had involvement of three or four limbs and none had single limb involvement: two or more extremities were involved in 62.5 per cent in the Army series[30], and in 91.5 per cent in Java series[31]. If the patient continues to smoke, three- or four-limb involvement might be the regular course of the disease with the lapse of time.

In the lower extremities, there was no difference in the frequency of involvement in the extremities between left and right, though Graves reported that the left was involved three times more frequently than the right.[32] Although the upper limb was involved in the majority of the patients, ischemic symptoms of the fingers were recognized in the minority of them. In 56 of the 255 patients, the initial ischemic symptom was noticed in the fingers. Our results showed a marked trend toward quadrilateral extremities involvement, when the disease first manifested itself in the fingers.

Impaired arterial pulsations

Absent arterial pulsation is one of the most important signs suggestive of arterial occlusive lesions in the extremities. Absence of the pulsation usually indicated that the palpated artery is not occluded but the more proximal segment to the artery examined by touch is obstructed, as long as the pulseless artery is not palpated as a solid cord.

At the first examination, one or both femoral pulses were impalpable in 20 (8%) of the 255 patients; normal femoral pulses with absent popliteal pulse were in 83 (32%), and normal popliteal pulses with absent posterior tibial and/or dorsalis pedis pulses in 152 (60%). From the status of the impaired arterial pulsations, it may be given as a conclusion that the proximal site of arterial occlusion was the aortoiliac region in 8%, the femoropopliteal in 32% and the infrapopliteal in 60%. In 60% of the patients, the arterial occlusive lesions remained below the knee. In other word, the obstructive lesions had progressed to the suprapopliteal region in 40% of all the patients until the first examination at our hospital. Compared with European series,[33] a higher incidence of the iliofemoropopliteal involvement in our series suggests that patients at an advanced stage predominated in the Nagoya series.

In case of arterial occlusion below the ankle at early stage of the disease, namely, with palpable ankle pulses, the patient with the disease very rarely consults a physician, because of an indefinite sign. The incidence of absence or hypoplasia of the anterior tibial and the posterior tibial artery was $7.1 \pm 0.73\%$ and $4.9 \pm 0.98\%$ in Japanese; $3.3 \pm 0.52\%$, $8.4 \pm 1.42\%$ in European respectively.[34] These fact should be taken into consideration on the occasion of pulsation of the ankle pulses.

The necrotic lesions in Buerger's disease do not usually appear on more than two extremities simultaneously. In 1937 Littauer and Wright[35] reported the case history of a patient suffering from the disease with acute simultaneous quadrilateral gangrenous lesions shortly after the first ocurrence of an ischemic ulcer on the finger.

Clinical presentation and progression

The patients do not think much of such ischemic symptoms as coldness, paresthesia or claudication, but they have themselves carefully examined when remarkable skin color changes or painful trophic changes occurred. Although it remains unknown whether the initial inflammatory lesion might occur simultaneously in multiple places of mainly the acral region of the extremities or at succesive intervals, progression of the arterial occlusions to the forearm or the lower leg in addition to those in the hand or the foot seems to be necessary for the occurrence of an unmistakable symptom of the disease. Fifty-six of the 255 patients in our series had ischemic symptoms of the fingers as an initial symptom, such as coldness, color changes, numbness or trophic changes. Of the 56 cases, 37 (66%) had four-limb involvement, 17 (30%) three-limb, and 2 (4%) 2-limb. Of the 199 cases with no initial finger ischemia, four limbs were affected in 65 (33%), three in 92 (46%), and two in 42 (21%). Compared the patients with the ischemic symptoms of the fingers as an initial symptom to the patients who had no initial symptoms of the fingers, the former had a tendency to have four-limb involvement more frequently than the latter.

The major initial symptoms were paresthesia, coldness, or cyanosis in 94 of the 255 patients (37%), foot claudication in 38 (15%), calf claudication in 42 (16%), rest pain in 26 (10%), gangrene or ulceration in 47 (19%), and thrombophlebitis in 8 (3%). The chief complaints at the first examination at the author's hospital were paresthesia, coldness, or cyanosis in 18 patients (7%), foot claudication in 20 (8%), calf claudication in 33 (13%), rest pain in 34 (13%), gangrene or ulceration in 145 (57%), and thrombophlebitis in 5 (2%).

While paresthesia, coldness or cyanosis accounted for 37% of the initial major symptoms, and claudication and critical ischemia (rest pain, gangrene or ulceration) amounted to about 30% of the symptoms respectively, the critical ischemia accounted for 70% of the major symptoms at the first visit to our hospital and the percentage of claudication, sensory disturbances, coldness or color changes remarkably decreased. As in the time elapsed from the onset to the first consultation at the author's institution, the necrotic lesions occurred in the majority of the patients, the painful gangrenous lesions distracted the patients' attention from the pervious symptoms, though foot or calf claudication, neuropathy, clod sensitivity or color changes persisted still. As the patient's attention was attracted by intractable gangrene or ulceration and his walking was circumscribed within narrow bounds, he became forgetful of the foot claudication for which he had been very concerned at onset of the disease. Therefore, after the ischemic ulceration healed, the foot claudication arouses the patient's attention again.

In case of progression of the infrapopliteal arterial occlusion to the suprapopliteal region, foot claudication was superseded by calf claudication, and the calf pain attracted the patient's attention in the first place during walking, because the calf muscles work most actively in walking. Even after improvement in calf claudication by arterial reconstruction, foot claudication remained almost unchanged, because the proximal arterial reconstruction only returned the patients to the status quo ante, in the days of foot claudication.[36] Arterial reconstruction of the crural and plantar arteries enough to relieve foot claudication is usually not feasible. Although cold sensitivity, a sensation of numbness after exercise, or vasospastic phenomenon was often recognized as the earliest subjective manifestation of the disease, the ischemic symptoms not infrequently persisted after complete healing of the necrotic lesions. Severe microcirculatory disturbances once induced by multiple peripheral arterial occlusive lesions wouldn't be noticeably improved in spite of surgical or conservative treatment.

Considering these findings, while gangrene or ulceration is an inevitable consequence of the severe ischemia, the necrotic lesion is not an essential feature of the disease but a secondary phenomenon. The characteristic feature of the disease may be critical limb ischemia due to breakdown of the microvascular circulation in the periphery.

From the onset of symptoms to the end of follow-up, gangrene or ulceration occurred in 184 (72%) of the 255 patients, thrombophlebitis migrans in 109 (43%), and involvement of the upper extremity in 230 (90%). It is striking that the upper limbs were involved in 90 per cent of the patients with the disease. Of the 230 patients with upper limb involvement, however, only 94 (41%) had obvious ischemic symptoms of the fingers, such as paresthesia, coldness, Raynaud's phenomenon, gangrene or ulceration. Each individual symptom should be estimated in connection with clinical course of the disease.

REFERENCES

1. Buerger L. (I-45).
2. Buerger L. (I-49).
3. Goodman RM et al. (II-1).
4. Shionoya S, Ban I, Nakata Y, Matsubara J, Shinjo K, Hirai M, Kawai S, Suzuki S, Tsai WH. Diagnosis, pathology, and treatment of Buerger's disease. Surgery 1974 ; 75 : 695-700.
5. Fontaine R, Kim M, Kieny R. Die chirurgische Behandlung der peripheren Durchblutungsstörungen. Helv Chir Acta 1954 ; 21 : 499-533.
6. Sasaki H, Sato Y, Maeyama T, Okuma T, Ohara I. A plantar ischemia test after walking as an index of walking exercise in the patients with Buerger's disease. J Jap Coll Angiol 1980 ; 20 : 873-8 (in Japanese).
7. Buerger L. (I-48).
8. Fairbairn JF II. Clinical manifestations of peripheral vascular disease. In : (I-36), pp 3-49.
9. Nielsen SL et al. (V-10).
10. Lassen NA et al. (V-32).
11. Hirai M, Shionoya S. Clinical use of Xe-133 non-ischemic work method in obliterative arterial diseases of the leg. Jap Circul J 1974 ; 38 : 763-74.
12. Hirai M, Shionoya S. Intermittent claudication in the foot and Buerger's disease. Br J Surg 1978 ; 65 : 210-3.
13. Cranley JJ. Ischemic rest pain. Arch Surg 1969 ; 98 : 187-8.
14. Buerger L. (I-40).

15. Mozes M, Cahansky G, Doitsch V, Adar R. The association of atherosclerosis and Buerger's disease: a clinical and radiological study. J Cardiovasc Surg 1970; 11: 52-9.
16. Buerger L. (I-37).
17. Ueno A, Kajiura N. Phlebitis migrans with syetmic vascular diseases. In: (IV-13), pp 190-3.
18. Hirai M, Ban I, Nakata Y, Matsubara J, Shinjo K, Miyazaki H, Kawai S, Shionoya S. Buerger's disease and toe ulceration. Geka 1976; 38: 285-9 (in Japanese).
19. Szilagyi DE, DeRusso FJ, Elliott JP. Thromboangiitis obliterans: clinico-angiographic correlations. Arch Surg 1964; 88: 824-35.
20. McPherson JR, Juergens JL, Gifford RW. Thromboangiitis obliterans and arteriosclerosis obliterans: clinical and prognostic differences. Am Intern Med 1963; 59: 288-96.
21. Hirai M, Shionoya S. Arterial obstruction of the upper limb in Buerger's disease: its incidence and primary lesion. Br J Surg 1979; 66: 124-8.
22. Tanabe T, Kiyota N, Yokota A, Yasuda K, Homma H, Sugie S. Problems on diagnosis and treatment of upper limb lesions of Buerger's disease. In: (IV-13), pp 206-10.
23. Barker NW. Arterial occlusion in the hands and fingers associated with repeated occupational trauma. Proc Staff Meet Mayo Clin 1944; 19: 345-9.
24. Heidrich H, Hollatz F, Potthoff R. Thromboangiitis obliterans und psychodynamische Befunde. In: (II-17), pp 59-62.
25. Baker G, Massell TB. An exploratory study of personality factors in thromboangiitis obliterans: a study of 18 patients. Angiology 1956; 7: 319-30.
26. Cabezas-Moya R, Dragstedt LR II. An extreme example of Buerger's disease. Arch Surg 1970; 101: 632-4.
27. Isayama Y. A right of excluding smoke. Tokyo: Iwanamishoten, 1983 (in Japanese).
28. Laslett LJ, Ikeda RM, Mason DT. Female adolescent Buerger's disease: objective documentation and therapeutic remission. Am Heart J 1981; 102: 452-6.
29. Allen EV, Brown GE. Thrombo-angiitis obliterans: a clinical study of 200 cases. Ann Intern Med 1927; 1: 535-49.
30. Freeman N. The diagnosis and treatment of thromboangiitis obliterans in the vascular centers of army general hospitals. Am Heart J 1947; 33: 332-40.
31. Hill GL et al. (II-19).
32. Graves AM. Thromboangiitis obliterans: a review. 1931; 12: 489-98.
33. Kummer A, Widmer LK, Da Silva A, Hug B. Thromboangiitis obliterans-zum Morbus Winiwarter-Buerger. VASA 1977; 6: 384-91.
34. Adachi B. Das Arteriensystem der Japaner Band II. Kyoto: Kyoto University Press, 1928, pp 215-41.
35. Littauer D, Wright IS. Simultaneons quadrilateral acute ulcerations in thrombo-angiitis obliterans: report of a case. Am Heart J 1937; 14: 466-73.
36. Shionoya S, Hirai M, Ohta T. A prospective study of hemodynamic changes associated with distal arterial bypass in the leg. Thorac cardiovasc Surgeon 1980; 28: 200-5.

CHAPTER VII
ANGIOGRAPHIC FINDINGS

A. The Dawning of Angiography

Although angiography is almost as old as roentgenology itself,[1] the earliest good vasograms of the living person were published in 1923 by Berberich and Hirsch.[2] Femoral angiography was at first performed by Brooks[3] in 1924, and he said that arteriography was of great value not only in determining the necessity of amputation and the amputation level but also in evaluation the site and extent of the collateral circulation.

A detailed angiographic investigation on the occlusive lesion in patients with Buerger's disease, with special reference to collaterals, was reported by Saito[4] in 1932: he used emulsion of iodine preparation, made by Yanagisawa, the chief apothecary of Nagoya University Hospital. The contrats medium consisted of emulsified Lipiodol in glycerine, alcohol, gum aradic, and lecithin, and the emulsion received the poetic name, "L'ombre," the shadow.[5] It contained oil particles smaller than red blood cells and it did not have any hemolytic action, and careful histological examination did not reveal any embolization or irritating effect. Saito and his colleagues obtained nice carotid angiograms and proved the usefulness of the contrast material in extremities as well.

Saito made a surgical method out of his approach. He injected his contrast material into one of the small branches of the artery he wanted to visualize. In doing so he avoided injury to the particular artery he wanted to see (Fig. VII-1 and 2). In case of femoral angiography, the contrast medium was injected into the external pudendal artery; in case of brachial angiography, it was injected into the superior ulnar collateral artery. On the occasion of infrapopliteal visualization, the medial superior genicular artery or the lateral superior genicular artery was used as the entry for the injection. The contrast medium was injected into the branch artery under clamping the femoral or brachial artery proximal to the orifice of the branch artery into that the needle was inserted. At that time, the arteriography produced a good visualization under such a blockade of the local circulation.

The arteriographic findings obtained from 15 patients with Buerger's disease in his series were as follows:

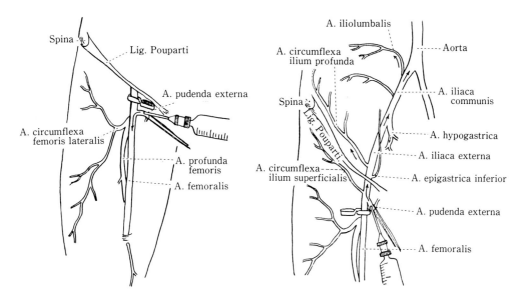

Figure VII-1. Femoral arteriography by puncture into the external pudendal artery through skin incision. (From Saito M, et al. J Jpn Surg Soc 1932 ; 32 : 1513-51.)

Figure VII-2. Retrograde pelvic arteriography by puncture into the external pudendal artery through skin incision. (From Saito M, et al. J Jpn Surg Soc 1932 ; 32 : 1513-51.)

Occlusion of the arm arteries
In 2 cases with the disease, the radial and ulnar arteries were occluded and the anterior and posterior interosseous arteries performed the duties of a collateral circulation to the hand and fingers : the former played a more important role in the formation of collaterals in case of occlusion of the forearm arteries than the latter.

In 21 limbs of 14 patients with the disease, the site of the arterial occlusion was the iliac region in one, the iliac and femoral in one, the femoral in 12, the popliteal in 2, the crural in 4, and the foot in one.

Occlusion of the iliac arteries
In case of occlusion of the external iliac artery, a collateral circulation to the femoral artery was mediated with the deep circumflex iliac and the inferior epigastric artery.

In case of occlusion of both the external iliac and femoral arteries, a collateral circulation to the lower leg was maintained through the internal iliac, inferior gluteal, obturator, medial circumflex femoral, and deep femoral arteries.

Occlusion of the femoral artery
In case of occlusion of the femoral artery between the inguinal ligament and the orifice of the deep femoral artery, a collateral pathway developed via the internal iliac, inferior gluteal, obturator, medial and lateral circumflex femoral, and deep femoral arteries. However, such a localized occlusion in this segment was rarely

seen, and on the occasion of obstruction of this segment due to a rapid proximal progression of the lesion in addition to distal femoral occlusion, ischemic symptom was the most severe. In case of occlusion of the femoral artery between the orifice of the deep femoral artery and the origin of the descending genicular artery, the descending branch of the lateral circumflex femoral artery and the perforating arteries of the deep femoral artery played an important role in the collateral circulation.

In case of occlusion of the femoral artery below the origin of the descending genicular artery, development of collaterals was dependent on the state of the popliteal artery. On the occasion of the consecutive occlusion of the popliteal artery, collaterals were produced through the descending genicular artery and muscular branches. The muscular branches played more important role in the formation of collateral to the infrapopliteal region than the deep femoral and descending genicular arteries. In the event of no occlusion of the popliteal artery, sufficient collaterals were developed through the descending genicular artery and muscular branches.

In short, the femoral artery was most frequently occluded between the origin of the deep femoral artery and the orifice of the descending genicular artery, and the descending branch of the lateral circumflex femoray artery and the most distal perforating artery of the deep femoral artery participated most in the development of collaterals. In case of occlusion of the femoral artery below the origin of the descending genicular artery , the collaterals were mainly produced through the descending genicular artery and muscular branches.

Occlusion of the popliteal artery
In case of occlusion of the popliteal artery below the origin of the sural arteries, the collateral were developed through the sural arteries and muscular branches of the femoral artery.

Occlusion of the crural arteries
Collateral circulation was attributed to one or two of the three main crural arteries, and a perforating branch and a communicating branch of the peroneal artery were the key point: the former connects the peroneal artery with the anterior tibial artery and the latter connects the peroneal artery with the posterior tibial artery.

In general, the development of collaterals in the lower leg was less sufficient than in the thigh, because the mein crural arteries are separated by the interosseous membrane.

Arterial occlusion in the foot
In case of occlusion of the dorsalis pedis artery, collaterals were developed mainly through the anterior lateral malleolar artery and the lateral tarsal artery. In case of occlusion of the medial plantar artery, the compensation was fulfilled by the lateral plantar artery. In case of occlusion of the lateral plantar artery, the

collaterals were developed through the medial plantar artery and the perforating branches of the dorsalis pedis artery.

In sum, collateral development was dependent on the location of the occlusion, its anatomic relationship to effluent and reentering collaterals, and the course and distribution of the collateral vessels. In case of occlusion of the femoral artery, the descending branch of the lateral circumflex femoral artery, the third perforating artery (the terminal part) of the deep femoral artery, and the descending genicular artery mainly contributed to the collateral supply. In case of occlusion of the popliteal artery, the muscular branches and the sural arteries had a play in collateral development. In case of occlusion of the crural arteries, the collaterals to the foot was developed through the perforating or communicating branches of the peroneal artery. In case of arterial occlusion in the foot, the collateral supply between the dorsal and plantar arteries of the foot was formed through the ramus plantaris profundus and perforating branches. In case of occlusion of the forearm arteries, the anterior interosseous artery participated in the formation of the collateral supply to the hand.

These general rules of collateral development on the occasion of the arterial occlusion is applicable not only to Buerger's disease, but also to other peripheral arterial occlusive diseases. As the degree of the ischemia due to arterial occlusion rests on the compensatory function by the collateral circulation, the extensive arteriographic study on the collateral supply in Buerger's disease was valuable for understanding pathologic physiology in arterial occlusive disease. While noninvasive diagnostic techniques for evaluating circulatory disturbances developed before angiography, for example, skin temperature measurement, oscillometry, Moszkowicz's reactive hyperemia method, skin color recovery time and so on, they were all inaccurate and subjective. Angiography brought arterial occlusive lesions in a living body into relief.

Standards of judgment of a normal arteriogram are prerequite for the arteriographic diagnosis. The characteristics of normal arteries in the arteriograms were noted by Allen and Camp[6] as follows: first, the smooth and uninterrupted contour of their lumen; secondary, the direct course of the vessels; and thirdly, the presence of no more than a minimum of collateral circulation. They thought that the chief value of arteriogrsphy lay not in the direction of diagnosis but in that of pathogenesis.

In 1935 Edwards[7] reported the arteriographic comparison of Buerger's disease and arteriosclerosis. In arteriosclerosis the arteriogram showed complete occlusion of segments but in addition showed eccentric filling defects in the other segments. The arteries also showed a more tortuous course than normally; and the collateral circulation was greatly increased. In Buerger's disease the arteriogram showed a varying extent of thrombosis, with smooth-walled segments above the occluded segments. The course of the vessels was less likely to be toutuous; and the collaterals, though increased in number above the normal, were yet fewer than in the arteriosclerotic. The difference between the irregular lumen of arteriosclerosis and the smooth appearing lumen of Buerger's disease, he said, could be explained by the occurrence of localized atheromata in the former disease, and their absence, in uncomplicated cases, in the latter. While discrete areas of proliferative thickening of the vessel wall might occur in Buerger's disease, the process was more apt to be one involving the entire circumference of the lumen, giving the lumen a reduced but regular outline.

Furthermore he commented that the blood stream tolerated localized atheromata well, thrombosis occurring late in arteriosclerosis. In Buerger's disease, however, even a small extent of involvement was quickly followed by thrombosis. In this way the arteriogram of an arteriosclerotic vessel may show atheromatous changes in outline, with or without occlusion; wheareas in Buerger's disease it is almost an "all or none" proposition, i.e., as soon as the artery is involved more than a very little, it is apt to be thrombosed, and show abrupt loss of its lumen up to the normal part of the artery. Concerning the fewer collaterals in Buerger's disease, he suggested that it might be to some extent a matter of time. That is, if the duration of the process were as long as in the arterioscleoric, the collaterals might gradually develop to the some extent. His paper touched the core of the subject and brought the difference in the arteriographic features between TAO and ASO into relief.

Arteriography visualizes only the segments escaped from the arterial occlusion, and we do not know about the real state of the not visualized regions in the arteriograms. An "all or none" proposition is adept in delineating a distinctive feature of the occlusion due to Buerger's disease.

B. Angiographic Characteristics in Buerger's Disease

In 1940 Kumamoto[8] regarded abrupt occlusion and coil-like collaterals characteristic for TAO. In 1958 Hershey and his colleagues[9] found abrupt and tapering occlusions, threadlike lumen due to recanalization and no calcification, intimal irregularity, or plaques in the arteriograms of three legs amputated because of Buerger's disease.

In 1962 Mckusick et al.[10] reported characteristic features from 14 brachial arteriograms in 10 patients and 17 femoral arteriograms in 12 patients with Buerger's disease as follows:
Brachial arteriogram
    1. No evidence of atheroma.
    2. Occlusion of the ulnar or radial artery, or both, at or above the wrist.

3. Persistence of the interosseous arteries, with terminal collaterals to the radial or ulnar arteries.
4. Marked tortuosity of recanalized radial or ulnar arteries.
5. "Spiderlegs" or "tree roots" configuration of collateral vessels at the point of previous obstruction of the artery.
6. Abnormal tortuosity in arteries to thumb and to other arteries in the hand.
7. Pruning of digital arteries.
8. Attenuation or interruption of 1 or both palmar arches.

Femoral arteriogram
1. Absence of significant changes that suggest atheroma in large vessels.
2. Smooth-lined vessels of even caliber down to a point of abrupt obstruction.
3. A segmental rather than diffuse involvement.
4. Minimal and probably earliest lesions in arteries of the feet and lower leg.
5. Often striking bilateral symmetry.
6. Spiderlegs or tree roots configuration of vessels around the point of focal disease.
7. Corkscrew tortuosity of superficial femoral and peroneal arteries which apparently had been occluded at their origin and subsequently recanalized.
8. Some tendency for lesser involvement of the peroneal artery as compared to the anterior tibial and posterior tibial arteries.

They emphasized the focal, or segmental, nature of the process in Buerger's disease and the diffuse character of the process in atherosclerosis.

In 1964 Szilagyi et al.[11] described the angiographic images in 22 patients with Buerger's disease under three headings: 1) Disseminated segmental occlusion. In these cases the angiograms showed occlusion of discontinuous portions of the primary and secondary branches of the popliteal or brachial artery; the occlusive change was located at various levels but was generally in the distal portions of the branch; at times branches of the plantar arches alone were involved. The segments of localized narrowing or occlusion would at times coalesce and cause obliteration of an entire arterial trunk or branch; 2) Distal infrapopliteal occlusion. The primary branches of the popliteal artery displayed a narrowing of the lumen that usually commenced in the middle third and became accentuated distalward, fading into complete lack of filling in their distal reaches; and 3) "Rippling" or "corrugated" appearance. The X-ray image consisted of ring like circular segments of stenosis 2 to 3 mm in width alternating at very constant intervals with segments of normal diameter, principally in the femoropopliteal axis and its primary divisions. They emphasized that the presence of obliterative lesions in the infrapopliteal arterial tree in complete absence of occlusive involvement of the femoral artery was a finding quite specific to the disease, and it was never seen in arteriosclerosis. Further they said that "corrugated" appearance might be specific to the disease, though the title to this claim was tenuous, since it was entirely statistical.

On analyzing the angiographic observations in patients with Buerger's disease in Israel, in 1965 Goodman et al.[12] reported that the most common site of arterial occlusion in the upper extremities was in the digital arteries (21 of 34 cases), the next most common was occlusive changes in the ulnar artery (15 of 34 cases). Other sites of arterial occlusion involved the palmar and radial arteries, respectively. In no case was occlusion of the interosseus artery observed.

In 1970 Lambeth and Yong[13] reported arteriographic findings in 16 patients with Buerger's disease in Malaysia. Diffuse arterial narrowing, occlusions, and a segmental pattern of arterial involvement were the most frequent observations, and apparently uninvolved arteries were smooth walled with regular contour. Femoropopliteal occlusions tended to be abrupt, while the more distal occlusions were frequently tapered. Collaterals at the sites of the distal occlusions occasionally presented a typical tree-root appearance; the more proximal collaterals around segmental occlusions in the larger vessels at times had the characteristic tortuous, corkscrew configuration. Early venous opacification, presumably evidence of arteriovenous shunting, and standing waves were infrequently demonstrated. The most striking feature of their study was the high incidence of femoropopliteal disease: localized dilatations and irregularities, stenoses, and occlusions were demonstrated in one-half of the lower limbs examined. From the presence of distal arterial occlusions in every instance of femoropopliteal involvement, they infered that the stenoses, dilatations, and irregularities of the femoropopliteal segment might represent early stages in the proximal progression of the inflammatory process and presage large vessel occlusion, though the validity of this prediction should await the results of serial arteriography in selected patients.

On the basis of analysis of arteriograms in 40 patients with Buerger's disease in Spain, Rivera[14] regarded the following arteriographic characteristics as typical for the disease:

1. Absence of arteriosclerotic lesions, with smooth arterial walls.
2. In general, slightly narrowed arterial lumen.
3. Multiple segmental occlusive lesions, localized predominantly in the forearm and hand, leg and foot, less frequently in the arm and thigh.
4. A progressive but regular reduction in width of the arterial tract above the thrombosed segments.
5. The collateral circulation was established primarily through the vasa vasorum surrounding the thrombosed segment (direct type of collateral circulation); "corkscrew" appearance.
6. In distal occlusions, the artery terminates with a series of small branches displayed as "tree roots" or "spider's jegs."
7. A localized narrowing of the lumen with regular margins in the femoropo-

plitea segment, possibly representing the early stage of the disease with only inflammatory lesions of the arterial wall.

Description of arteriographic features

In 1976 the Buerger's Disease Research Committee of the Ministry of Health and Welfare of Japan reported the arteriographic finding in 1367 patients: Buerger's disease (TAO) in 809 cases (26 females), arteriosclerosis obliterans (ASO) in 548 (35 females), and miscellaneous in 10.[15]

The arteriographic findings were obtained from 731 lower limbs and 78 upper limbs in Buerger's disease; from 528 lower limbs and 20 upper limbs in arteriosclerosis obliterans.

The arteries from the aorta to the digital arteries were consecutively numbered from 1 to 24 in the upper limb; from 1 to 26 in the lower limb for computerization. For instance, the proximal segment of the radial artery was numbered 11, the middle 12, and the distal 13: the proximal segment of the posterior tibial artery was numbered 15, the middle 16, and the distal 17[15].

All the arteriographically occlusive lesions were described according to the criteria as follows (Fig.VII-3):

1. Occlusion
    Abrupt
    Tapering
2. Stenosis: reduction in diameter of more than 50%
    Moth-eaten
    Localized
3. Irregularity: reduction in diameter of less than 50%
4. Collaterals
    Bridging: bypass-like collateral
    Corkscrew: coil-like collateral along the occluded vessel
    Tree root: root-like configuration of vessels around the point of abrupt occlusion
5. Kinking: bending of the artery at angle of more than 20° with the original course of the artery
6. Dilatation
7. Accordion: accordion-like or corrugated appearance
8. Diffuse smooth narrowing: narrowing of the artery just above occlusion.
9. Anomalous course: anatomical anomaly of the main artery
10. Early venous filling: localized early venous filling seen mainly in the thigh and foot
11. Fine thread: abnormally narrowed main artery below occlusion

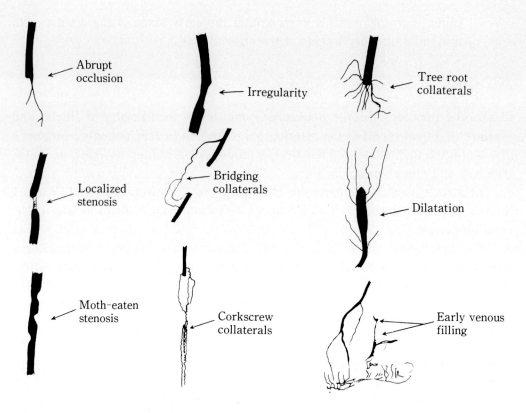

Figure VII-3. Sketches of angiographic features. (From Sakaguchi S. Junkankika 1977 ; 1 : 190-205.)

12. Miscellaneous.

These criteria of the description of arteriographic findings are useful for understanding and evaluating of the occlusive lesions in arteriograms of patients with arterial occlusive disease.

Lower extremity

Abrupt occlusion was most frequently recognized in the anterior and posterior tibial arteries. However, this type of occlusion was frequently seen in the iliofemoral region in ASO, and it did not appear that this type of occlusion was typical for TAO. Tapering occlusion was most frequently observed in the anterior tibial artery, and was seldom seen in the suprapopliteal region. This types of occlusion was much more frequently seen in TAO than in ASO, and it might be a characteristic finding for TAO.

Infrapopliteal arteries were diffusedly occluded and it was a great contrast to ASO. Although the anterior tibial artery, the posterior tibial artery and the peroneal artery were arranged in order of rate of occlusion, there was no significant difference in the incidence among them. As the dorsal and plantar arteries of the foot were the most frequently occluded, the arterial occlusion in TAO seemed to be centered around the ankle[15]. While stenosis and irregularity were frequently seen in the aortoiliac and femoropopliteal regions in ASO, irregularity was demonstrated mainly in the popliteal artery in about 1-3% of the cases with TAO.

Coil-like and root-like collaterals were frequently seen mainly in the posterior tibial artery and they were regarded as typical for TAO.[15] Kinking was frequently seen in the external iliac artery and the posterior tibial artery in ASO, but it was also recognized in the external iliac artery in TAO. The external iliac artery showed a marked tendency toward kinking. Accordion-like appearance was frequently seen in the anterior tibial artery in TAO. Early venous filling was the most frequently seen in the deep femoral artery in both TAO and ASO. Although it was also recognized in the lateral plantar artery in TAO, it did not seem to be typical for TAO. However, it remains unknown why early venous filling is observed only in such restricted arteries. Fine thread was much more frequently seen in the crural arteries and foot arteries in TAO than in ASO. This finding seemed to be typical for TAO, but detecting whether the abnormally narrowed main artery below the occlusion means arterial spasm or recanalization remains an unsolved problem[15].

Comparing the arteriographic findings of the lower extremity in females with those in males, neither stenosis nor irregularity was seen and fine thread was seldom recognized in the former. In short, the characteristic lesions for ASO were mainly distributed in the suprapopliteal region, and those for TAO were exclusively seen in the infrapopliteal region.

Upper extremity
Occlusion was restricted in the forearm arteries and the more distal arteries in TAO. Tapering occlusion was frequently seen in the digital arteries, but differentiating it from normal appearance seemed to be not easy. Occlusion was more frequently seen in the distal than in the proximal segment of the radial and ulnar arteries, and the superficial and deep palmar arches were frequently occluded. The arterial occlusions in TAO seemed to be centered around the wrist. Localized stenosis was seen in the brachial and forearm arteries.

Coil-like collaterals were frequently seen in the forearm and palmar arteries, and corkscrew type of collateral was typical for TAO. Kinking was recognized more frequently in ASO than in TAO. Dilatation and accordion-like appearance were rarely seen in TAO. Diffuse smooth narrowing was more frequently seen in the forearm arteries in TAO than in ASO. As no early venous filling was recognized in the brachial arteriograms, this finding seemed to be not characteristic for TAO, but to be found only in some restricted arteries. Fine thread was seen frequently in the palmar arteries, and it seemed to be typical for TAO.[15]

The proximal segment of the ulnar artery (ulnar trunk) was infrequently affected; it might be in accord with the fact that the proximal segment of the posterior tibial artery (tibioperoneal trunk) often escaped the occlusion. The anterior interosseous artery was rarely occluded. All the detailed arteriographic findings in patients with Buerger's disease might have been exhaustively described by this study.[15]

Although there is no absolutely pathognomonic angiographic finding which is recognized only in Buerger's disease and is never seen in other disease, a combination of several features is characteristic for the disease, namely, infrapopliteal and infrabrachial sites of the main occlusive lesions, abrupt and tapering occlusion, corrugated configuration, fine thread-like appearance, corkscrew-or tree roots-like collaterals, and no calcification or moth eaten stenosis.

C. Typical Arteriographic Figures of Occlusive Lesions

Sites of initial lesions

The initial lesions may be detected with angiographic examination in an asymptomatic limb of the patients who have characteristic features for Buerger's disease in the other affected limbs.

Upper limbs
In 1979 Hirai and Shionoya[16] compared arteriographic findings in 33 upper limbs with obvious ischemic symptoms with those in 45 upper limbs who underwent the examination irrespective of ischemic symptoms in the fingers. All the cases with occlusions of the palmar and more proximal arteries had occlusion of the digital arteries, excepting only one. As the digital arteries were most frequently occluded in the patients without ischemic symptoms of the fingers, the pathological process seems to start in the digital arteries (Fig. VII-4 and 5). However, the fact that segmental occlusions are observed in the arteries of the hand and forearm suggests that the disease might begin in not only in the fingers but also in these parts independently.

Lower limbs
In 137 (70%) of 195 femoral arteriograms obtained from the patients with Buerger's disease at our hospital from 1967 to 1976, the occlusive lesions were localized in the infrapopliteal region: the anterior tibial artery was occluded in 107 limbs, the posterior tibial artery in 102, and the peroneal artery in 66: the femoropopliteal segment was also involved in 58 limbs (30%) of them, in addition to the infrapopliteal lesions[17]. In 1974 Kusaba et al.[18] found angiographically the occlusion of the deep femoral artery in 10.7% of 75 limbs with Buerger's disease, the superficial femoral artery in 17.3%, the popliteal artery in 34.6%, the anterior tibial artery in 78.6%, the posterior tibial artery in 77.3%, the peroneal artery in 60.0%, the dorsalis

C. TYPICAL ARTERIOGRAPHIC FIGURES OF OCCLUSIVE LESIONS 129

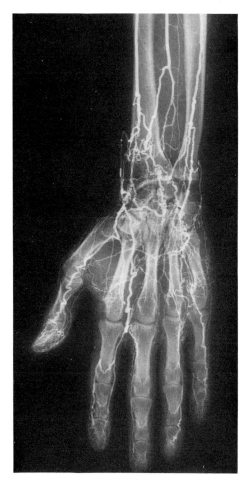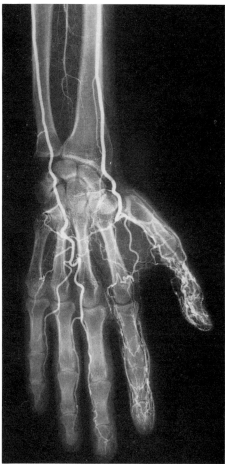

Figure VII-4. Right brachial arteriogram of a 46-year-old man with Buerger's disease. Despite of multiple occlusions of the arteries of the forearm and hand, the right upper extremity is asymptomatic.

Figure VII-5. Left brachial arteriogram of the same patient as in Figure VII-4. Despite of multiple occlusions of the palmar arch, the metacarpal and the digital arteries, the left hand is asymptomatic.

pedis artery in 83.8% and the plantar artery in 88.2%.

In 1975 Takao and his colleagues[19] demonstrated angiographically localized occlusive lesions around the ankle in 9 patients with Buerger's disease, in addition to occlusions in the foot and digital arteries, with a newly developed technique.[20] As there was no occlusion in the main arteries above the ankle, they considered these occlusive lesions around the ankle as the initial lesions due to the disease (Fig. VII-6). In 1981 Yano and his colleagues[21] examined the arteries of the feet and toes in 22 patients with TAO, ASO, collagen disease or miscellaneous with the direct geometric magnification arteriography. They clearly demonstrated a thrombus in

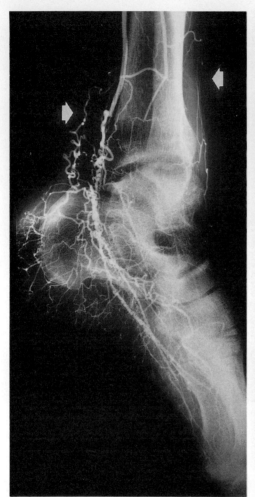 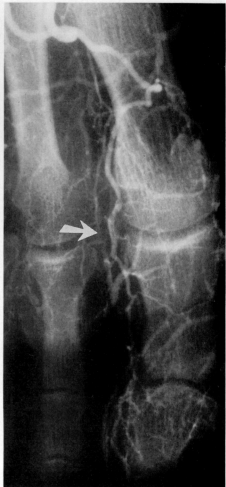

Figure VII-6. Left femoral arteriogram of a 34-year-old man with Buerger's disease. Multiple arterial occlusive lesions are seen around the ankle. The posterior tibial artery and the peroneal artery are abruptly occluded above the ankle (arrows). The medial and lateral plantar arteries show a corkscrew appearance (recanalization). The anterior tibial artery and the dorsalis pedis artery are occluded almost over their length.

Figure VII-7. Magnification arteriogram of the right foot arteries of a 46-year-old man with Buerger's disease.
The first plantar metatarsal artery is occluded with thrombus (arrow). (From Yano T, et al. In: Fukuda Y ed. Annual Report of the Vacular Lesions of Collagen Disease Research Committee of the Ministry of Health and Welfare of Japan; 1980, pp 313-8.)

the metatarsal artery in addition to occlusions in the digital and metatarsal arteries[22](Fig. VII-7). In a patient with periarteritis nodosa the occlusive lesions were observed in more distal vessels than those in TAO. Their results would confirm Buerger's opinion that the process does not originate in the capillaries or smallest arterioles, but begin in branches of moderate size. Judging from these

C. TYPICAL ARTERIOGRAPHIC FIGURES OF OCCLUSIVE LESIONS 131

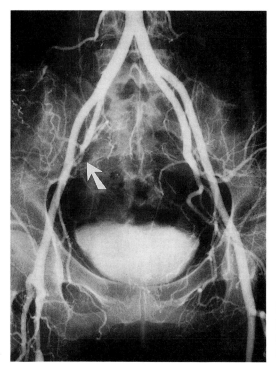

Figure VII-8. Pelvic arteriogram of the same patient as in Figure II-3. The superior and inferior gluteal arteries are occluded at their origin (arrow).

studies, the disease might commence in the digital, metatarsal, tarsal, calcaneal, arcuate, arcus plantaris, dorsalis pedis, and lateral and medial plantar arteries or their branches.

Aortoiliac region

Although the peripheral arteries are mainly affected with the disease, an involvement of the iliac artery is not rarely seen in addition to the occlusive lesions in the leg. Twenty-one (8%) out of 259 patients with Buerger's disease at our hospital from 1967 to 1977 showed aortoiliac occlusion: juxtarenal aortic occlusion in two, common iliac occlusion in one and external iliac occlusion in 18[17].

Pelvic angiography revealed localized occlusive lesions in the branch vessels of the internal iliac artery, and biopsy of the branch artery showed typical histological feature of Buerger's disease[23](Fig. VII-8). Judging from the arteriographic findings that localized occlusive lesions were recognized in the arteries mainly supplying the skeletal muscles such as the deep femoral and sural arteries, the disease might occur in the branch arteries of the proximal main arteries, independent of the initial lesions in the periphery of the extremities.

Occlusion

Occlusion is classified into some types by the state of visualization of the arteries

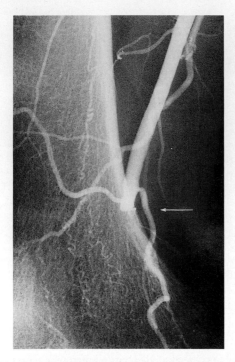

Figure VII-9. Right femoral arteriogram of a 45-year-old man with Buerger's disease. The superficial femoral artery is abruptly occluded near the exit of the adductor canal (arrow).

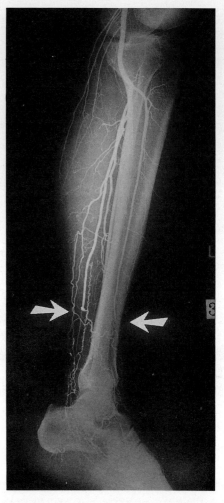

Figure VII-10. Left femoral arteriogram of a 39-year-old man with Buerger's disease. The anterior and posterior tibial arteries are abruptly occluded at the lower one-third of the leg (arrows).

just proximal and distal to obstruction of the lumen.

Abrupt occlusion

The smooth column of contrast medium is abruptly interrupted. The abrupt loss of its lumen means that the occluded segment due to thrombosis ends at the normal part of the artery (Fig. VII-9). It suggests the high frequency of infrapopliteal localization of the occlusive lesions that the abrupt occlusion was most frequently seen in the anterior and posterior tibial arteries in the disease, though this type of occlusion occurs in any artery (Fig. VII-10).

Tapering occlusion

The smooth column of dye reduces its diameter taperingly just like the end of a

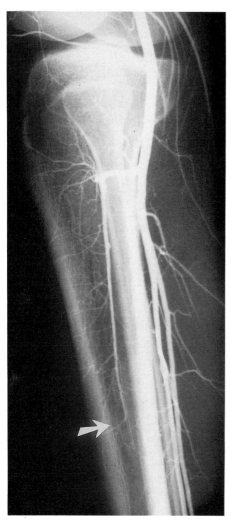

Figure VII-11. Right femoral arteriogram of a 43-year-old man with Buerger's disease. The anterior tibial artery shows a tapering occlusion at the middle of the leg (arrow).

radish. The feature implies that a narrowing of the lumen due to intimal thickening in the artery above the point of occlusion becomes accentuated distalward, fading into complete lack of filling in its distal reach. The high frequency of the tapering occlusion in the anterior tibial artery might be related with the hypoplastic anomaly of the artery (Fig. VII-11). Hershey et al.[9] reported a case in whom the anterior tibial artery was hypoplastic and did not extend to the foot, and the dorsalis pedis artery was an extension of the peroneal artery. They said that absence of an artery or an anomalous course of the artery was easily differentiated from an occlusion because in the latter collateral vessels were obvious.

As above described[24], the incidence of absence or hypoplasia of the anterior tibial artery in Japanese was higher than that in European (7.1±0.73% vs. 3.3± 0.52%). On the contrary, the incidence of absence or hypoplasia of the posterior tibial artery in Japanese was lower than that in European (4.9±0.98% vs. 8.4± 1.42%). Judging from that the incidence of the tapering occlusion in the mid tibial artery was 14.4% ; the mid posterior tibial, 8.2% ; and the distal peroneal, 6.7%, in the Annual report of the Buerger's Disease Research Committee[15], it might be unreasonable to attribute this type of occlusion entirely to the hypoplastic anomaly of the affected artery.

Segmental occlusion

Segmental occlusion has been said to be one of the most characteristic features for Buerger's disease[5](Fig. VII-12). However, the arteries have many places susceptible

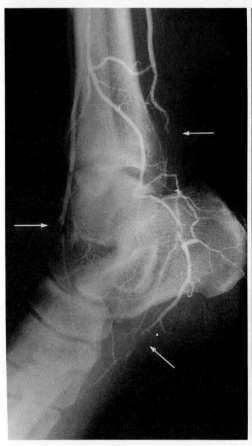
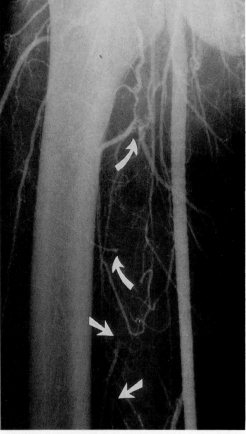

Figure VII-12. Right femoral arteriogram of a 42-year-old man with Buerger's disease. Segmental occlusions of the anterior tibial, the posterior tibial and the plantar artery are seen around the ankle (arrows). (From Shionoya S. In : Rutherford RB, ed. Vascular Surgery 3rd ed, W. B. Saunders, 1989, pp 207-17.)

Figure VII-13. Right femoral arteriogram of the same patient as in Figure VII-12. Multiple segmental occlusions are seen in the deep femoral artery and its branch arteries (arrows). The superficial femoral artery shows a corrugated appearance.

to arteriosclerotic lesions such as the orifices of branch arteries or the segments liable to traumatic injury, and the arteriosclerotic lesions are also segmental at the early stage.

Segmental arterial occlusions not only in the hand and foot but also in the skeletal muscles in Buerger's disease suggest a multicentric occurrence of the initial lesion (Fig. VII-13). Multicentric genesis or not, systemic factors might act in cooperation with local factors. When the regions lying between the segmental occlusions become obstructed, the finished picture is a continuous widespreading occlusion. Angiography at intervals may reveal the evolution and fusion of the initial lesions.

Stenosis and irregularity

While the main arteries proximal to the occlusion are smoothlined and of even caliber as a rule, stenosis or irregularity is sometimes seen mainly in the popliteal artery(Fig. VII-14). There are two manners in which proximal progression of the disease occurs; continuous and skip progression. The two types may occur in combination. The skip lesion in the popliteal artery, stenosis or irregularity, has been regarded as a result of the proximal progression of the inflammatory process[13]. The preexisting lesion in the popliteal artery favors occurrence of the thrombotic occlusion (skip progression) (Fig. VII-15).

The specimen harvested from the skip lesion of the popliteal artery of a patient with Buerger's disease who underwent arterial reconstruction because of complete occlusion of the preexisting stenotic lesion of the popliteal artery showed fresh thrombus with typical giant cell foci and inflammatory cell infiltration throughout the vessel wall, on the basis of proliferative thickening of the intima.[25] The same agent that elicits vascular inflammation with obstructive thrombus in the small arteries in the periphery of the extremities may involve the medium-sized or large arteries and provoke a parietal thrombus which results in various intimal changes. If the thromboangiitic process recurs at the precursory lesion, the lumen will be completely occluded with a thrombus.

While stenosis or irregularity of the vessel wall was recognized in about 1 to 3% of almost every main artery of the lower extremity[15], it is unknown whether the localized stenotic lesion was caused by the inflammation due to Buerger's disease or by hemodynamic changes or traumatic injuries, because the intimal thickening would result from various causing factors.

In 1977 Takao and his colleagues[26] found skip occlusions in 26 (19%) of 137 patients with Buerger's disease, and observed stenoses and irregularities (skip lesions) near the bifurcation of the femoral artery and the Hunter's canal, and at the popliteal artery. They regarded those regions as liable to be injured by the

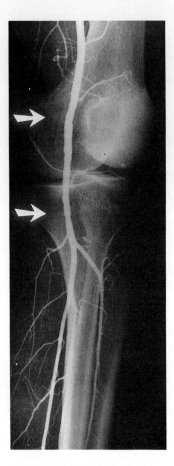 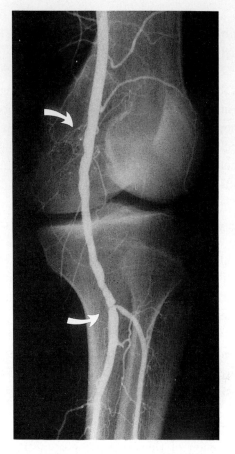

Figure VII-14. Left femoral arteriogram of a 33-year-old man with Buerger's disease. The popliteal artery shows irregularities of the vessel wall (skip lesion) (arrows). The anterior tibial artery shows a tapering occlusion with a corrugated appearance.

Figure VII-15. Left femoral arteriogram of a 51-year-old man with Buerger's disease (onset at the age of 42). The popliteal artery shows irregularities and a remarkable narrowing at the bifurcation (skip lesion) (arrows).

movement of the hip joint, compression from the adductor muscles or movement of the knee joint. Further they[27] examined histopathologically those narrowed but unoccluded segments, and recognized parietal thrombus, destruction of the internal elastic membrane and inflammatory cell infiltration in the vessel wall. They attached importance to the damage of the internal elastic lamina and suggested that the site of the destruction of the internal elastic membrane probably due to traumatic injury might favor the occurrence of the inflammation as Buerger's disease. They concluded[27] that skip progression might be due to a secondary thrombosis originated at the skip lesion.

Annotation: skip lesion is defined as stenosis, dilatation or irregularity of the vessel wall localized in the main patent artery above the peripheral occluded segment; skip occlusion is defined as the obstruction lying between the apparently normal segments. Elucidation of the pathogenesis of the skip lesion in the main artery in Buerger's disease is a topic for further discussion.

Dilatation

Although dilatative lesion is sometimes demonstrated associated with the stenotic skip lesion, true aneurysmal change is rarely seen in such artery as the radial, ulnar, anterior tibial, popliteal and extracranial arteries[28-31](Fig. VII-16).

As pathologic examination revealed no marked destruction or necrosis of the muscle fibers in the media of the affected artery, in spite of inflammatory cell infiltration throughout the vessel wall, it is hardly thinkable that an aneurysmal

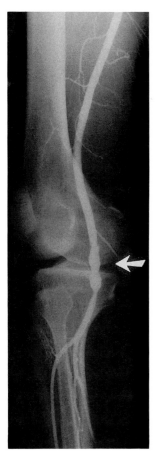

Figure VII-16. Right femoral arteriogram of a 41-year-old man with Buerger's disease. The second portion of the popliteal artery shows a dilatative lesion (skip lesion) (arrow). (from Shionoya S. World J Surg 1983; 7: 544-51.)

change of the vessel wall would result from the damaged media, as a rule. However, the media of the main artery affected with Buerger's disease showed not a little destruction in a rare case (Fig. IV-6), and there is no denying the possibility of occurrence of the aneurysmal lesion due to the disease.

Diffuse smooth narrowing

Diffuse smooth narrowing of the artery just above the site of occlusion is relatively frequently seen in the forearm arteries (Fig. VII-17), but the external iliac artery shows sometimes similar feature (Fig. VII-18).

In a patient with the disease with occlusion of bilateral femoral arteries in

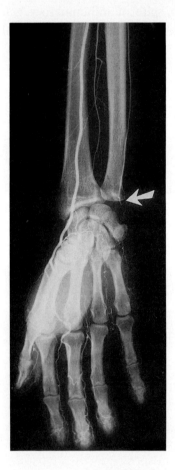

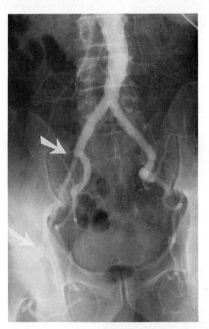

Figure VII-18. Translumbar aortogram of a 49-year-old man with Buerger's disease. The left external iliac artery is occluded at its origin, and the right external iliac artery is diffusely narrowed. The narrowed vessel seems to represent an early stage in the proximal progression of the inflammatory process and to presage occlusion of the segment (arrows). (From Shionoya S, et al. J. Cardiovasc Surg 1978 ; 19 : 69-76.)

Figure VII-17. Right brachial arteriogram of 51-year-old man with Buerger's disease (onset at the age of 46 years). The ulnar artery shows a diffuse narrowing and is abruptly occluded at the wrist (arrow). The palmar arch, the metacarpal and the digital arteries are diffusely occluded. (From Shionoya S. In : Rutherford RB, ed. Vascular Surgery 3rd. ed. W. B. Saunders, 1989, pp 207-17.)

addition to the infrapopliteal obstructive lesions, an unilateral external iliac artery was diffusedly narrowed and appeared as a tiny vessel, while the contralateral external iliac artery was completely blocked.[23] From the comparison between the angiographic features of the bilateral external iliac arteries, the former vessel seemed to represent an earlier stage than the latter and to presage complete occlusion of the segment in the future. The diffuse narrowing of the artery throughout its entire length, above the point of obstruction, might imply an intimal thickening due to the disease. It remains to be determined whether such a lesion always precede the complete occlusion of the affected artery, like the skip lesion in the popliteal artery.

Considering the very rare occurrence of occlusion of the brachial artery in patients with Buerger's disease, the preexisting stenotic lesion of the brachial artery and diffuse narrowing of the forearm arteries would more rarely favor progression of the occlusion, compared with the skip lesion in the lower extremity. Difference in collateral circulation and hydrokinetics between the upper and the lower extremity might be related with the different clinical course.

Fine thread

Fine thread means abnormally narrowed main artery below the site of occlusion, and the feature was seen mainly in the hand and in the infrapopliteal region : the incidence ascended distalward in the upper and the lower extremity.[15] The pathogenesis of the finding might be arterial spasm, recanalization or diffuse intimal thickening due to reduction in inflow (Fig. VII-19).

Accordion-like appearance

"Rippling" or "corrugated" appearance is by far frequently recognized in the femoropopliteal segment and the crural arteries in TAO compared with ASO (Fig. VII-20). The accordion-like appearance is seen not only in the femoropoliteotibial axis but also in the its primary divisions such as the sural arteries (Fig. VII-21).

In 1955 Ratschow[32] reported at first a particular form of contraction of the arterial wall in the arteriograms of the femoropopliteal segment, and he named it "Perlschnurarterie" (beads-like artery). In 1957 Wickbom and Bartley[33] called the feature in the femoral artery circular constrictions ; Ito and Takeuchi[34] described it as beads-like artery at first in Japan, and in 1961 Morioka et al.[35] named it accordion-like arterial shadow.

In 1970 Hara[36] found the feature in 38 of 347 cases(45 of 521 lower limbs) : the incidence was 15.9% in TAO, 21.4% in chronic arterial occlusive disease (cases not identified TAO or ASO), and 5.4% in miscellaneous. He summarized as follows : 1)

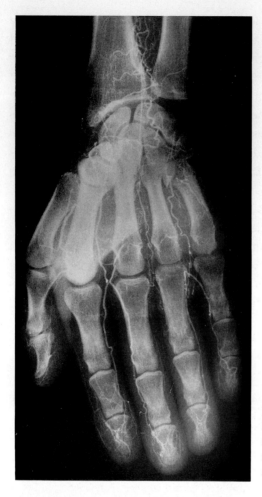

Figure VII-19. Right brachial arteriogram of a 52-year-old man with Buerger's disease (onset at the age of 40 years). The arteries of the forearm and hand are extensively obstructed, and the remaining vessels look as fine threads.

the shadows were observed more frequently by femoral arteriography performed under spinal anesthesia than by that under local anesthesia; 2) a rectangular position of the examining knee joint was more favorable for producing the shadows than a straightly extended or an extremely flexed position; 3) the shadows were found more frequently in males of the thirties without arterial sclerosis than in elder subjects; 4) it was observed mostly in the femoropopliteal and the anterior tibial arteries, exclusive of curving portions (femoro-popliteal junction and the portion of the anterior tibial artery immediately distal to the orifice); 5) the wave lengths of the shadows had a positive correlation with diameters of the arteries involved; 6) wavy contour of the shadows was static on the serial arteriograms. The shadows were usually reproduciable and involved the same artery in repeated study; 7) the involved segment seemed to be rather in a dilated state than in a constricted one, compared with another segments; 8) whether lumbar sympathectomy and vaso-

C. TYPICAL ARTERIOGRAPHIC FIGURES OF OCCLUSIVE LESIONS

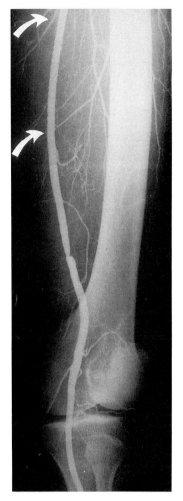
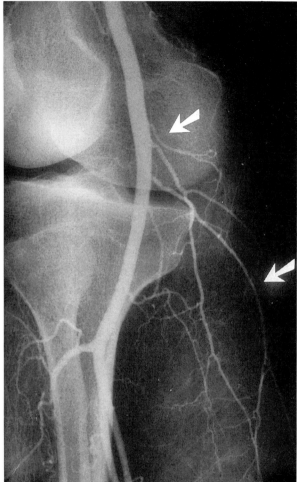

Figure VII-20. Left femoral arteriogram of a 48-year-old man with Buerger's disease. The superficial femoral artery shows a corrugated appearance (arrows) and there is a localized narrowing near the opening of the adductor canal (skip lesion).

Figure VII-21. Right femoral arteriogram of the same patient as in Figure VII-14. The sural arteries show an accordion-like appearance (arrows).

dilating drugs influenced on occurrence of the shadow was still controversial; and 9) the following factors seemed to have no relation to the occurrence of the accordion-like shadows: puncture of the arterial wall, concentration of the contrast medium, and injection mode of the contrast.

In 1973, based on clinical and experimental studies, Ishikawa and his colleagues[37] reported that the shadows did not indicate the presence of a pathological state of the arterial wall, but presumably appeared in a physiologic one, and concluded that a delicate arterial state of longitudinal constriction might be a cause of the accordion-like shadows. They based their hypothesis on following facts: 1) the shadows were observed mainly on the femoral, popliteal, and tibial arteries, especially in rectangular position of the knee joint; 2) the shadows were usually reproducible and the contour of the shadows was stationary; 3) the artery in vivo was physically in moderately stretched state especially in young persons, and the longitudinal tension would be altered with position of the knee joint; 4) the muscles of the arterial wall was slightly relaxed under spinal anesthesia; 5) the shadows frequently appeared in males of thirties; 6) experimental arteriograms of the excised canine artery demonstrated a pattern similar to the accordion-like shadows under a delicate condition of intraluminal pressure and of longitudinal traction; and 7) the constricting waves were shown experimentally in the spiral strip of the human artery suspended in the Magnus apparatus.

Although the accordion-like shadow appears even in a physiologic state, the feature may be regarded as characteristic for TAO, in view of its higher incidence in TAO compared with that in ASO. The accordion-like appearance is different from arterial spasm caused by puncture and catheterization,[38] and it seems to touch on the fringe of the peculiar character of the arterial wall of muscular type.

Early venous filling

Early venous filling due to arteriovenous shunt was the most frequently seen in the deep femoral and lateral plantar arteries[15](Fig. VII-22).

It remains unresolved why the arteriovenous shunt is so frequently seen in such arteries supplying blood for the muscles. Ohara[39] attributed the early venous filling in the foot to the collateral vessels with arteriovenous fistula. As the finding is also recognized in ASO, the pathogenesis might be related with a congenital arteriovenous communication (microvascular malformation).

Figures at venous phase

Very few investigations about the angiographic figures at the venous phase in TAO have been reported, though some venographic examinations were carried out in the days of Buerger in order to detect a possibility of arterialization of the deep veins in ischemic legs.

In 1976 Chopra et al.[40] laid an emphasis on venous involvement on the basis of venographic investigation of 25 patients with TAO. Venograms were interpreted as "normal," "abnormal" or "suspicious." They were interpreted normal if they

C. TYPICAL ARTERIOGRAPHIC FIGURES OF OCCLUSIVE LESIONS

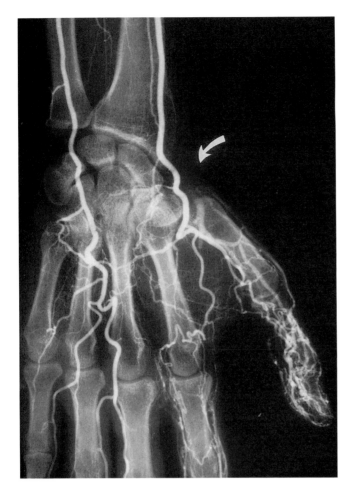

Figure VII-22. Left brachial arteriogram of the same patient as in Figure VII-4 (enlargement of Figure VII-5). Early venous filling is seen near the distal wrist crease (arrow).

satisfied the following criteria : 1) visualization of the anterior tibial, posterior tibial, peroneal, popliteal and superficial femoral veins ; 2) normal valves, contour and regular smooth vein walls ; 3) no filling defect ; 4) no incompetent perforators ; and 5) good post-exercise clearance. Thrombosis was diagnosed : 1) filling defect ; 2) irregular venous walls and valves ; and 3) incompetent perforators and abnormal collaterals. "Suspicious" venogram was classified : 1) non-visualization of a vein with abnormal collaterals ; 2) incompetent perforators and abnormal collaterals ; 3) persistent narrowing of the caliber of the vessel ; and 4) inadequate postexercise clearance. Combining the clinical evidence with phlebographic and histopathological investigations, the incidence of the venous involvement in their series was about 60%. This figure was significantly higher compared to the previous studies[41,42]. They thought that the low incidence of the venous involvement in the other series was due to the lack of venographic studies.

Interpretation of venographic findings as normal compares poorly with that of arteriograms. Furthermore, occlusions of the crural veins below the knee result in no clinically significant disturbance of venous return as a rule, and venographic examination is not directly concerned in diagnosis and treatment of Buerger's disease.

However, it is interesting that Yano et al.[21] found atonic dilatation of the toe veins in a patient suffering from intractable ischemic ulcers of the toes by magnification arteriography at venous phase. As the microcirculatory stagnation is closely bound up with the formation of intractable necrotic lesions in critical ischemic limbs, such an atonic dilatation of the toe veins is suggestive of participation of the venous stagnation in the ischemic ulceration.

Collaterals

The degree of ischemia in chronic arterial occlusive disease rests on the extent of collateral circulation. There are two types of collaterals in view of the mechanism of development[4,43] : 1) by revascularization of the occluded vessels, and 2) by vessels bypassing the occluded segment. The former is formed by recanalization of the occluding thrombus in the affected artery and development of the vasa vasorum in the occluded artery: the latter is produced by anastomosis between the vessels branching off above and below the occluded segment of the artery.

The direct type of collateral circulation is established primarily through the vasa vasorum surrounding the occluded segment and recanalization of the thrombus; this accounts for "corkscrew" appearance of the collaterals (Fig. VII-23). The indirect type of collateral circulation consists of an inflow artery and an outflow artery; this accounts for "bridging" appearance of the collaterals (Fig. VII-24). "Tree roots" configuration may be built up with a combination of the direct and indirect types of collateral circulation (Fig. VII-25).

Considering that the thrombus is much earlier and better organized with recanalization in TAO than in ASO, it is understandable that "corkscrew" or "tree roots" configuration of collateral vessels is more frequently seen at the point of obstruction of the artery in TAO than in ASO. Reduction in activity to recanalize the thrombus and atheromatous intimal thickening at the orifice of the branching vessels in ASO impede the development of collateral circulation. Contrary to the previous reports[7], the visualized collaterals seem to be much more in number in TAO than in ASO.

There were some patterns of development of collateral circulation according to the sites of occlusions, judging from the angiographic findings in 128 limbs with TAO in our series.[43]

Occlusions of the crural arteries

In 85 of the 128 limbs the occlusions were localized below the knee.

C. TYPICAL ARTERIOGRAPHIC FIGURES OF OCCLUSIVE LESIONS   145

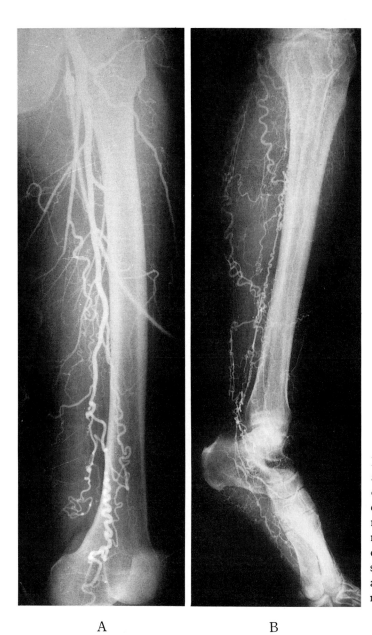

Figure VII-23. Left femoral arteriogram of a 48-year-old man with Buerger's disease. The superficial femoral, the popliteal and the crural arteries are extensively occluded, and collateral vessels show a corkscreew appearance. A: Above knee region. B: Below knee region.

A   B

1) Occlusion of the anterior tibial artery (60 limbs)
Although the collaterals originated in the popliteal, the posterior tibial or the peroneal artery, the collateral circulation was poor. It might be attributable to scarce preexisting anastomoses between the other crural arteries and the anterior tibial artery from which the anterior tibial muscle derives its chief blood supply.

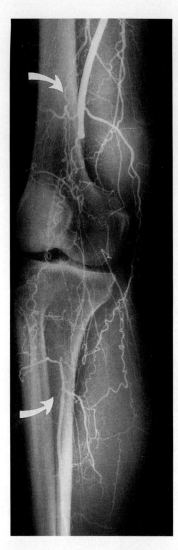 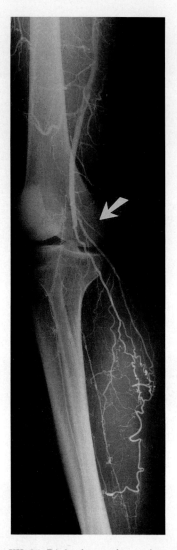

Figure VII-24. Right femoral arteriogram of a 38-year-old man with Buerger's disease. The popliteal artery is occluded, and the collateral circulation through the descending genicular artery between the femoral artery and the peroneal artery shows a bridging appearance (arrows).

Figure VII-25. Right femoral aretriogram of a 38-year-old man with Buerger's disease. The popliteal artery is occluded at the second portion, and the collateral vessels through the sural arteries show a tree roots appearance (arrow).

2) Occlusion of the posterior tibial artery (60 limbs)

The collateral vessels originated from the peroneal and sural arteries. The more proximally the posterior tibial artery was occluded, the more frequently the sural arteries anastomosed with the muscular branches in the posterior crural muscles, but there was no enlargement of the diameter of the sural arteries.

3) Occlusion of the peroneal artery (40 limbs)

In case of occlusion of the peroneal artery at its origin, no development of collateral circulation was recognized, when the posterior tibial artery was patent. The development of collateral circulation in case of occlusion of the crural arteries was dependent on patency of the peroneal artery. Potent collaterals were formed through the peroneal artery, and no effective direct communication was developed between the anterior tibial and the posterior tibial artery.

The reason why "corkscrew"-or"tree roots"-collaterals are the most frequently seen in the posterior tibial artery is as follows: 1) the incidence of absence or hypoplasia of the posterior tibial artery is much lower than that of the anterior tibial artery; 2) muscular branches of the posterior tibial artery supply soleus and the deep muscles on the back of the leg, but those of the anterior tibial artery are mainly distributed to the anterior tibial muscle; and 3) the posterior crural muscles exceed in the quantity of muscle and motion than the anterior tibial muscle.

As the branches of the posterior tibial artery are superior in the number and function to those of the anterior tibial artery, the former favors the formation of collateral circulation compared with the latter. While some muscular branches of the anterior tibial artery pass through the interosseous membrane to anastomose with branches of the posterior tibial and peroneal arteries, the collateral communication between the anterior crural and the posterior crural muscles develops poorly as a rule, as Saito already mentioned.[4]

Occlusions of the femoropopliteal Segment

In 43 of the 128 limbs the occlusion progressed to the suprapopliteal region in addition to the infrapopliteal occlusions: continuous occlusions (29 limbs); the suprapopliteal occlusion continued successively from the infrapopliteal occlusion (A group); and skip occlusions (14 limbs); the suprapopliteal occlusion skipped a part (mainly the bifurcation) or most of the popliteal artery (B group). In view of development of collateral circulation, the saphenous branch of the descending genicular artery and the sural arteries were the keys to the development of collateral circulation.

1) Occlusion below the orifice of the sural arteries (10 limbs)

In both groups, the saphenous branch and sural arteries developed as collateral vessels, especially the latter.

2) Occlusion below the orifice of the saphenous branch (8 limbs)

In both groups the saphenous branch became the main collateral vessel. Although the sural arteries sometimes were visualized from the middle of the course and extended distalward, the extent was poorer than in case of occlusion below the orifice of the sural arteries.

3) Occlusion beyond the orifice of the saphenous branch (23 limbs)

In A group, collateral vessels originating in the deep femoral artery ran into the saphenous branch or sural arteries, through which the collateral circulation extended more distally. In B group, collateral vessels originating in the deep femoral artery anastomosed with the genicular network, because the bifurcation of the popliteal remained patent. Therefore, there was little scope left the saphenous branch and sural arteries for further activities as collaterals.

4) Skip occlusion above the orifices of the saphenous branch and sural arteries (2 limbs)

Collateral vessels originating in the deep femoral artery anastomosed with the genicular network, because there was no need of collaterals bypassing the popliteal segment. However, the saphenous branch and sural arteries may develop as collateral pathway according the site and extent of occlusive lesions in the crural arteries.

Occlusions of the aortoiliac region

The proximal progression of the occlusion due to TAO terminated at the external iliac artery as a rule[23]. The external iliac artery was usually occluded throughout its entire length, and collateral circulation was formed mainly via the branches of the internal iliac artery (the inferior gluteal and the obturator artery) and of the deep femoral artery (the lateral and the medial circumflex femoral artery).

On the basis of the iliac occlusion, a secondary thrombotic process rarely reached just below the orifices of the renal arteries.[17] While collateral circulation in case of the juxtarenal aortic occlusion due to TAO developed in the same manner as in case of the juxtarenal aortic occlusion due to atherosclerosis, the compensatory function of the collaterals in the former seemed to be poorer than in the latter, because of more widespread obstruction in the iliofemoral segment.

Occlusions of the forearm arteries

In the brachial arteriographies performed in the patients with TAO at our hospital from 1967 to 1978, the arteriograms of 78 limbs were fit for the diagnosis of occlusive lesions[16].

Thirty-three of them were carried out before February 1977, being performed mainly in patients with severe digital ischemia. During this period, obstruction of both the radial and the ulnar artery was overwhelmingly prevalent. The remaining 45 arteriograms were carried out after March 1977, irrespective of the presence of ischemic symptoms or signs in the fingers. In the latter group, obstruction of the more distal arteries was detected with increased frequency. In 39 hands without clinical evidence of ischemia the most common site of occlusion was the digital artery: the segmental type of obstruction accounted for 36% of cases in which occlusive lesions were detected only in the digital artery. In the arteries of the hand, diffuse occlusion associated with an involved radial or ulnar artery was a common finding, but segmental occlusion was also seen in this area. In all but one of 59 cases that were found to have obstructions in the arteries of the hand, or in the radial or the ulnar artery, occlusive lesions of the digital artery were also observed.

The interosseous arteries remained patent in the majority of the patients with TAO, and they played the most important role in the development of collaterals in case of occlusions of the forearm arteries. Although the bridging type of collateral was the most frequently seen in the forearm, hand and digital arteries, "corkscrew" or "tree roots" configuration of collateral vessels was also recognized. Marked tortuosity of recanalized vessels was conspicuous. While the occlusive lesion progressed to the brachial artery in five out of the 255 cases in our series, no case with proximal progression of the occlusion to the axillary artery was observed.

REFERENCES

1. Doby T. Development of angiography and cardiovascular catheterization. Littleton: Publishing Sciences Group, 1976.
2. Berberich J, Hirsch S. Die Röntgenographische Darstellung der arterien und Venen am lebenden Menschem. Klin Wschr 1923; 2: 2226-8.
3. Brooks B. Intra-arterial injection of sodium iodid: preliminary report. JAMA 1924; 82: 1016-9.
4. Saito M, Kamikawa K, Yanagizawa H. Arteriographic findings in patients with Buerger's disease: with special reference to development of collateral circulation. J Jpn Surg Soc 1932; 32: 1513-51 and 1759-96 (in Japanese).
5. Saito M, Kamikawa K, Yanagizawa H. A new method of blood vessel visualization (arteriography; veinography; angiography) in vivo. Am J Surg 1930; 10: 225-40.
6. Allen EV, Camp JD. A roentgenographic study of the peripheral arteries of the living subject following their injection with a radiopaque substance. JAMA 1935; 104: 618-24.
7. Edwards EA. The arteriographic comparison of thrombo-angiitis obliterans and arteriosclerosis. N Engl J Med 1935; 213: 616-7.
8. Kumamoto M. Arteriography as a special diagnostic method of spontaneous gangrene. Jitchiikatorinsho 1940; 17: 584-601 (in Japanese).
9. Hershey FB, Aikman WO, Ackerman LV, Stamp WG. Pathologic and radiographic studies of amputated extremities. Surgery 1958; 44: 1008-23.
10. McKusick VA et al.(I-71).
11. Szilazy DE et al.(VI-19).
12. Goodman RM et al.(II-1).
13. Lambeth JT, Yong NK. Arteriographic findings in thromboangiitis obliterans: with emphasis on femoropopliteal involvement. Am J Roentgenol Rad Ther Nucl Med 1970; 109: 553-62.
14. Rivera R. Roentgenographic diagnosis of Buerger's disease. J Cardiovasc Surg 1973; 14: 40-6.
15. Sakaguchi S. Angiography in Buerger's disease. Junkankika 1977; 1: 190-205 (in Japanese).
16. Hirai M, Shionoya S.(VI-21).
17. Shionoya S. Buerger's disease. In: Sakaguchi S ed. Arterial occlusive disease. Tokyo: Kaneharashuppan, 1979, pp 170-83 (in Japanese).
18. Kusaba A, Kiyose T, Moriyama M, Furuyama M, Inokuchi K. Arteriographic characteristics of Buerger's disease. In: lshikawa K ed. Annual report of the Buerger's Disease Research

Committee of the Ministry of Health and Welfare of Japan, 1974, pp 80-7 (in Japanese).
19. Takao T, Ooiwa S, Naiki K, Yano T. Angiographic findings: with special reference to initial occlusive features. In: (IV-55), pp 41-9.
20. Kato K, Takao T, Ooiwa S, Naiki K, Yano T. Arteriography of the foot. J Jap Coll Angiol 1973; 13: 287-92 (in Japanese).
21. Yano T, Naiki K, Kato R, Kazui H, Terasawa T, Tsuchioka H. Occlusion of the arteries of the toes in the patients with vascular diseases by magnification arteriography. In: Fukuda Y ed. Annual Report of the Vascular Lesions of Collagen Disease Research Committee of the Ministry of Health and Welfare of Japan, 1981, pp 322-7 (in Japanese).
22. Yano T, Naiki K, Kato R, Kazui H, Nagata M, Kobayashi M, Terasawa T, Nakai T. An angiographic study on occlusive lesions of metatarsal and digital arteries of Buerger's disease. In: (IV-50), pp 313-8 (in Japanese).
23. Shionoya S, Ban I, Nakata Y, Matsubara J, Hirai M, Kawai S. Involvement of the iliac artery in Buerger's disease: pathogenesis and arterial reconstruction. J Cardiovasc Surg 1978; 19: 69-76.
24. Adachi B.(VI-34).
25. Shionoya S.(I-79).
26. Takao T. et al.(IV-13).
27. Takao T. et al.(IV-14).
28. Takao T. et al.(IV-54).
29. Sakaguchi S.(IV-55).
30. Uchida H. et al.(IV-56).
31. Giler Sh. et al.(IV-57).
32. Ratschow M. Die Perlschnurarterie. Z Neurochir 1955; 15: 154-9.
33. Wickbom I, Bartley O. Arterial spasm in peripheral arteriography using the catheter method. Acta Radiol 1957; 47: 433-48.
34. Ito T, Takeuchi Y. Angiographically bead-like vessel. Jap Circul J 1958; 22: 190 (in Japanese).
35. Morioka Y, Ishikawa K, Mishima Y, Sugaya Y. Bead-like appearance in arteriograms of the lower extremity. Jap Circul J 1961; 25; 476 (in Japanese).
36. Hara K. Accordion-like arterial shadows observed on the arteriograms of the lower extremities. J Jap Coll Angiol 1970; 10: 461-74 (in Japanese).
37. Ishikawa K, Mishima Y, Morioka Y, Hara K. Accordion-like arterial shadows observed on the arteriogram. Angiology 1973; 24: 398-410.
38. Lindbom Å. Arterial spasm caused by puncture and catheterization. Acta Radiol 1957; 47: 449-60.
39. Ohara I. Angiographic and pathohistologic study of the etiology of Buerger's disease. In: (VII-18), pp 15-8 (in Japanese).
40. Chopra BS et al.(IV-37).
41. Abramson D. Diagnosis and treatment of thromboangiitis obliterans. Geriatrics 1965; 20: 28-41.
42. Schatz IJ, Fine G, Eyler WR. Thromboangiitis obliterans. Br Heart J 1966; 28: 84-91.
43. Shionoya S, Hirai M. Collateral circulation in Buerger's disease. J Jap Coll Angiol 1976; 16: 525-7 (in Japanese).

CHAPTER VIII
CLINICAL COURSE

The traits characteristic of Buerger's disease consist in the clinical course. The clinical course of the disease is decidedly influenced by the patient's smoking habits. The worsening of the disease does not occur if the patient completely stops smoking, but it does recur if the patient resumes smoking. This is an established and undeniable fact. The disease usually starts at the small vessels of the periphery in the extremities, mainly in the arteries of the digits, hand and foot. Within a given period after the onset of the disease, the occlusive lesions might progress to the forearm or the leg arteries, and the pattern of the infrabrachial or the infrapopliteal occlusions seems to follow the patient as a shadow.

A. Pattern of Arterial Occlusion

Information on manner and rate of progression of the obstructive lesion has considerable prognostic and therapeutic significance in Buerger's disease. Although there have been many studies of arteriographic feature of occlusive lesion in the disease, knowledge of arteriographic pattern and manner of progression in Buerger's disease remains limited, because repeated angiography bore some risk and was uncomfortable for the patient. In 1954 Hashimoto et al.[1] repeated angiographic examination in 8 patients with Buerger's disease: proximal progression of the occlusion in the main arteries in 3 cases and no progression in 5. They posed a question whether one group with progression of arterial occlusion was pathogenetically different from the other group with unchanged pattern of arterial occlusion.

From 1967 through 1980 one hundred eight patients with Buerger's disease underwent simultaneously bilateral femoral arteriography at our hospital[2]. With the exception of three patients who had already undergone below knee amputation unilaterally, arteriographic patterns were analyzed in 210 limbs of 105 patients.

Site of arterial occlusion

The site of arterial occlusion is given in Table VIII-1. There were no differences

Table VIII-1. Sites of arteriographic occlusive lesions in 210 limbs with Buerger's disease. (From Shionoya S, et al. Angiology 1982 ; 33 : 375-84.)

	Right	Left
Femoralis superficialis	14	7
Poplitea	28	25
Tibialis anterior	95	87
Tibialis posterior	84	85
Peronea	59	46

in the morbidity of each artery between the right and left sides. Regarding frequency of obstruction of the crurual arteries, the anterior tibial artery was occluded in about 90% of 210 limbs ; the posterior tibial artery, in about 80% ; and the peronesl artery, in about 50%.

In 42 of 105 patients, the femoropopliteal segment was affected in addition to the infrapopliteal occlusions ; the disease progressed to the suprapopliteal region in about 40% of all the patients in this series. The patients with occlusive lesion of the femoropopliteal segment in addition to the infrapopliteal obstruction were named the femoropopliteal group ; the patients with only infrapopliteal occlusive lesions, the infrapopliteal group.

Pattern of crural arterial occlusion

Regarding the pattern of the crural arterial occlusion, the bilateral arteriograms were classified into three types as follows : 1) similar : the same arteries were occluded in both legs as seen in Figure VIII-1 ; 2) different : the affected arteries were different in both legs as seen in Figure VIII-2 ; and 3) unilateral : obstructive lesion was seen in only an unilateral leg.

When the pattern of the crural arterial occlusion in the femoropopliteal group was compared with that in the infrapopliteal group, the "similar pattern" was recognized in about 40% of each group (Table VIII-2). The case in which a patent crural artery was smoothly continuous with the dorsalis pedis or the plantar artery was named "continuous"(Fig. VIII-3) ; the case in which a crural artery revisualized via a collateral channel was connected with the foot artery was named "discontinuous"(Fig. VIII-4).

A. PATTERN OF ARTERIAL OCCLUSION

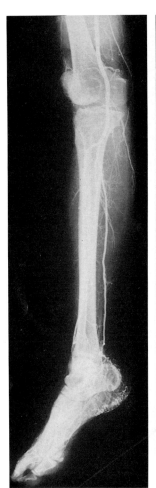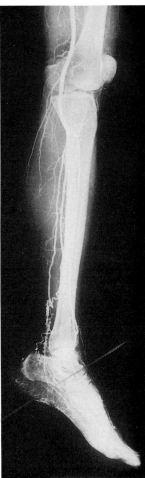

Figure VIII-1. Bilateral femoral arteriograms of a 44-year-old woman with Buerger's disease. The peroneal arteries are patent, and the anterior and posterior tibial arteries are abruptly occluded just above the ankle in both legs (similar pattern). (From Shionoya S, et al. Angiology 1982 ; 33 : 375-84.)

Table VIII-2. Pattern of crural arterial occlusion by bilateral arteriography in 105 patients with Buerger's disease. (From Shionoya S, et al. Angiology 1982 ; 33 : 375-84.)

	Femoropopliteal group	Infrapopliteal group
Similar	19(45%)	26(41%)
Different	21	30
Unilateral	2	7
Total	42	63

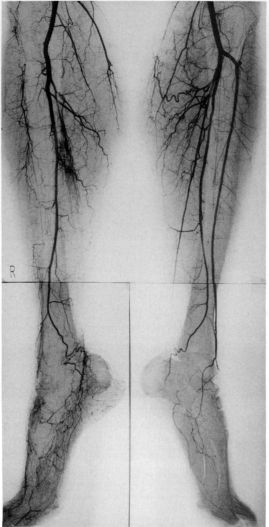
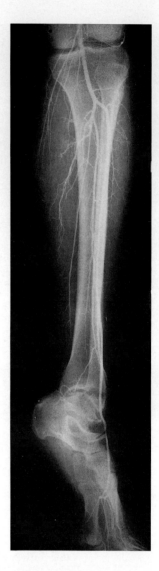

Figure VIII-2. Bilateral femoral arteriograms of a 31-year-old man with Buerger's disease. While the anterior and posterior tibial arteries are occluded and the peroneal artery is patent in the right leg, only the posterior tibial artery is occluded and the anterior tibial artery and the peroneal artery are patent in the left(different pattern).

Figure VIII-3. Left femoral arteriogram of the same patient as in Figure II-3. While the posterior tibial artery shows a tapering occlusion, the anterior tibial artery is continuous with the dorsalis pedis artery(continuous arterial flow).

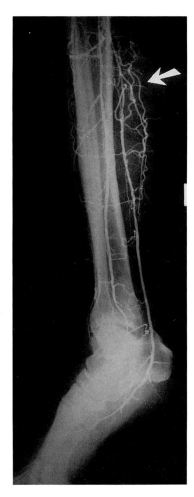

Figure VIII-4. Right femoral arteriogram of a 45-year-old man with Buerger's disease. The popliteal artery is occluded, and the posterior tibial artery visualized at the middle of the leg by collaterals is continuous with the plantar artery(discontinous arterial flow)(arrow).

Crural arterial occlusion pattern and necrotic lesion

Nectoric lesions were seen in 68 of the 105 patients. While gangrene or ulceration occurred bilaterally in 10 of 28 patients with the similar pattern, bilateral necrotic lesions were observed in 12 of 40 patients with the different pattern : the incidence of occurrence of bilateral necrotic lesions in the former group was not significantly higher than that in the latter group. On analyzing a relationship between the continuity of arterial pathway and the trophic lesion, the toe was ulcerated in 4 of 58 limbs with the continuous arterial pathway, but ulceration occurred in 86 of 152 limbs with discontinuous one : there was no comparison between the two groups.

Affection of the popliteal artery

In 4 of 15 limbs with stenosis, irregularity or dilatation of the popliteal artery(skip lesion) in this series, the popliteal artery was occluded within the follow-up period. Repeated arteriography revealed skip progression in 2 cases with stenosis and continuous progression in the other 2 cases with dilatation of the popliteal artery: the preexisting runoff vessels below the knee in the former cases remained patent in spite of the progression of the occlusion, while the runoff vessels in the latter were occluded concurrently with the proximal progression of the lesion. In the former cases thrombotic occlusion probably occurred at the site of the skip lesion, accompanied with no extensive secondary thrombosis; in the latter cases secondary thrombosis contiguous to the skip occlusion might have progressed proximally and distally. Concurrent thrombotic occlusion of the infrapopliteal runoff vessels with the skip occlusion at the popliteal artery might rest on the compensatory function of the collaterals to the crural arteries escaped from occlusion.

The fact that the initial pattern of the infrapopliteal arterial lesions remained comparatively unchanged after the occlusion progressed to the suprapopliteal region means that the distal arteries escaped from the disease (runoff vessels) could be saved from the involvement notwithstanding exacerbations producing progression of the thromboangiitic process. Whether the compensatory function of the collateral circulation is good or bad would be related with maintaining a stabiltiy of the runoff vessels. While foot claudication is typical for the infrapopliteal arterial occlusion, calf claudication usually occured when the occlusion progressed above the orifices of the sural arteries. Therefore, the point of time at the onset of calf claudication in the patient who had complained foot claudication up to that time indicates the more proximal progression of the lesion.

Manner and rate of progression

While the similar pattern of the crural arterial occlusion was recognized in 45 of the 105 patients, it is interesting that there was no difference in the incidence of the similar pattern of the crural arterial occlusion between the femoropopliteal group and the crural group. This implies that the original pattern of the infrapopliteal arterial lesion did not frequently change even when the thromboangiitis lesion progressed to the suprapopliteal region on the basis of the skip lesion of the popliteal artery.

In the another series at our hospital, femoral arteriography was repeated in 34 limbs of 25 patients with Buerger's disease whose ischemic symptoms deteriorated during the last 9 years.[3] There was no more proximal progression of the occlusive lesion in the main arteries in 10 limbs; progression within the same main artery in 8 limbs, and the more proximal progression beyond the first affected main artery in 16 limbs. In 8 of 12 limbs which showed proximal progression from the crural to the femoropopliteal segment, the pattern of the crural arterial occlusion did not change after the exacerbation.

Although the pathogenesis of the skip lesion remains unknown, the localized stenosis, dilatation or irregularity of the femoropopliteal segment might be due to ascending progression of the obstructive lesion in its branch artery: the skip lesion of the popliteal artery was deemed to be induced by ascending progression of the thromboangiitic lesion in the sural arteries in some cases.[4] Contrary to arteriosclerosis obliterans, block in the main stream does not seem to protect the deterioration of occlusive lesions in the distal segment below the block.

Progression of arterial occlusion and trophic lesion

The fact that multiple severe occlusions of the distal arteries are essential in Buerger's disease has been substantiated not only by angiographic features but also by hemodynamic changes associated with distal arterial reconstruction; the foot or the toe blood pressure frequently did not return to normal after such successful arterial revascularization as femoropopliteal or femorotibial bypass grafting[5]; i.e., improvement of inflow did not bring about normalization of the distal blood pressure because of multiple arterial occlusive lesions below the ankle. Therefore, it was a natural consequence that smooth connection of a crural artery with the dorsalis pedis or the plantar arch was seen only in 58 of the 210 limbs. The result that the necrotic lesion of the toe was far more frequently noticed in the discontinuous group than in the continuous group means that anastomosing collateral channels were not enough to compensate the impaired arterial insufficiency due to the disease.

The most distal region of the extremities might be ready to fall into gangrene if the more proximal arteries were blocked in addition to the preexisting occlusive lesions in the foot and toes. Deterioration of ischemia in case of no progression of the occlusive lesion of the main artery in arteriograms might be attributable to aggravation of microcirculation due to the disease, which could not be detected by the conventional angiography. The observation that there was no difference in the incidence of bilateral necrotic lesion between the group with the similar arterial occlusion pattern and the group with the different pattern implies that arteriography does not disclose the compensatory function of collaterals.

Initial pattern of arterial occlusion and the course of the disease

Judging from the retrospective and follow-up study of the patients with Buerger's disease, the pattern of arterial occlusion in the lower leg seemed to be fixed within relatively a short span of time after the onset of symptoms. Thereafter, the worsening of ischemic symptoms was not always accompanied with the more proximal extension of the obstructive lesion in the main artery, rather it was due to the circulatory deterioration at the microvascular level, which could not be recognized by usual angiography, in more than half number.

In view of the natural course of the disease, it is also interesting that the pattern of the crural arterial occlusion remained unchanged after the progression of the lesion to the suprapopliteal region in no small numbers. These facts suggest that an essential process of Buerger's disease consists in the peripheral small vessels, and pathogenesis of the more proximal progression of the lesion in the main artery might be different from that of the earlier lesion before fixation of the pattern of arterial occlusion in the lower leg. A preexisting lesion in the femoropopliteal segment was favorable to occurrence of the thrombotic occlusion, and occlusion of the proximal artery might be not infrequently due to ascending and/or descending extension of the secondary thrombosis originating in the skip lesion[6].

It is difficult to predict the natural course of the patient with the disease on the basis of the initial pattern of the arterial occlusion at the early stage. Although smoking is the most important determinant of the clinical course of the disease, the susceptibility and response to smoking of the patient is not uniform. While the continuous progression to the proximal segment resulted in ischemic gangrene or ulceration within a short period in some smokers, only the microcirculatory disturbance in the acral region was gradually aggravated, with a minute necrosis in the finger tip for a long period in other smokers. On the basis of the pattern of arterial occlusions in the foot and lower leg, it is no easy to predict the clinical course of a patient with the disease and his reponse to smoking. However, if the pedal arch remains patent via the peroneal artery escaped from the involvement in case of occlusion of the anterior and posterior tibial arteries, the patient's clinical course would be more favorable compared with the others with no visualization of the pedal arch.

B. Correlation Between the Vessel Involved and Its Clinical Course

The initial lesions of Buerger's disease might originate in the multiple regions of the peripheral vessels, and remission and relapse of the disease are intimately related to cessation and resumption of smoking. The correlation between the vessel involved and the rate and manner of the progression is discussed.

Involvement of the arteries of the upper extremities

In about 500 cases of thrombo-angiitis obliterans observed from 1909 to 1922, Buerger[7] gave attention to involvement of the upper extremities: coldness and a feeling of numbness and deadness of the fingers might be the first symptoms in one or both hands simultaneously, trophic disturbances soon following. He noticed that the circulatory manifestations in the upper extremities did not bear the same relationship to posture as in the lower limbs, for ischemia would be absent on elevation, or if present, would be very slight. From a survey of many histories he thought that the upper extremities might be clinically involved in the following ways: 1) without subjective symptoms; 2) with vasomotor symptoms predominating; 3) with lesions simulating the results of neurogenic disturbances; 4) with trophic disturbances alone; 5) with trophic and vasomotor phenomena; 6) with gangrene of slight extent; 7) with extensive gangrene threatening the viability of the extremity; 8) with extensive atrophy of the hand and forearm; 9) with changes simulating scleroderma and sclerodactyly; and 10) cases with acute arteritis of portions of the radical or ulnar artery (migrating arteritis).

In 1929 Allen[8] devised the method detecting arterial occlusions distal to the wrist (Allen test), and it has been shown that asymptomatic occlusion of the ulnar artery was often encountered in chronic arterial occlusive disease. In case of the ulnar artery occlusion alone, digital ischemia was caused by occlusive lesions in the palm or digital arteries, depending on the completeness of the palmar arches as well as on collaterals from the terminal branches of the radial artery.[9]

In 1977 Tanaka et al.[10] found 7 cases of only upper limb involvement out of 309 cases of Buerger's disease, and emphasized to differentiate the disease from occlusion of the arteries of the forearm and hand after repeated blunt trauma (hypothenar hammer syndrome) from the following viewpoints: bilateral involvement, no relation between the traumatically affected area and the site of arterial occlusion, the existence of migrating phlebitis, and extensive occlusions including the arteries, of the digit, hand and forearm. Tanabe and his colleagues[11] recognized the upper limb involvement alone in 8 of 152 cases of Buerger's disease in their series: no phlebitis migrans was present in all the cases and four of them did their work attended with repeated blunt trauma. Twenty-eight of the 152 cases suffered from involvement of both the upper and lower extremities and ischemic ulceration was seen in 18 of the 28 cases (57%). In 1979 Hirai and Shionoya[12] compared the brachial arteriographic findings in 26 limbs with severe digital ischemia to those in 32 limbs, carried out irrespective of the presence of ischemic symptoms or signs in the fingers.

While obstruction of both the radial and the ulnar artery in addition to the occlusion of the arteries of the hand and fingers was overwhelmingly prevalent in the former, the most common site of occlusion was the digital artery in the latter.

The existence of a patient with Buerger's disease in whom the disease remains restricted only in the upper extremity all the time is a topic for further discussion. In virtue of prohibition of smoking at the early stage, it might be not unreasonable that the thromboangiitic process in the upper extremity could come to complete remission before the disease manifests itself in the lower extremity. Trauma is closely related with pathogenesis of Buerger's disease, and it is suggested that repeated blunt injury to the hand or fingers is involved in the development of the disease as well as in the manifestation of symptoms.

Involvement of the foot arteries

In 1988 Kato et al.[13] found angiographically occlusion of the dorsalis pedis, the lateral plantar, the medial plantar, the tarsal, the plantar arch, and the digital arteries in 70.3%, 62.0%, 62.9%, 73.6%, 71.8%, and 84.3% respectively, of 239 lower extremities with Buerger's disease. The incidence of ischemic ulceration was 40% of 84 limbs with occlusion of all the plantar arch, the dorsalis pedis and the plantar arteries; the recurrence rate of the lesion was 23%.

Aggravation of ischemic symptoms in the digits and foot with no obvious evidences of the proximal progression of the occlusive lesion verified by angiorgaphy or palpation of the main artery is not an uncommon episodic exacerbation of the disease. It may be the worsening of arterial occlusion at the microvascular level or the rheological deterioration induced by neurogenic, hormonal or hematogenous factors.

Delineating how the digital arteries are involved with the thromboangiitic process is not easy, but a distinct visualization of the thrombus in the dorsal metatarsal artery by magnification arteriography has thrown an objective light on the manner of the progression of the disease[14](Fig. VII-7).

Femoropopliteal involvement

In 1948 Kinmonth[15] classified the clinical types of Buerger's disease into three groups according to the initial site of the disease, for it sometimes started in large vessels, sometimes in the small vessels, and sometimes in both simultaneously. He emphasized the main criterion of differentiation was the presence or absence of the popliteal pulse, and prognosis varied in the three groups as regards alleviation of symptoms by sympathectomy and survival of the limb: 1) Obstruction of a main vessel: thrombosis occurred in the femoral or in the popliteal artery, the popliteal pulse was not palpable, and the main symptom was intermittent claudication in the calf. When the thrombosis did not extend downwards into the smaller distal vessels, the collateral circulation was usually adequate to prevent gangrene of the foot(type I); 2) Obstruction of small vessels: when the smaller vessels were the first to be attacked, the popliteal pulse remained palpable, but the pulses at the ankle were diminished or absent. Symptoms appeared in the foot — claudication in the sole, rest pain, constant erythrocyanosis of the skin, and coldness followed by ulceration or gangrene of the toes. Some of the patients in this group had claudication in the calf, which, in the presence of a popliteal pulse, must be attributable to obstruction of the muscular branches of the main vessels (type II); and 3) Mixed type: the disease attacked the main and the smaller arteries simultaneously, and so claudication in the calf, loss of the popiteal pulse, and rest pain in the foot (type III).

His clinical observation was precise and much to the point. His type II corresponds to the infrapopliteal occlusion type, which is more than half of all the patients with Buerger's disease; type I, to femoropiliteal occlusion type due to the skip progression, and type III, to femoropiliteal occlusion type due to the continuous progression. Description of calf claudication attributed to obstruction of the muscular branches of the crural arteries was the result of his keen insight into pathophysiology of the disease.

Angiographic studies on the pattern of occlusion and the rate of progression in femoropopliteal arteriosclerosis obliterans revealed the preponderance of progression in the segment proximal to the block as compared with the segment distal to the block of the artery.[16] It is tempting to theorize that this protective effect of the block on the distal segment results from the lowering of the distal arterial pressure. Detecting whether a lower than normal pressure (or flow) can protect against the deposition and progression of the atheromatous lesion deserves further inquiry.

Judging form the rate and manner of progression of the occlusive lesion in Buerger's disease, the block of the main artery seems to have no protective effect on the deterioration of the lesion in the segment distal to the block, contrary to arteriosclerosis obliterans. Reduction in blood pressure or flow in the distal vessels below the block of the main artery does not result in decreasing the incidence of recurrence of the thromboangiitic lesion in a locality of low pressure or flow.

In 1976 Hirai and et al.[17] reported the rate and manner of femoropopliteal involvement in Buerger's disease, in view of arteriographic findings in 135 limbs of 101 patients as follows: 1) in 83 limbs the occlusions were localized below the popliteal artery, and 10 of them (12%) showed the skip lesion in the popliteal artery; 2) in 20 limbs the segmental occlusion in the femoropopliteal segment was seen in addition to the infrapopliteal occlusions; 3) in 32 limbs the femoropopliteal occlusion was contiguous to the occlusion of the crurunal arteries; 4) only one of 81 limbs with infrapopliteal occlusion showed the progrssion of the lesion to the suprapopliteal segment during a 5.3 year-follow-up-period on the average ; and 5) in 78% of 45 limbs with femoropopliteal occlusion in addition to infrapopliteal ones, calf claudication occurred shortly after the onset of initial ischemic symptoms. Based on the results above described, the femoropopliteal involvement might occur at early stage of the disease and progression from the crural arteries to the suprapopliteal segment was relatively rare after pattern of the infrapopliteal arterial occlusion had been fixed.

In 1986 Sasaki et al.[18] angiographically found progression of the occlusion from the crural to the popliteal artery in 15 limbs (11 patients) of 55 limbs (40 patients with Buerger's disease) during the follow-up-period. The time elapsed from the initial examination to the occlusion of the popliteal artery was 2 to 3 years in 7 limbs, 3 to 4 years in 2, 4 to 5 years in 2, 5 to 6 years in 2 and longer than 6 years in 2 (average : 3 years 7 months). Discrepancy in the incidence of the progression and the time elapsed from onset to the progression between the two series might be caused by difference in the time elapsed from the onset of symptoms to the first examination at each hospital. If the pattern of the infrapopliteal arterial occlusions was probably fixed at the patient's first visit at the hospital, the further clinical course would be dependent on his smoking habits.

Although the disease starts not only at the small vessels of the toe and foot but also at the small branch arteries of the femoropopliteal segment, initial ischemic symptoms owe their occurrence mainly to the infrapopliteal arterial occlusions. There are two types of manner of the more proximal progression in the main artery : 1) within about one year after the onset of symptoms the femormopopliteal involvement might be encountered in patients who continue smoking in disregard of advice ; and 2) more than two years after the onset of symptoms the suprapopliteal progression might be observed in case of intermittent prohibition of smoking.

The skip lesion may play an important role in each type of the femoropopliteal progression. As in 7 limbs of Sasaki's series the skip lesion was seen at the distal segment of the superficial femoral artery (inside the adductor canal), at the middle part of the popliteal artery (between the heads of the gastrocnemius muscles) and at the distal part of the popliteal artery (under the arcus tendineus m. solei)[18], the skip lesion was deemed to be formed on the basis of the damaged arterial wall due to repeated movement of the knee joint. In the medium-sized or large artery such as the femoropopliteal segment, the thromboangiitic inflammation might make a raid into the weak spot of the vessel.

In 1977 Nakata et al.[19] found remarkable inflammatory cell infiltration in the small vessels in the soleus muscle in one of 11 cases of muscle biopsy, and small muscular branch vessels of the femoropopliteocrural main arteries were obstructed angiographically in 23 of 151 limbs (13.2%), though the main arteries were patent. From these findings, the disease might start in the small muscular branch vessels of the leg arteries, independently of the initial lesion in the digit and foot. Through the proximal progression of the occlusion in the branch vessels, the skip lesion of the main artery might be formed.

In 1984 Shigematsu et al.[20] angiographically found occlusive lesions of the femoral arterial bifurcation in 34 of 123 patients (28%) with Buerger's disease : in 18 of the 34 cases, obstructive lesions were recognized at the main segment or the branch vessel of the deep femoral artery. While the site of occlusion in the superficial artery was localized around the Hunter's canal in case of no occlusion of the deep femoral artery, the extent of occlusion progressed to the more proximal area of the superficial femoral artery in case of obstruction of the deep femoral artery in their series. Mavor[21] considered that progression from a block in the adductor canal was in a proximal direction rather than distal in ASO, and he pointed out that there might be a logical reason for proximal, as opposed to distal, extension from the adductor canal, namely, that the branches in the superficial femoral artery between the adductor canal and the bifurcation of the common femoral are more scanty than those in the popliteal artery. This relation of the hemodynamic state and the progression of occlusion applies to the manner of the progression of occlusion in TAO.

The deep femoral artery is the nutrient artery to the thigh muscles and anastomoses with the genicular net work in case of occlusion of the superficial artery. Obstruction of the deep femoral artery causes the blockade of the collateral circulation via the femoral arterial bifurcation, and it might be closely related with the proximal progression of the occlusion in the superficial femoral artery (Fig. VIII-5). As the deep femoral artery and its branches were occluded in addition to the infrapopliteal occlusions in 12 (22%) of 54 limbs of 30 patients with Buerger's disease in our recent series and the superficial femoral and the popliteal artery were patent in 6 of the 12 limbs, the disease might start in the muscular branches of the thigh.[22]

Persistence of the pattern of the infrapopliteal arterial occlusion after the suprapopliteal progression due to the skip lesion may be related with a tendency of the femoral artery to the proximal progression of occlusion, as opposed to distal. Contrary to ASO, the initial occlusive lesion in the muscular branches of the deep femoral artery as well as the crural arteries deserves more attention as a feature representative of Buerger's disease (Fig. VIII-6).

Aortoiliac involvement

Although Buerger's disease primarily affects the medium and small arteries of the muscular type, large arteries of the elastic type are sometimes involved.

The external iliac artery

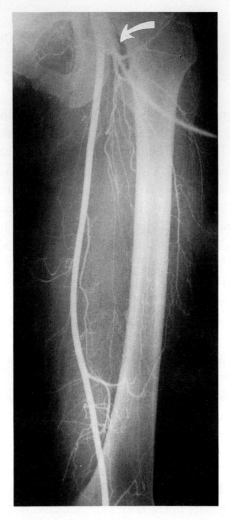 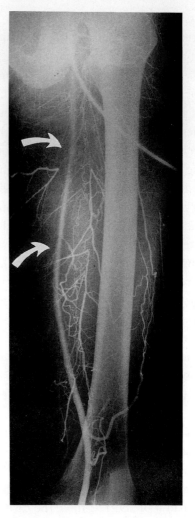

Figure VIII-5. Left femoral arteriogram of the same patient as in Figure II-3. The deep femoral artery is occluded except the lateral circumflex femoral artery(arrow).

Figure VIII-6. Left femoral arteriogram of a 45-year-old man with Buerger's disease. The deep femoral artery and its muscular branches are segmentally occluded(arrows).

In 1973 Abu-Dalu et al.[23] in Israel reported two cases of TAO of the external iliac artery confirmed by histology, notwithstanding the common femoral artery was quite normal in appearance. Later Haddad et al.[24] added a case of obstruction of the external iliac artery to the Israel series. In 13 of 216 patients with Buerger's disease at our hospital from 1967 to 1976, the external iliac artery was occluded but the common iliac artery remained open: in 12 of the 13 cases, the common and superficial femoral arteries were obstructed. Occlusion of the external iliac artery occurred 2 to 8 years after the onset of symptom[25](Fig. VIII-7).

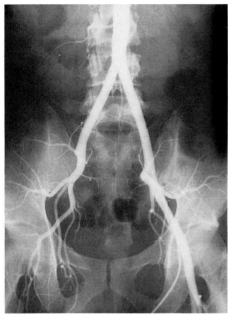

Figure VIII-7. Aortogram of a 26-year-old man with Buerger's disease. The right external iliac artery and the right femoral artery are occluded, and collateral circulation is formed through the branches of the internal iliac artery.

The external iliac artery was most frequently involved with the disease in the pelvic region, and the end of ascending progression of the occlusive lesion in the lower extremity was counted as the external iliac artery. Of 16 limbs with aortoiliac involvement, Shigematsu et al.[20] found occlusion of the deep femoral artery in 10 limbs, and occlusion of the superficial femoral artery in 3 limbs: the deep and/or the superficial femoral arteries were occluded in 13 of the 16 limbs. They considered that occlusion of the deep femoral artery took part in progression of the occlusive lesion to the aortoiliac region. Because of scanty branch vessels of the external iliac artery, the occlusive process originating in the femoral artery might progress at a stretch to the iliac bifurcation.

Before the complete occlusion a diffuse narrowing of the external iliac artery throughout its entire length, probably due to an intimal thickening caused by thromboangiitic inflammation of the artery, was sometimes observed, and the preexisting lesion was deemed to favor the iliac occlusion. Histologically characteristic features of Buerger's disease were observed in the thrombotic occlusion of the external iliac artery in the reported cases: the involvement of the external iliac artery with the disease has been substantiated.[25] The hip joint movement might participate in the pathogenesis of the skip lesion in the external iliac artery.

The internal iliac artery

In case of occlusion of the external iliac artery, the internal iliac artery was frequently escaped from the affection and took an active part in collateral circulation to the thigh through the anastomosis between its branches and the medial and lateral circumflex femoral arteries. While the trunk of the internal iliac artery was rarely involved with the disease, its branch vessels were not infrequently affected, though the diagnosis of occlusive lesion in the pelvic arteriogram was not always easy.

In the pelvic arteriograms, Taguchi et al.[26] found occlusive lesion of the superior gluteal, the obturator or the middle rectal artery in 6 of 22 patients with Buerger's disease (Fig. VIII-8). In examining the angiographic finding, the following points should be taken into consideration to avoid the misinterpretation: 1) diagnosis based on serial angiorgams; 2) comparison with the contralateral arterial course; 3) discrimination between vasospasm and occlusive lesion; and 4) existence of collaterals.[19]

Ischemic symptoms due to occlusion of these branch vessels do not manifest themselves as a rule, though the penile blood pressure may be decreased in case of occlusion of the internal pudendal artery. A 30-year-old patient with the disease in our series showed segmental occlusion of the inferior gluteal and the obturator artery, in addition to occlusion of the superficial and deep femoral arteries. Biopsy of the branch artery of the obturator artery revealed organized thrombus with inflammatory cell infiltration throughout the vessel wall, indentified as Buerger's disease[25]. Although relationship of the skip lesion of the branch arteries of the internal iliac artery with that of the leg arteries remains unknown, the disease might begin in the branch vessels of the pelvic region, independently of the small

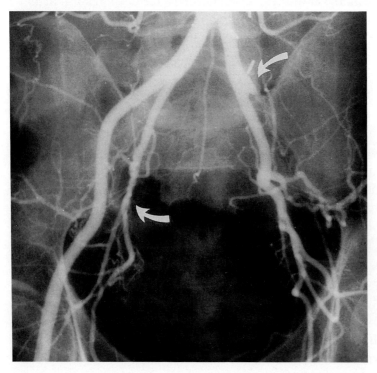

Figure VIII-8. Pelvic arteriogram of the same patient as in Figure VIII-4. While the left external iliac artery is occluded at its origin, the right external iliac artery is patent and the right superior gluteal artery is obstructed (arrows).

vessels of the periphery of the extremities.

As above described, Buerger[7] observed the acute lesions of the disease in the spermatic artery and veins of the spermatic cord, and old lesions in the branches of the gastric artery in a case of gastric ulcer. In spite of very rare involvement of the spermatic cord, the acute typical histological feature for Buerger's disease was recognized in the affected vessels, but the case report was silent on the limb ischemia of the two patients[27]. It might be attributable to earlier removal of the diseased portion, under the suspicion of being tuberculosis, thrombosis of the pampiniform plexus or neoplasm of the epididymis.

The common iliac arteries

In case of complete occlusion of the external iliac arteries, the common iliac arteries were usually escaped from the disease. During these 30 years at our hospital, only two cases showed occlusion of the common iliac artery, except cases with juxtarenal aortic occlusion. All the cases with occlusion of the common iliac arteries belonged to a juxtarenal aortic occlusion or a failure of arterial reconstruction such as iliofemoral bypass grafting, and no characteristic histologic feature was recognized in the occluded common iliac arteries.

In the overwhelming majority of cases with occlusion of the external iliac arteries, no continuous proximal progression of the disease occurred. A very rare involvement of the common iliac arteries might be related with sufficient outflow via the internal iliac arteries. Although the small branches to the peritoneum, the psoas major, the ureter, and the surrounding areolar tissue besides the iliolumbar artery might be affected with the disease, no clear angiographic evidence of the involvement was obtained.

The abdominal aorta

Of 513 patients with Buerger's disease at our hospital from 1967 through 1988, six showed complete occlusion of the infrarenal abdominal aorta (juxtarenal aortic occlusion) (Fig. VIII-9). The affected abdominal aorta wall showed no inflammatory features and the aortic lumen was obstructed with thrombus developing no tendency to organization.

Judging from that the common iliac arteries remained patent if the internal iliac arteries were open in case of occlusion of the external iliac arteries, secondary stagnant thrombosis might have occurred on the basis of blockade of the outflow vessels, when the internal iliac arteries were occluded in addition to obstruction of the external iliac arteries. The operative finding that thrombectomy of the abdominal aorta was usually easily performed in the same way as in juxtarenal aortic occlusion due to arteriosclerosis may illustrate the hypothesis. Three of the six patients with the juxtarenal aortic occlusion died of mesenterial infarction due to ascending progression of the infrarenal thrombosis.

Based on the pathological examination of the amputataed limb because of

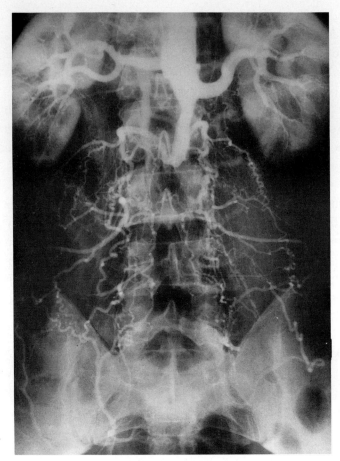

Figure VIII-9. Aortogram of a 39-year-old man with Buerger's disease. The abdominal aorta is occluded below the renal aretries (juxtarenal aorticocclusion). Nineteen years elapsed after onset of the disease.

Buerger's disease, Weber[28] reported that all the arteries appeared small (hypoplastic) in relation to the patient's size and there appeared to have been a certain degree of congenital hypoplasia, or deficient development, of the affected arteries. As the angiographic appearance of the aortoiliac region sometimes looked small for the patient's size, the diameter of the abdominal aorta was measured at the level of above the orifices of the renal arteries and of the aortic bifurcation in the aortograms of 13 cases with the disease : the average diameter was 20.6 ± 2.05mm and 16.2 ± 1.77mm respectively.[26] The mean diameter of the abdominal aorta above the bifurcation was 11 mm in 12 patients with hypoplastic aortoiliac system and 19.7mm in 20 patients without evidence of vascular disease[29].

As the abdominal aorta seemed to taper the diameter as it descends distalwards, the reduction rate of the diameter between the two levels was calculated by following formula :

$$\text{Reduction rate} = \frac{a-b}{a}$$

a : diameter at the level of above the orifices of the renal arteries
b : diameter at the level of the aortic bifurcation.

The reduction rate in the patients with Buerger's disease in our series was 21.4%[26]; that in Japanese adult corpses without arterial disease was 11.2%.[30] From these results, the infrarenal abdominal aorta in Buerger's disease seems to have a tendency to taper its diameter as it descends. Relatioship of the tapering reduction in diameter of the infrarenal abdominal aorta with the juxtarenal thrombotic occlusion in Buerger's disease remains unsolved.

In 1973 Gilkes and Dow[31] reported a case with Buerger's disease who showed juxtarenal aortic occlusion nine months after the left thigh amputation; at the amputation the aortoiliac region was normal in the angiogram. They did not think that their case represented simple propagation of bland thrombus in normal arteries, but considered that the aortic occlusion was another manifestation of the Buerger's disease. Mishima and his colleagues[32] recognized occlusion of the aortoiliac region in 20 of 410 patients with Buerger's disease in their series: the site of occlusion was the terminal abdominal aorta in 3 cases, the common iliac in 1, the internal iliac in 6, and the external iliac in 5. The mean duration from the onset of symptoms to the aortoiliac involvement was 5 years: the older the age at the onset of symptoms was, the earlier the high occlusion developed. As angiography showed localized irregularity of the aortoiliac segment in 7 of the 20 cases, they regarded the finding as the skip lesion due to the disease or arteriosclerosis.

Three of the 10 pelvic arteriograms in our series showed occlusion of the lumbar arteries. Yamaguchi[33] found angiographically occlusion of the lumbar arteries in 3 of 14 patients with Buerger's disease. Oshima and Ueno[34] reported a patient with Buerger's disease whose right fifth lumbar artery was occluded during the follow-up period. Aortotomy at aortopopliteal bypass grafting revealed a fresh thrombus at the orifice of the affected lumbar artery. These reports suggest that the disease might start in the lumbar arteries and result in thrombus formation at the orifices (Fig. VIII-10). Apart from the participation of the lumbar arteries in the development of the high aortic occlusion, the role of the lumbar arteries, giving off the vasa vasorum to the abdominal aortic wall, in the pathogenesis of localized intimal thickening inclusive of parietal thrombus of the abdominal aorta might be undeniable.

While the occluded abdominal aorta with thrombus showed no distinct inflammatory changes suggestive of Buerger's disease as a rule, the obstructed infrarenal abdominal aorta looked a cord-like appearance in 2 of the 6 cases with juxtarenal aortic occlusion in our series. The peculiar feature suggested that a congenital hypoplasia of the abdominal aorta might have taken part in development of the high

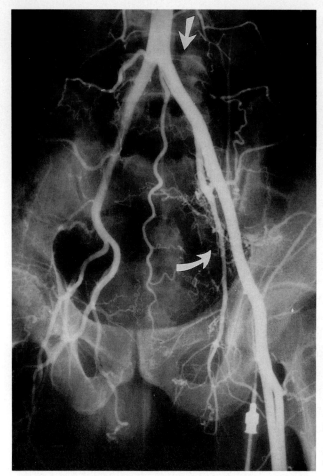

Figure VIII-10. Aortogram of a 33-year-old man with Buerger's disease. The external iliac artery and the femoral artery are occluded in the right side; the fourth lumbar aretry and the superior and inferior gluteal arteries are obstructed in the left (arrows).

aortic occlusion in these cases. Because the kidneys receive a large quantity of blood enough to prevent thrombus formation near the orifices, the incidence of the more proximal progression of thrombosis to the suprarenal region has been regarded low. However, in 3 of the 6 cases with juxtarenal aortic occlusion in our series, the thrombosis progressed beyond the orifices of the renal arteries, and the incidence of the lethal complication seemed much higher than previously expected.

C. Extraperipheral Arterial Involvement

Since Buerger reported the acute lesions of the disease in territories other than the vessels of the extremities, many papers on the visceral organ involvement with Buerger's disease outside the extremities have been reported.

Cerebral involvement

Buerger[7] experienced a lethal case with cerebral symptoms in addition to ischemia of the upper and lower extremities. In 1933 Foerster and Guttmann[35] reported two cases studied only clinically in which repeated attacks of transient weakness, numbness, aphasis and monocular blindness had occurred before ischemic symptoms of the extremities manifested themselves.

In 1935 Spatz[36] presented the first case of the cerebral form of Buerger's disease. The patient was a 43-year-old man, nonsmoker, who for several years had been subject to transient episodes of headache, scotoma, weakness and numbness of the right arm and difficulty in finding words. Dementia and paralysis of the right arm and bilateral legs supervened, and he died of circulatory insufficiency. The left cerebral cortex showed so-called "granular atrophy." Over the cerebral convexity, many of the branches of the middle cerebral artery were occluded and reduced to white "worm-like" string. The lumen of the diseased vessels was occluded with endothelial proliferation and thrombus. The stem of the middle cerebral artery and the internal carotid artery distal to the petrous bone were solidly occluded, but patent vessels intervened between the occlusion at the base and the white vessels over the convexity.

In 1939 Lindenberg and Spatz[37] classified the cerebral form of the disease into two types, from the standpoint of the localization of the vascular process in 22 cases. The distinguishing feature of Type I (8 cases) was the irregular distribution of the process in the territory of one or more major arteries or their branches. The proximal part of an artery was often normal and blood-containing, but on being traced distally, the vessel might abruptly became a white string which then extended to the finest vascular twigs. The tissue within the region of infraction was not totally destroyed as in cerebral embolism, and this irregular and incomplete destruction of the cortex and white matter was regarded a characteristic feature of cerebral Buerger's disease. The vessel changes in Type II (14 cases) were distributed more uniformly and symmetrically and involved the terminal branches of the three large brain arteries. In this type, so-called "granular atrophy" of the cortex was found and its unusual distribution was highly characteristic in that it involved the watershed regions where the most distal branches of each of the three major cerebral arteries bordered on those of its neighbor. Granular atrophy, which consists of multiple discrete tiny infarcts, gave the surface of the brain a pitted appearance. The lumen of the occluded white vessels was filled with a fresh loosely-arranged connective tissue in which entrapped endothelial-lined spaces represented attempts at recanalization. Although they emphasized endothelial proliferation (endarteriitis) and thrombosis, they finally left open the question as to which process was primary, endothelial proliferation or thrombosis. While clinical symptom in Type I was featured by its laterality such as hemiparesis or hemianopsis, there was no laterality of clinical picture in Type II. The keystone of their diagnosis of cerebral thromboangiitis obliterans was the pressence of white vessels occluded by fine connective tissue (worm-like vessels), but whether it was correct to assume that the occurrence of this change in the cerebral vessels overlying brain infarction indicated the same basic disease process which caused similar changes in the limb arteries remained an unanswered question.

Rosenhagen[38] discussed the clinical features of 8 cases of cerebral form of Buerger's disease including 7 cases of Lindenberg and Spatz, dividing them into two groups : 1) those in which cerebral manifestations occurred in association with disturbances in other parts of the body ; and 2) those with predominantly cerebral signs. In 1940 Hausner and Allen[39] found clinical evidence of cerebrovascular involvement in two per cent of 500 cases of Buerger's disease at the Mayo Clinic : the outstanding symptom was hemiplegia and in some cases there were such symptoms as confusion, disorientation, aphasia, loss of memory and hemianopia.

Thereafter, controversy continued regarding the existence of the white worm-like vessels associated with cerebral infarction and its pathogenetic significance. Although the internal carotid artery was occluded in several of Lindenberg and Spatz's cases, Antoni[40] in 1941 found occlusion of the internal carotid artery on the side of the infarct in his reported all three cases with Buerger's disease in the brain. In 1944, from a histological study of one case of cerebral thromboangiitis obliterans, Scheinker[41] considered the occurrence of small intramural hemorrhages to be the earliest vascular change : the change was followed by a reactive cellular proliferation of the subendothelial connective tissue, resulting in scar formation and occlusion.

In 1946 Davis and Perret[42] reported 11 cases of cerebral thrombo-angiitis obliterans in 9 of whom operation was performed. The most common symptoms were headache, paresthesia, pareses, aphasia, and visual defect. The anatomical diagnosis was made by the presence of the characteristic small, white, worm-like obliterated vessels, the granular atrophy of the cortex, and of thrombi associated with proliferation of the endothelial cells of the intima and subitimal layers of the vessels. However, only 3 of their patients had evidence of peripheral circulatory disturbances.

In 1952 Lippman,[43] reviewing the entire literature on cerebral thrombo-angiitis obliterans, would accept 30 cases as proved examples of the disease, and to these he added nine cases of his own. There was no proved characteristic anatomic picture of cerebrovascular involvement in Buerger's disease, and most patients suffering from the disease who actually developed cerebral complications had thromboses of one or several cerebral arteries and some had cortical granular atrophy. The most frequent site of cerebral arterial occlusion was the left middle cerebral artery (in 41% of the 39 cases); the right middle cerebral artery, in 23%; the left internal carotid artery, in 5.2%; the left common carotid artery, in 2.6%; the right common carotid artery, in 2.6%; and the left and right vertebral arteries, in 2.6%. The clinical course was characterized by frequent recurrences and remissions of the same focal cortical signs which terminated in permanent damage. The most frequent signs were hemiparesis or hemiplegia and partial or complete aphasia. The natural course for life was favorable provided the initial damage to brain tissue had not been too extensive and the use of tobacco had been discontinued. Aphasia and hemiparesis tended to persist with slight or no improvement. In 22 of the 39 cases, first developed peripheral vascular and then cerebravascular disease within a few years; in other 12 cases first developed cerebrovascular and then peripheral vascular disease in fairly short order. He concluded that the diagnosis of cerebral Buerger's disease was justified only if peripheral thromboangiitis obliterans was pressent.

In 1957 Fisher[44] reported a critical review of cerebral thromboangiitis obliterans and of the existence of Buerger's disease in addition, based on his observations of five cases, in which the pathologic findings conformed to Type I of Lindenberg and Spatz, and concluded as follows: 1) there was a lack of agreement as to the pathologic picture described by Spatz and others as the cerebral form of Buerger's disease; 2) the affected vessels showed white occlusion of multiple branches of a major cerebral artery but in addition an occlusion lying in the proximal part of the internal carotid or middle cerebral artery; and 3) it was suggested that the proximal occlusion was primarily and that the distal white obliterated arterial branches were the result of stagnation of blood flow consequent to failure of the cerebral circulation locally. The process was termed "stagnation thrombosis." Fisher, who took a skeptical view of the existence of Buerger's disease, considered that peripheral Buerger's disease might represent atherosclerotic occlusion of the aortic, iliac or femoral vessels associated with distal thrombosis due to slowed collateral blood flow with subsequent organization of the thrombus, on the analogy of the fact of cerebral thromboangiitis obliterans.

On reviewing the previously reported cases, when a patient with Buerger's disease in the extremities showed signs of neurological deficit, the disease process in the brain was liable to be regarded as due to the same cause as in the extremities. The question is how to identify the pathologic process in the vessels of the extremity in typical Buerger's disease with that found in the cerebral vessels of the cases under discussion. In the cerebral arteries, the internal elastic membrane is well developed but the adventitia is poorly organized, and in addition the media is absent at the birfurcation. Is the white worm-like occluded vessels in the brain attributable to a different response of the cerebral vessels with these peculiar structure to the same etiological agent, compared with that of the vessels of the extremities?

Although it is conceivable that Buerger's disease may start in the visceral vessels and later manifest itself in the extremities, the question arises whether all these vascular accidents might not be due to one underlying condition[45]. Considering that the over-all incidence of cerebrovascular complications in Buerger's disease amounted to less than 0.5%[43], the cerebrum might be well protected against external influences[46].

Coronary involvement

In 1910s Buerger[27] experienced two cases with the disease who died suddenly after the thigh amputation: the both showed marked atherosclerotic occlusion of the coronary arteries, but there was no evidence of thrombo-angiitis obliterans in the vessels examined. Based on the pathological examination of the autopsy materials that the lesions of thrombo-angiitis obliterans were confined to the vessels of the extremities, he considered that local predisposing factors must needs be requisite for the special susceptibility of these vascular territories. That the arterial channels affected by thrombo-angiitis become, or are inherently predisposed to atherosclerotic changes as well, seemed proven both by autopsy material as well as through their studies of the amputated limbs. Where reamputation was done years after the more distal part of the limb had already been removed, more marked atherosclerosis was found. Or, when the second lower extremity required amputation years after the first, atherosclerotic changes might be found that were absent during the earlier years of life; they might be slight or marked in degree.

In 1925 Perla[47] reported an analysis of 41 cases of Buerger's disease, with a case involving the coronaries and the aorta: the patient received the amputation of the left hand and bilateral legs and died at his age of 44 years. Autopsy revealed thrombotic occlusion of the abdominal aorta just below the renal arteries and the left coronary artery: the disease process in the coronary artery resembled that in the vessels of the extremities. He concluded that a careful follow-up of all cases of Buerger's disease would reveal more instances of such fatal complications, and the possible association of coronary disease with the disease threw a new light on Buerger's disease.

In 1929 Allen and Willius[48] found clinical evidence of disease of the coronary arteries in seven out of an unselected series of 225 cases of Buerger's disease observed at The Mayo Clinic: the age of seven patients was 40, 40, 43, 44, 45, 47, and 48 years, respectively. Almost all the patients suffered from severe retrosternal pain and their electrocardiograms showed significant ischemic changes. One of them died suddenly after a severe attack, but autopsy was not permitted. As to the coronary involvement in th patient with Buerger's disease they presented three explanations: 1) Buerger's disease of the extremities caused predisposition to sclerotic changes in the coronary arteries; 2) the disease of the coronary arteries was typical of Buerger's disease; or 3) sclerosis of the coronary arteries and Buerger's disease of the peripheral arteries occurred in the same patients because they were inherently susceptible to arterial disease.

In 1930 Samuels and Feinberg[49] presented 5 cases with definite cardiac symptoms and electrocardiographic evidence of myocardial damage, out of 50 cases with Buerger's disease at the Mount Sinai Hospital. In 1934 Averbuck and Silbert[50] reviewed the causes of death of patients with Buerger's disease. The causes of death were operative intervention in 7 cases; intercurrent disease, accidents and suicide in 12; asthenia and cachexia in 6, and extraperipheral occlusive vascular accidents and sudden death in 22. In 11 of the 19 autopsy cases vascular thromboses occurred in arteries other than those of the extremities: the hepatic in 1, the coronary in 6, the celiac axis in 2, the mesenteric in 3, the abdominal aorta in 3 and the cerebral in 2. From the frequency of such vascular involvement they concluded that a bona fide association doubtless existed and that the thrombotic occlusive manifestations outside the extremities were related to the established disease process. In 1936 Saphir[51] reviewed thirty cases with Buerger's disease in which coronary lesions were found at autopsy: an analysis of these cases revealed that in a vast majority the lesions of the coronary arteries were arteriosclerotic, with or without coronary thrombosis. He reported an instance of sudden death. The autopsy revealed severe thromboangiitis obliterans of the coronary vessels and vessels of the lower extremities, in addition to arteriosclerosis: the myocardium showed a diffuse fibrosis with multiple old and organizing infarcts.

In common with cerebral thromboangiitis obliterans, the question arose as to whether the arteriosclerosis of the coronary arteries was a coincidental occurrence in no way related to thromboangiitis obliterans, whether the coronary sclerosis was merely a different stage (end stage) of thromboangiitis obliterans, or whether the coronary sclerosis developed as an entirely different entity on the basis of Buerger's disease. Judging from the age of the patient with the coronary involvement and the fact that in other vessels thromboangiitis obliterans predominated, Saphir[51] suggested that Buerger's disease produced the initial changes which resulted in arteriosclerosis. As the specific changes for Buerger's disease became less characteristic with the lapse of time and only fibrosis and hyalinization remained, but the giant cell foci could be seen in the region of the atheromatous ulcer in the case where the causative agent of Buerger's disease apparently persisted, he concluded that a primary inflammatory lesion of the artery might be at least one factor in the causation of arteriosclerosis.

In 1972 Inada and his colleagues[52] reported a 30-year-old man with Buerger's disease in whom ischemic symptoms of the extremities manifested themselves after attacks of the precordial pain (myocardial infarction) at his age of 27 years: the patient died suddenly at thirty-six. Reviewing the reported cases with the coronary involvement in the literature, the high incidence of sudden death and relatively premature death in them is worth notice.

As already stated, Doerr[53] classified modes of development of arteriosclerotic lesions into four types. The fourth type is characterized by active cell capacity, namely, monoclonal cellular plaques, and is mainly observed in the coronary artery at the second or the third decade of life: it is considered one of the most important causes of sudden death in the younger generation. Albertini[54] named the coronary sclerosis as "arteriitis stenosans coronariae" with a formation of small thrombi on intimal cushions, and considered it a coronary manifestation of Buerger's disease. Judging from the clinical course and the pathological features of the cases of sudden death, the majority of them seemed to belong to the fourth type by Doerr.

This type of arteriosclerosis is not concerned with transport and perfusion of the blood constituents, contrary to ordinary arteriosclerosis. In case of the juvenile coronary sclerosis, it is "a play in one act," and it is called "malignant" type, because of its high mortality.[55]

The "malignant" type of arteriosclerosis appears as disseminated, polytope intimal proliferations without lipoprotein-incorporation at first, and they become necrotic because of tumefaction, i.e., edema with a high concentration of proteoglycanes. The malignant, juvenile sclerosis most frequently affects the coronary arteries rich in cells. Although it remains unsolved whether the patients with Buerger's disease significantly more frequently suffer from this type of coronary sclerosis compared with a normal population of the same age, the existence of the coronary involvement requires serious attention in the treatment of the patients with Buerger's disease.

Visceral involvement

The renal arteries
The subject has been referred to cursorily in the item of the abdominal aorta involvement. In case of juxtarenal aortic occlusion, the renal arteries sometimes were occluded by the proximal, continuous progression of the infrarenal thrombus.

Buerger[26] reported a lethal case with thrombotic narrowing of the left renal artery, contiguous to juxtarenal aortic occlusion, after repeated amputation of the lower limbs because of Buerger's disease. Sprunt[56] found renal arterial involvement in eight cases, in a review of all autopsies on cases of Buerger's disease reported in the literature up to 1934. In 1951 Malisoff and Macht[57] reported a case with renovascular hypertension who had showed clinical features of Buerger's disease in the lower extremity and her blood pressure returned to normal after nephrectomy. The right renal artery was occluded with thrombus, and the pathohistological examination revealed typical lesions of Buerger's disease.

While several cases with renovascular hypertension due to Buerger's disease have been reported, controversy continued regarding the identification of the lesion of the renal artery, just like in case of cerebral or coronary involvement with Buerger's disease. The question about alternative judgement, Buerger's disease or arteriosclerosis, won't be repeated here again.

Recently 5 cases with renovascular hypertension due to Buerger's disease were reported in Japan[58-61] : 4 of the 5 cases had juxtarenal aortic occlusion and the remanining one showed stenosis of the right renal artery without occlusion of the abdominal aorta, though the lesion of the renal artery was not identified histologically with thromboangiitis obliterans. In the majority of the cases with renovascular hypertension due to the disease, the proximal, continuous extension of thrombosis based on the juxtarenal aortic occlusion might play the most important role in the pathogenesis.

The coeliac and mesenteric arteries

Buerger[26] found bland thrombosis in the coeliac trunk and the superior mesenteric artery in one of four lethal cases with Buerger's disease : microscopic examination of the affected arteries showed the typical lesions of arteriosclerosis with varying degrees of thrombosis, nowhere lesions of thromboangiitis obliterans. Thereafter several dozens of cases with occlusion of the coeliac trunk, the superior mesenteric artery, the inferior mesenteric artery or their branches, during the course of Buerger's disease, have been reported.[62-70]

Although some patients suffered from chronic intestinal ischemia (abdominal angina) or chronic mechanical obstruction due to strictured bowels, the majority of the cases showed severe abdominal pain due to gangrene or perforation of the intestine caused by occlusion of the mesenteric arteries. While the former were generally improved by arterial reconstruction or resection of the affected intestine, more than about 50% of the latter died of a serious morbid state or postoperative complications such as anastomotic insufficiency after operation.

In the follow-up period, from 1977 through 1988, of the 255 patients with Buerger's disease in our series, three patients with juxtarenal aortic occlusion died of massive intestinal gangrene due to acute occlusion of the mesenterial vessels : because of a sudden and rush course of the disease no emergency operation was of use. Reviewing the lethal cases of acute mesenterial occlusion, almost all the cases showed juxtarenal aortic occlusion before the attack or were regarded to have occlusion of bilateral iliofemoral segments, judging from bilateral limb amputation in their past history. Of the 11 autopsy cases with arterial occlusion beside the extremities by Averbuck and Silbert,[50] three cases with involvement of the celiac trunk and the mesenterial vessels had received above or below knee amputation due to occlusion of the iliofemoral segment, without exception.

As to the visceral involvement with Buerger's disease, it seems to be important to differentiate the cases with the preexistent occlusion of the aortoiliac region from the cases without such the lesion. The former should be managed and followed up with a mind to the lethal visceral involvement, but it is impossible to predict such a discrete involvement of the branch vessel of the coeliac or mesenteric arteries in the latter. In 1988 Saito et al.[71] reported a 44-year-old female with Buerger's disease who received left hemicolectomy because of stricture and ulceration of the transverse and the descending colon. It is striking that her small subserosal artery of the resected specimen showed the typical histological features for Buerger's disease, granulomatous reaction with giant cells in the thrombus. In the same manner as in the extremities, an acute lesion of the small vessel of the intestine might be most characteristic at early stage.

Rosenberger et al.[72] said the differential diagnosis between atheromatous and thromboangiitic occlusion of the coeliac and mesenterial arteries from angiographic standpoint of view as follows: 1) in atherosclerosis the aorta and the common iliac arteries were almost always involved, while in Buerger's disease these vessels remained normal up to the death of the patient with almost all splanchnic arteries being occluded; 2) in atherosclerosis the occlusion of the superior mesenteric artery was usually abrupt and close to its origin, while thromboangiitic occlusion generally occurred at the point of branching, and might show partial recanalization. The first criteria is merely a general consideration, and it is not applicable to the case of visceral involvement with Buerger's disease. The second paragraph is understandable in view of the mode of progression of thromboangiitic lesion, and Borlaza et al.[73] also indicated that the arterial occlusion, which occurred at the branches of the vessels rather than at the origins, was an angiographic feature characteristic of Buerger's disease.

In 1979 Sobel and Ruebner[74] reported a case of Buerger's disease involving the coeliac trunk: the coeliac artery showed an isolated, severe focal stenotic lesion, 1 cm from the aortic takeoff, which resulted in hepatic, splenic, and pancreatic infarction. Based on bland, noninflammaroty, nonatherosclerotic thrombosis with organization and recanalization in the coeliac trunk, they regarded the coeliac artery involvement as an unusual manifestation of Buerger's disease. Apart from the question of the identification of the occlusive lesion in this case, thromboangiitis obliterans has been thought to involve the smaller branches of the coeliac and mesemteric arteries than the main stems: this means that symptoms suggestive of alimentary ischemia may arise in a patient with a normal arteriogram unless visualization is obtained of the smaller branches of the coeliac and mesenteric arteries.[62]

The majority of the reported cases of thromboangiitic lesions of the small and large intestine showed "segmental" infarction of the bowel due to thrombosis in the terminal mesenterial vessels: on the contrary, thrombotic occlusion of the stem of the superior mesenteric artery, related with continuous progression of the juxtarenal aortic occlusion, generally caused massive gangrene of the small and large intestine. If the association between thromboangiitis obliterans in the extremities and visceral involvement is not an accidental one and the incidence is much higher than in a group of normal individuals, why have we rarely encountered the patients with visceral involvement due to Buerger's disease? The reason might be attributable to difficulty of detecting the ischemic lesions in the intestine. In case of a localized involvement of some territories of the bowel, it is difficult to establish the presence of poor blood flow to the involved intestinal wall,[75] unlike the heart or the extremities. Furthermore, clinical abdominal manifestations such as pain, vomiting or diarrhea are no traits characteristic of thromboangiitic lesion.

Taube[76] reported a patient with recurrence of severe abdominal pain whose right leg had been amputated for Buerger's disease, and he considered the patient the first case presenting symptoms of intermittent claudication of the mesenteric vessels. However, without pathohistological verification, his conclusion is hard to understand. Undeniable pathological proofs of the widespread nature of the disease were sadly lacking in the literature, and the preponderance of purely presumptive case reports has borne out the contention. Nevertheless, pathohistological endorsement has posed a question to interpreting the significance of the thromboangiitic lesions found at autopsy, especially in the distant place, since intercurrent affections, atherosclerosis and secondary thromboses, with such changes as healing might induce, could play a role in producing the final histopathological picture, not at all typical of the disease.

Graves[77] pointed out that in Buerger's disease, when the lesion had existed for many years, a secondary thickening of the intima took place with corresponding proliferation of elastic fibres that must not be confused with the arteriosclrotic process: in Buerger's disease the more centrally situated arteries developed a tendency to arteriosclrotic lesions even though the arteries of the extremities showed but little sclerosis. Cohen and Barron[78] said that the histopathologic differentiation of thromboangiitis obliterans and arteriosclerosis in the extremities rested on the involvement of nerves and veins and the relatively spared internal elastic layers in the artery, typical of the former process: in the other organs of the body one usually encountered the nonspecific thrombosis typical of many types of occlusive vascular disease. Thus one was left with impression that even with definite thromboangiitic obliterans of centrally located vessels, the usual chronic course with recurrent inflammation and superimposed arteriosclerosis led to a histological picture at eventual examination uncharacteristic of thromboangiitis obliterans. One was forced therefore to define these distant areas of thromboangiitic involvement purely on an empirical basis; the clinical story, the concomitant process elsewhere, comparative yourth for arteriosclerosis, and the localization of the process, rather than the histopathological picture. With these thoughts in mind, the clinician should be better able to interpret vascular phenomena complicating any type of peripheral vascular disease and particularly Buerger's disease.[78]

In Buerger's disease involving the visceral organs it is after all a question of arterial thrombosis, because the disorder is a primary intraluminal thrombosis. Williams[79] found thrombus with vasculitis, thrombus without vasculitis, but never vasculitis in the absence of intraluminal thrombus, in the material from the extremity of a recent occlusion. The intense inflammatory reaction in the acute lesions and their subacute counterparts are not a feature of ordinary thrombi: their appearances suggest an inflammatory response to constituents of the thrombus, at first limited to the vascular lumen, then later spreading to involve the vessel coats and adjacent structures. If a typical inflammatory response were to be found in the affected vessels of the visceral organs, it would support the visceral involvement with Buerger's disease. The problem is to establish its place in idiopathic arterial thrombosis devoid of such an intense inflammatory response.

Judging from the segmental occlusive lesions of the extremities in Buerger's disease, the disease may not start from one special focus in a vessel, but rather arise at various levels, at different periods. However, there is little or no relationship between the state of the arteries in the visceral organs and that of the peripheral arteries regarding the distribution of the arteriosclrotic lesions, and the same rule may apply to thromboangiitic lesions. The question of thrombosis is closely linked with that of infarction, for it is infarction which gives rise to most of the symptoms resulting from thrombosis. Although the symptoms of intestinal infarction would show great variations in character and severity, depending upon the size and the location of the area of gut involved, almost nothing is known concerning the symptoms of small infarction of the spleen, pancreas and kidneys. The failure to recognize attacks of arterial thrombosis in the abdominal organs might be due to the unnoticed course of the acute occlusion and the inherent difficulties of diagnosis.

Taking these circumstances into consideration, the incidence of the visceral involvement in Buerger's disease might be greater than generally expected, but the proof has yet not obtained. In 1987 Ito et al.[80] reported a patient with Buerger's disease who developed severe left back pain with fever 10 days after left thoracic sympathectomy because of ischemic ulceartion of the finger. Laparatomy disclosed a large splenic pseudocyst including necrotic tissue: the splenic artery showed chronic inflammatory changes and the pseudocyst was considered to be due to an infarction of the spleen.

Controversy continues regarding the interpretation of the old thrombotic occlusion of the small vessels around the gastric or duodenal ulcer[81]. It means to go back into the time of Friedländer[82]: he proposed a concept of "arteriitis obliterans," cellular proliferation of the intima of the small arteries near the inflammatory lesion. "Arteriitis of obliterans" is essentially a secondary response to the surrounding interstitial inflammatory process, and the organization of thrombus was regarded to be analogous to "arteriitis obliterans." The thrombotic occlusion of the small vessels near gastric or duodenal ulcer, with or without remarkable endothelial cells, might be identified with thromboangiitis obliterans, if the lesion were proved to play an primary role in the pathogenesis of the ulcerative disease.

Harrington and Grossman[83] reported a case of involvement of the sigmoid colon who had numerous manifestations of peripheral vascular involvement sufficient to substantiate the diagnosis of Buerger's disease. On the fourteenth postoperative day after resection of th affected sigmoid colon, he suddenly developed thrombosis of the dorsal vein of the penis; this resulted in ganrene of the distal two thirds of that organ, and perforation of the urethra requiring extensive plastic and urologic procedures. This unique complication of penile thrombosis with Buerger's disease was thought to be the first such case.

The pulmonary artery

In 1940 Hausner and Allen[39] found in the literature reports of six cases suggesting thromboangiitis obliterans of the lung, but they regarded the diagnosis questionable in all instances, because there was no involvement of peripheral arteries in these cases. They reported a lethal case with involvement of pulmonary: the patient complained of nocturnal precordial pain about one year after swelling of bilateral legs; afterward gangrene of both feet and hemorrhage from the intestine developed and he died shortly. Autopsy disclosed that gangreneous enteritis and hepatitis, thrombosis of a pulmonary artery, infarction of the lung and thrombosis of the right iliac artery had been present. Microscopic study disclosed rather marked inflammatory reaction in the wall of the pulmonary artery, consisting of numerous histiocytes, fibroblasts, and fewer lymhocytes. There was a well-organized highly cellular mural thrombus attached to the wall and extensive fresh thrombosis with slight organization limited to a few regions. Autopsy of another case[84] of pulmonary involvement revealed fresh thrombus in the abdominal aorta and the pulmonary trunk and its branches: histology of the affected arteries showed inflammatory changes of the media and adventitia and intimal thickening. Although the possibility of pulmonary embolism originated in the deep vein thrombosis was not ruled out in the both cases, thrombosis of the aortoiliac segment and severe ischemia of the lower extremities were common to the two cases.

Generalized involvement

Reports of Buerger's disease affecting vascular territories other than the extremities are accumulating. In 1934 Birnbaum[85] et al. reported a 19-year-old man of generalized thrombo-angiitis obliterans in detail: the cerebral, retinal, pulmonary, coronary, mesenteric, suprarenal, pancreatic, duodenal, hepatic, renal and prostatic vessels and the vessels of the extremities were involved. The painful swelling in the calves was due to thrombophlebitis of the veins of the lower extremity. They considered the severe attack of cramplike abdominal pain, nausea and vomiting as a result of the involvement of mesenteric vessels with resulting ischemia of the bowel: the icterus to be on a basis of hepatic focal necrosis which might have been a result of the involvement of the heaptic vessels. The pleuritic pain followed by cough and hemoptysis was deemed to be related to the pulmonary thrombosis.

Based on clinical experience of 500 cases of Buerger's disease at the Mayo Clinic, in 1940, Hausner and Allen[39] emphasized that Buerger's disease might be a widespread disease and a serious disease, not only because it necessitated the amputation of extremities but also because it was associated with involvement of regions more vital than the extremities: the necessity for treatment in an attempt to cause quiescence or regression of the vascular lesions should be based upon this consideration, because amputation of both legs might not necessarily mean that the patient would be no longer subject to vascular lesions in other regions. However, beyond explanation by them was the repeated observation that the occlusive arterial lesion in regions other than the extremities was almost always degenerative in nature, whereas it was clearly inflammatory in nature in the extremities.

Reviewing 130,000 autopsy cases from 1966 to 1971 in Japan, Ooneda and Shinkai[86] found only one case of generalized Buerger's disease: a 38-year-old man died of acute suppurative peritonitis due to jejunal perforation caused by infraction 6 years after bilateral thigh amputation performed during about 4 years following the onset of peripheral ischemic symptoms. The thoracic and the abdominal aorta were occluded with thrombus in addition to the peripheral arteries, and infarction was seen in the heart, kidney, spleen and jejunum. Histologically, obliterating thromboangiitic changes were recognized in almost all the arteries and veins: some of the thrombi were relatively fresh, although the thrombi were mostly well organized.

In 1979 Akima et al.[87] reported a 33-year-old man with generalized Buerger's disease: the onset of the disease was at his age of 24 years. He underwent later left below knee and right foot amputation, and died of intestinal infarction. Autopsy revealed widespread intestinal necrosis, myocardial infarcts, thrombosis of the aortoiliac region and intimal thickening with organized thrombus in the small arteries of the lung, spleen, stomach, intestine and prostata.

In the majority of the reported cases of generalized Buerger's disease, the patients had already undergone the major leg amputation, and the histologic changes of their vascular lesions outside the extremities were always proved to be those of atherosclerosis or thrombosis rather than of thromboangiitis obliterans. While Saphir[51] considered the primary inflammatory lesion a factor in the development of visceral atherosclerosis in some patients, detecting whether the visceral arteries of the patients with Buerger's disease are somewhat more than normally susceptible to atherosclerotic and thrombotic occlusion remains an unsolved question.

In 1929 Barron and Linenthal[45] already collected 34 cases of general distribution of Buerger's disease: 27 cases from their series and 7 from the literature. From the review of these cases they concluded that the disease frequently involved the blood vessels of the brain, neck, thorax and abdomen, as well as of the extremities. If the disease may sttack any pary of the vascular system, why the vessels of the extremities are more frequently involved than others? They thought that the greater demand made on the circulatory channels of the lower extremities because of static conditions might favor the more rapid development of the lesion; moreover, the feet were more susceptible to slight injuries from deformities of the nails and from calluses, which were frequently the starting points of gangrene. They reported of a case with generalized distribution of the disease in full: he underwent a gastroenterostomy because of duodenal ulcer at first, and three years later an amputation below the knee was done on account of gangrene of the toe. Two months later he complained of bleeding hemorrhoids, and seven years later he suffered from a hemiparesis of the righ side. While it is true that a patient with Buerger's disease may have duodenal ulcer, bleeding piles and cerebral thrombosis, the question arises whether all these vascular accidents might not be due to one underlying condition. They answered their own question: in the absence of arteriosclerosis, cardiorenal disease or hypertension, it might be reasonable to suppose that there was a relation between the thrombo-angiitis obliterans of the lower extremities, the presence of which had been definitely proved, and other vascular accidents, and that they were all of the same pathology.

Advocates of generalized Buerger's disease emphasized that the disease might start in visceral vessels and not involve the periphery at all, or that it might affect the peripheral and central vessels simultaneously. If it were true, a patient suffering from visceral manifestation devoid of peripheral ischemia could be diagnosed as Buerger's disease for a while, and we go so far as to say that such a patient exists as only the visceral involvement with no arterial occlusion of the extremities through life. If it were true, how can the disease be disgnosed?

While autopsy not infrequently discloses thrombotic occlusion of some vessels in the visceral organs, it is difficult to detect or interpret the pathogenesis of such an occlusive lesion as simple thrombosis devoid of characteristics of systemic or local etiological factor, namely, arteriosclerosis, collagen disease, infection, trauma, hypercoagulable or prethrombotic state and the like. In that case, the coexistence or preexistence of Buerger's disease in the extremities might be quite attractive to the person concerned.

Buerger minutely described the pathologic changes of the affected vessels in the extremities in addition to the characteristic clinical feature and course, and the disease was established as a definite clinical and pathologic entity. However, no strict clinical diagnostic criteria was established, because scant attention was riveted on the clinical course characteristic of the disease. Moreover, it was a happy coincidence to a monist that the pathohistological feature was not pathognomonic : there was no absolutely pathognomonic finding by which the ultimate diagnosis could be determined without any objection, though the granulomatous reaction with microabscess including giant cells and inflammatory cell infiltration throughout the vessel wall lended a characteristic appearance to the thrombotic occlusion of Buerger's disease at the acute stage.

It is well known that the controlateral, completely asymptomatic leg shows not infrequently the almost same arterial occlusion pattern in arteriograms as that in the symptomatic leg due to Buerger's disease. However, it is not easy to detect such an asymptomatic arterial occlusive lesion in the visceral organs, by angiography or noninvasive diagnostic techniques.

A patient with Buerger's disease may suffer from another vascular accident in the whole course of his life, but the question is whether vascular occlusion in parts of the body other than the extremities is merely a coincidence or not. The propriety of the monistic interpretation that all the vascular accidents are of the same pathology might be estimated by the incidence of such vascular occlusions outside the extremities in Buerger's disease. If the incidence is significantly higher in patients with the disease than in a normal population, a conception of "generalized Buerger's disease" is justifiable, even though the pathology of the vascular occlusion indicates a simple thrombosis.

Judging from the clinical course of the disease, Buerger's disease may be classified into five types : 1) upper extremity type (arterial occlusion of the forearm and hand) ; 2) crural type (arterial occlusion of the leg and foot) ; 3) femoral type (progression of arterial occlusion to the femoropopliteal segment) ; 4) aortoiliac type (progression of arterial occlusion to the aortoiliac region) ; and 5) generalized type (visceral involvement in addition to extremities). The patients of the aortoiliac type, especially of juxtarenal aortic occlusion, are subject to progression of thrombosis into the suprarenal region of the aorta, but there is no predicting what will come as the result. While rare involvement of the visceral vessels is supported by the fact that the patients with Buerger's disease have a practically normal survival as compared with a normal population of the same age and sex distribution, detecting asymptomatic or latent occlusive lesions of the visceral organs is a topic for further discussion.

REFERENCES

1. Hashimoto Y, Kamiya K, Okada T. Treatment of spontaneous gangrene. Rinshogeka 1954 ; 9 : 359-65 (in Japanese).
2. Shionoya S, Hirai M, Kawai S, Seko T, Ban I. Pattern of arterial occlusion in Buerger's disease. Angiology 1982 ; 33 : 375-84.
3. Shionoya S, et al.(IV-16).
4. Shionoya S.(IV-4).
5. Shionoya S, et al.(VI-36).
6. Takao T, et al.(IV-14).
7. Buerger L.(I-48).
8. Allen EV. Thromboangiitis obliterans: methods of diagnosis of chronic occlusive arterial lesions distal to the wrist with illustrative cases. Am J Med Sci 1929 ; 178 : 237-44.
9. Hirai M. Ulnary artery occlusion and digital ischemia. VASA 1979 ; 8 : 298-302.
10. Tanaka T, Tada Y, Murakami K, Maruyama Y, Ueno A. Occlusion of the arteries of the forearm and hand after repeated blunt trauma. J Jap Coll angiol 1977 ; 17 : 363-7 (in Japanese).
11. Tanabe T, et al.(VI-22).
12. Hirai M, Shionoya S.(VI-21).
13. Kato R, Kondo M, Kazui H, Ohta T, Naiki K, Tsuchioka H. Distal crural and pedal angiographic findings and pedal ulcer in Buerger's disease. J Jap Coll angiol 1988 ; 28 : 383-7 (in Japanese).
14. Yano T, et al.(VII-22).
15. Kinmonth JB.(IV-11).
16. Warren R, Gomez RL, Marston JAP, Cox JST. Femoropopliteal arteriosclerosis obliterans—arteriographic patterns and rates of progression. Surgery 1964 ; 55 : 135-43.
17. Hirai M, Ban I, Nakata Y, Matsubara J, Shinjo K, Kawai S, Suzuki S, Shionoya S. Reconsideration of Buerger's disease in view of arteriographic findings. J Jap Coll Angiol 1976 ; 16 : 521-3 (in Japanese).
18. Sasaki H, Ohara I, Maeyama T, Ohkuma T, Ichiki M, Okuyama K, Moroboshi Y, Kasai M. Popliteal arterial occlusion and prognosis of affected limbs in Buerger's disease. J Jap Coll Angiol 1986 ; 26 : 15-9 (in Japanese).
19. Nakata Y, Ban I, Matsubara J, Kawai S, Shionoya S. Onset and course of Buerger's disease. J Jap Coll Angiol 1977 ; 17 : 465-8 (in Japanese).
20. Shigematsu H, Miyata R, Sasaki K, Morioka Y, Setoyama R, Ohashi S, Morioka Y. Occlusive lesions of the femoral arterial bifurcation in Buerger's disease. J Jap Coll Angiol 1984 ; 24 : 1225-9 (in Japanese).
21. Mavor GE. The pattern of occlusion in atheroma of the lower limb arteries: the correlation of clinical and arteriographic findings. Br J Surg 1956 ; 43 : 352-64.
22. Inoue H, Yamamoto K, Matsushita M, Kuriyanagi Y, Taguchi M, Alam S, Nishikimi N, Ohba Y, Ito A, Sakurai T, Yano T, Shionoya S. Significance of occlusive lesions of the deep femoral artery in Buerger's disease. JJCVS ; 1990 (in Japanese)(in press).

23. Abu-Dalu J, Giler Sh, Urca I. Thromboangiitis obliterans of the iliac artery. Angiology 1973 ; 24 : 359-64.
24. Haddad M, Zelikovski A, Sternberg A, Urca I. Buerger's disease of the great vessels. VASA 1978 ; 7 : 258-62.
25. Shionoya S, et al.(VII-23).
26. Taguchi M, Shionoya S. Lesions of the visceral vessels in Buerger's disease. In : Mishima Y, ed. Annual Report of the Research Committee on Systemic Vascular Disorders of the Ministry of Health and Welfare of Japan, 1989, pp 82-6 (in Japanese).
27. Nesbit R, Hodgson NB. Thromboangiitis obliterans of the spermatic cord. J Urol 1960 ; 83 : 445-7.
28. Weber FP.(I-44).
29. Ameli FM, Hoy F. Preoperative diagnosis and management of the hypoplastic vessel syndrome. J Cardiovasc Surg 1983 ; 24 : 654-7.
30. Naruo M, Iguchi S, Kimura T, Iwamoto S. Changes in diameter of adult arteries by age group. J Showa Med Ass 1976 ; 36 : 233-41 (in Japanese).
31. Gilkes R, Dow J.(IV-27).
32. Mishima Y, Shigematsu H, Oota I, Miyazawa Y, Iwatani M. Aortoiliac involvement in Buerger's disease. In : (IV-14), pp 390-4 (in Japanese).
33. Yamaguchi H. The figures of obstruction in early stage and their style of aggrevation in Buerger's disease. J Jap Coll Angiol 1980 ; 20 : 805-13 (in Japanese).
34. Oshima T, Ueno A. A young patient with Buerger's disease suffering from a solitary thrombus in the abdominal aorta. In : Mishima Y, ed. Annual Report of the Resarch Committee on Systemic Vascular Disorders of the Ministry of Health and Welfare of Japan, 1986, pp 63-5 (in Japanese).
35. Foerster O, Guttmann L. Cerebrale Komplikationen bei Thromboangiitis obliterans. Arch Psychiat Nervenkrank 1933 ; 100 : 506-15.
36. Spatz H. Über die Beteiligung des Gehirns bei der v. Winiwarter-Buergerschen Krankheit (Thrombo-endangiitis obliterans). Dtsch Z Nervenheilk 1935 ; 136 : 86-132.
37. Lindenberg R, Spatz H.(IV-19).
38. Rosenhagen H. Bemerkungen zur Klinik der cerebralen Form der Thrombo-andarteriitis obliterans (v. Winiwarter-Buergerschen Krankheit). Virchows Arch path Anat 1939 ; 305 : 558-66.
39. Hausner E, Allen EV.(IV-28).
40. Antoni N.(IV-20).
41. Scheinker IM.(IV-21).
42. Davis L, Perret G. Cerebral thrombo-angiitis obliterans. Br J surg 1946 ; 34 : 307-13.
43. Lippman HI.(IV-29).
44. Fisher CM.(I-57).
45. Barron ME, Linenthal H. Thrombo-angiitis obliterans : general distribution of the disease. Arch Surg 1929 ; 19 : 735-51.
46. Zülch KJ. The cerebral form of von Winiwarter-Buerger's disease : does it exist ? Angiology 1969 ; 20 : 61-9.
47. Perla D.(I-50).
48. Allen EV, Willius FA.(IV-22).
49. Samuels SS, Feinberg SC. The heart in thrombo-angiitis obliterans. Am Heart J 1930 ; 6 : 255-

63.

50. Averbuck SH, Silbert S. Thrombo-angiitis obliterans IX : the cause of death. Arch Intern Med 1934 ; 54 : 436-65.
51. Saphir O.(IV-23).
52. Inada K, Hirose M, Okabe K, Okada A. Visceral lesions in Buerger's disease : a case with myocardial infarction. Rinshotokenkyu 1972 ; 49 : 692-6 (in Japanese).
53. Doerr W.(IV-33).
54. Albertini A.(IV-35).
55. Doerr W.(IV-34).
56. Sprunt TP. Thrombo-angiitis obliterans as a generalized vascular disease. South Med J 1934 ; 27 : 698-703.
57. Malisoff S, Macht MB. Thrombo-angiitic occlusion of the reanl artery with resultant hypertension. J Urol 1951 ; 65 : 371-9.
58. Maekawa M, Sawami H, Iguchi M, Saimyoji H, Murai A, Hirakawa S, Kakei Y, Tamura T, Kishitani M. Human hypertension of Goldblatt type caused by Buerger's disease. Jap Circul J 1959 ; 23 : 681-80.
59. Hirakawa T, Fukushige M, Shiraishi T, Fujimoto Y. A case of renal hypertension due to Buerger's disease. Hinyokiyo 1968 ; 14 : 867-71 (in Japanese).
60. Tsuchiya M, Matsuo M, Daijo K. A case of renal hypertension due to Buerger's disease. Kitanobyoinkiyo 1971 ; 16 : 69-72 (in Japanese).
61. Gomi T, Ikeda T, Yuhara M. Renovascular hypertension due to Buerger's disease. Jap Heart J 1978 ; 19 : 308-14.
62. Rob C. Surgical diseases of the celiac and mesenteric arteries. Arch Surg 1966 ; 93 : 21-32.
63. Guay A, Janower ML, Bain RW, McCready FJ. A case of Buerger's disease causing ischemic colitis with perforation in a young male. Am J Med Sci. 1976 ; 271 : 239-40.
64. Sachs IL, Klima T, Frankel NB. Thromboangiitis obliterans of the transverse colon. JAMA 1977 ; 238 : 336-7.
65. Deitch EA, Sikkema WW. Intestinal manifestation of Buerger's disease : case report and literature review. Am Surgeon 1981 ; 47 : 326-8.
66. Soo KC, Hollinger-Vernea S, Miller G, Pritchard G, Frawley J. Buerger's disease of the sigmoid colon. Aust N Z J Surg 1983 ; 53 : 111-2.
67. Ohtaka H, Katsumata T, Takemiya M, Okabe H, Osakabe T, Nemoto H, Igarashi M, Atari H, Toyama K. A case of ischemic stricture of the small intestine associated with Buerger's disease. Jap J Gastroenterol 1984 ; 81 : 2588-93 (in Japanese).
68. Setoh K, Nishio Y, Shoji Y, Ashida T, Nomura H, Nakamura M, Inoue K, Tanaka T, Kashiwagi H, Fujita S. Ischemic and necrotic lesions of the small and large intestine resulting from Buerger's disease. Rinshogeka 1985 ; 40 : 555-60 (in Japanese).
69. Rosen N, Sommer I, Knobel B. Intestinal Buerger's disease. Arch Pathol Lab Med 1985 ; 109 : 962-3.
70. Iwai T, Sato S, Yamada T, Muraoka Y, Sakurawa K, Kinoshita H, Taenaka T, Endo M, Nakajima H, Nasu M, Kamiyama R, Isohisa I. Uniovular twins and Buerger's disease : two cases with abdominal angina or popliteal artery aneurysm. Gekashinryo 1987 ; 29 : 95-7 (in Japanese).
71. Saito O, Tei H, Matsumoto H, Hayashi K, Orino S, Hirata I, Ohshiba S, Takeda Y, Fujiwara

A, Okajima K. A case of ischemic lesion in the large intestine associated with Buerger's disease. Jap J Gastroenterol 1988 ; 85 : 738-42 (in Japanese).
72. Rosenberger A, Munk J, Schramek A, Arieh JB. The angiographic appearance of thromboangiitis obliterans (Buerger's disease) in the abdominal visceral vessels. Br J Radiol 1973 ; 46 : 337-43.
73. Borlaza GS, Rapp R, Weatherbee L, Demetropoulos K. Visceral angiographic manifestation of thromboangiitis obliterans. South Med J 1979 ; 72 : 1609-11.
74. Sobel RA, Ruebner BH. Buerger's disease involving the celiac artery. Hum Pathol 1979 ; 10 : 112-5.
75. Williams LF, Wittenberg J. Ischemic colitis : an useful clinical diagnosis, but is it ischemic ? Ann Surg 1975 ; 182 : 439-48.
76. Taube N. Mesenteric involvement in Buerger's disease (thromboangiitis obliterans) : report of two cases. JAMA 1931 ; 96 : 1469-72.
77. Graves AM.(VI-32).
78. Cohen SS, Barron ME.(IV-24).
79. Williams G.(III-36).
80. Ito K, Kawada T, Ohgi S, Tanaka K, Hara H, Mori T. Buerger's disease accompanied by a splenic pseudocyst caused by splenic arterial occlusion—a report of a case—. J Jpn Soc Clin Surg 1978 ; 48 : 1013-6 (in Japanese).
81. Loh BC, Hatano R, Sugihara K, Inoue K, Kudoh G, Iwai T, Satoh S, Menju M, Takizawa T, Aoki N. Buerger's disease in the right gastric artery associated with duodenal ulcer and minute early gastric cancer. Jap J Gastroenterol 1980 ; 13 : 68-72 (in Japanese).
82. Friedländer C.(I-6).
83. Herrington JL, Grossman LA. Surgical lesions of the small and large intestine resulting from Buerger's disease. Ann Surg 1968 ; 168 : 1079-87.
84. Kanazawa S, Takahashi S, Toshiba Y, Inoh T, Yorifuji S, Suzuki A, Funabiki N, Masumoto D. A case of Buerger's disease associated with the thromboangiitis of pulmonary vessels. Jap Circul J 1969 ; 33 : 1038-9 (in Japanese).
85. Birnbaum W, Prinzmetal M, Connor CL. Generalized thrombo-angiitis obliterans : report of a case with involvement of retinal vessels and suprarenal infarction. Arch Intern Med 1934 ; 53 : 410-22.
86. Ooneda G, Shinkai H.(IV-30).
87. Akima M, Ichimori S, Masuda H, Nomura T, Narayama S, Mitagawa S. A case of generalized Buerger's disease. Junkankika 1979 ; 5 : 473-9 (in Japanese).

CHAPTER IX
DIAGNOSIS

Diagnosis of Buerger's disease should not be made for the reason that the case is left in the basket. While the ultimate criterion for the diagnosis of thromboangiitis obliterans is said to rest on the finding of the typical histologic changes in the arteries of the extremities, it involves a risk to give too much importance to the histologic changes of the affected vessels, though the materiality of the histologic findings is undeniable. As the specify of the disease is derived from its clinical characteristics, the overemphasis of the microscopic identification associated with impractical histopathologic criteria tends to return to the period of the misconception.

Clinical diagnostic criteria

In order to make the clinical diagnosis of Buerger's disease, it is the starting point of the diagnostic procedure to ascertain the fact that the patient has occlusive peripheral arterial occlusions. The evidences necessary for this are absence of arterial pulsations, skin color changes, temperature changes, trophic changes and significant decrease in distal arterial blood pressure of the affected limb. Our clinical criteria for the diagnosis of Buerger's disease are 1) smoking history; 2) onset before the age of 50 years; 3) infrapopliteal arterial occlusive lesions; 4) either upper limb involvement or phlebitis migrans; and 5) absence of atherosclerotic risk factors other than smoking[1]. The clinical diagnosis of Buerger's disease is made when all five requirements are met.

Smoking

Although an outbreak of Buerger's disease in nonsmokers who are always exposed to environmental tobacco smoke is understandable in view of a higher pH, smaller particles and higher concentrations of carbon monoxides in sidestream smoke than in mainstream smoke, the relation between involuntary smoking and Buerger's disease remains an unsolved issue.

Apart from the etiological role of smoking, an intimate relation between smoking and progression of the disease is a unique event observed in the patients with Buerger's disease. If the patient is a nonsmoker, the diagnosis of Buerger's disease requires circumspection.

Age at onset

Buerger's disease may affect men in their 50s, but they might be expected to respond in a different manner to etiologic factors of the disease than younger men, according to the degree of arterial degenerative changes by ageing.

The initial lesion of Buerger's disease as well as arteriosclerosis might be triggered by an interaction between the blood and the intima. In the former, however, the lumen is occluded by thrombus without remodeling of the vessel wall and the entire pathological process is influenced by the mesenchymal activity of the vessel wall[2]. In the latter, there is a remarkable alteration of the vessel wall due to a defect in removal of plasma constituents from the artery, i.e., a disturbance of perfusion in the arterial wall[3]. In man in his fifties, the diagnosis can only be considered presumptive at first. Activated mesenchymal system is indispensable to provoke such a variegated inflammatory reaction as thromboangiitis obliterans, and the mesenchymal activity of the vessel might subsist up to the forties.

Sex

The prevalence of women with Buerger's disease in our series was 2%. While young women with normal ovarian function may be affected with the disease, it has been known as a fact that young female smokers lacking in the sex hormone were not rarely involved with the disease. In case of peripheral ischemia due to organic arterial occlusive lesion in females, the cause may be attributable to collagen disease in the majority of the cases.

Because the clinical course of collagen disease is completely different from that of Buerger's disease, differential diagnosis should be carefully made: prohibition of smoking has no definite influence on the natural history of the collagen disease unlike Buerger's disease. The clinical presentation and histopathology of Buerger's disease in women differ in no way from that in men, and there is no evidence that the disease is milder in women, since gangrene or ulceration occurred in the majority of the female patients. Viewing the matter from a different standpoint, the incidence of asymptomatic females with Buerger's disease might be more higher than expected, but there is no facts to endorse the speculation.

Infrapopliteal arterial occlusive lesions

Although the disease is distributed not only in the infrapopliteal region but also in the upper limb, the thigh and the pelvic area, the main feature of the disease is the infrapopliteal arterial occlusive lesions. The most frequent occurrence of ischemic lesions in the lower extremities may be ascribed to the greater vascular demands, to static conditions, and to exposure of the vessels to mechanical and thermal irritations. Judging from the asymptomatic involvement in the contralateral leg and in the upper limb, an incomplete type of Buerger's disease in which no apparent ischemic symptoms manifest themselves in the lower extremities might exist. It may well be that the disease process would be arrested through abstaining from smoking before the ischemic symptom appears in the foot.

The most characteristic ischemic symptoms in case of the infrapopliteal arterial occlusion are rubor and foot claudication. Abnormally red tinged skin color of the toes and foot, particularly on dependency, is due to a stagnant peripheral circulation caused by poor inflow, multiple occlusion of the distal arteries and veins, atony of the microcirculatory vessels, and an increase in blood viscosity. Persistence of the skin color change even after proximal arterial reconstruction and/or sympathetic denervation is peculiar to the disease.

Hirai and Shionoya[4] divided 41 patients with Buerger's disease only involving the infrapopliteal arteries into two groups: 1) 30 limbs with foot claudication; and 2) 20 limbs without foot claudication. The blood pressure at the foot and the toe in the former was significantly lower than that in the latter, though there was considerable overlapping between the two groups. The severe muscle circulatory insufficiency in the foot with claudication might result from occlusion of the nutrient arteries supplying the plantar muscles as well as poor development of collaterals of the foot in limbs with occlusion of the posterior tibial and/or the plantar arteries. Foot claudication is considered to be nearly specific to Buerger's disease and a useful item in the clinical diagnosis of the disease, as is generally accepted with other manifestations such as upper limb involvement and migrating phlebitis. Foot claudication often persisted after the proximal arterial reconstruction in case of the ascending progression of occlusion into the iliofemoral segment, because the infrapopliteal arterial occlusions remained unchanged after the proximal revascularization.

Migrating phlebitis

Mozes and his colleagues[5] called migrating phlebitis, Raynaud's phenomenon and upper extremity involvement "systemic manifestations" to distinguish them from the local signs and symptoms in the leg that were directly related to arterial insufficiency, namely, claudication, rest pain, ulceration and gangrene. Therefore, in their series, the clinical diagnosis of Buerger's disease was made when in addition to ischemic manifestation in the legs two or more of the systemic manifestations were present.

Migrating phlebitis is the most characteristic symptom representative of an inflammatory nature of the disease. However, the existence of thrombophlebitis migrans is obliged to be depent on the patient's interest and understanding about the symptom, particularly in case of its earlier occurrence than the onset of ischemic symptoms. If migrating phlebitis is considered one of the requirements for the diagnosis of the disease, the diagnostic criteria are placed in an awkward situation that they rely on the patient's memory. As typical Raynaud's phenomenon occurs not so frequently as generally expected in Buerger's disease, it is not appropriate to add Raynaud's phenomenon to the requirement of the diagnostic criteria. In view of the conception of the disease that Buerger's disease is a systemic arterial occlusive disease, the systemic manifestations are indispensable for the diagnostic criteria. In the author's series, phlebitis migrans developed in 43 per cent and involvement of the upper extremity occurred in 90 per cent; both upper limb involvement and phlebitis migrans occurred in 33 per cent.

In our preceding series of 193 patients with Buerger's disease, both upper limb involvement and phlebitis migrans occurred in 65 patients; either upper limb involvement or phlebitis migrans occurred in 128 patients. Patients with both involvements were compared to those with either, and no significant difference in the site of arterial occlusion, the number of the affected limbs, the ischemic symptoms, and the clinical course was found between the two groups[6]. Therefore, either upper limb involvement or phlebitis migrans seems sufficient to support the clinical diagnosis of Buerger's disease.

Absence of atherosclerotic risk factors

Hypertension, diabetes mellitus, and hyperlipidemia, particularly atherogenic lipoprotein must be routinely examined. In case of the succeeding occurrence of the atherosclerotic risk factors during the course of Buerger's disease, such an association of atherosclerosis and Buerger's disease is not against the diagnostic criteria.

Whether this is a coincidence or whether atherosclerosis becomes superimposed on Buerger's disease through a predisposition of the arterial tree to the disease is uncertain. It must be admitted that a predisposition to vascular diseases, as it manifests itself in certain cases, seems to express itself both in a susceptibility to thrombotic lesions as well as to degenerative ones. Autopsy findings in cases of Buerger's disease showed that the more centrally situated arteries developed a tendency to arteriosclerotic lesions even though the arteries of the extremities showed very little sclerosis[7].

A point of diagnostic importance

Addiction to smoking, to put it strong, "nicotine deficiency[8]," presenile onset of arterial occlusion, severe ischemia of the lower extremity (rubor and foot claudication), systemic manifestation (phlebitis migrans or upper limb involvement), and absence of atherogenic risk factors are the noteworthy points in the clinical diagnosis of Buerger's disease.

Arteriographic findings such as tapering or abrupt occlusion, corkscrew or root-like appearance of collaterals, and corrugated appearance serve as supporting evidence, and characteristic pathohistologic findings, giant cell foci in the thrombus at acute stage and well-organized thrombus with considerably preserved general architecture of the vessel wall at chronic stage, corroborate the existence of the disease. The true nature of Buerger's disease consists in the characteristic clinical features and course, and the diagnosis should be based principally upon knowledge of the natural history of the disease[9].

Differential diagnosis

The differential diagnosis of Buerger's disease is usually not difficult if the typical clinical features are kept in minds.

Arteriosclerosis obliterans

The history of Buerger's disease was a history of the contention against arteriosclerosis obliterans, about the clinicopathological independence[10]. If the diagnostic criteria of Buerger's disease are turned inside out, it will be changed into the diagnostic criteria of arteriosclerosis obliterans. As the differential diagnostic features in Buerger's disease and arterioscleosis obliterans have been already described, it needs no repetition here.

Although arteriosclerosis is a generalized disease, it has a predilection for some areas at early stage. In its simplest form the distribution of lower extremity disease is segmental, involving either the aortoiliac or the femoropopliteal segments. However, 20% to 69% of patients will have various combinations of multisegmental disease; combined segmental arterial disease(CSAD)[11]. Haimovici[12] found femoral-popliteal-tibial and iliac occlusion in 3 per cent of 189 patients with arteriosclerotic lesions of the lower extremity.

Chronic atherosclerotic occlusive disease of the extremities starts most frequently in the iliofemoral segment. As the infrapopliteal arteries remain infact at early stage, the initial ischemic symptom is usually calf claudication: no necrotic lesion occurs from the beginning. If the localized disease progresses to multisegmental involvement, rest pain, gangrene or ulceration may occur. In patients with arteriosclerosis obliterans who have diabetes mellitus, the infrapopliteal arteries were liable to be involved[12].

With few exceptions, symptoms are confined to the lower extremities, but asymptomatic occlusion of a subclavian artery may be discovered by means of abnormally low blood pressure in an affected arm: the left subclavian artery is more frequently affected than the right. In case of occlusion of the subclavian artery, no necrotic lesion of the finger occurs and the degree of arm claudication is slight, if any. When the onset of ischemic symptoms in the lower extemity occurs after 50 years of age, patients should be studied carefully with arteriosclerosis obliterans in mind.

Collagen disease

In female patients with extremity ischemia, Buerger's disease must be distinguished from collagen diseases, such as scleroderma or systemic lupus erythematosus, because not only the digital arteries but also the infrabrachial and infrapopliteal arteries may be occluded in collagen diseases.

If the typical clinical symptoms, such as sclerodactyly, gastrointestinal involvement, facial erythema, arthritis, and Raynaud's phenomenon and immunologic abnormalities are all present, an accurate diagnosis of collagen disease is not difficult. However, before the characteristic clinical features appear all together, a long-term follow-up study is indispensable to make an accurate diagnosis. It should be kept in mind, in this regard, that the natural course of Buerger's disease is uneventful unless smoking continues, wheareas the natural history of collagen diseases has no connection with smoking. Buerger's disease is apparently a self-limiting disease, as the obstructive process eventually stops if smoking is strictly inhibited, but this intimate relationship between smoking and the disease process does not apply to collagen diseases.

Because sympathetic denervation not infrequently deteriorates sclerotic skin changes by inhibition of sweating, the differential diagnosis of Buerger's disease from collagen diseases is important from the viewpoint of treatment. On the basis of the clinical observation of ischemic symptoms of the upper extremities in thromboangiitis obliterans, Buerger[13] demonstrated cases simulating scleroderma in 1915: the vascular occlusion led, by virtue of the effects of malnutrition, to a condition of dystrophy, the clinical picture being akin to that of sclerodactyly. Scleroderma is characterized by colorful skin changes from edmatous thickening to atrophic induration of the fingers and typical severe Raynaud's phenomenon.

Occupational arterial occlusive disease of the hand

Arterial occlusive disease of the hand due to repetitive occupational trauma is confined to one hand. In case ischemic symptoms of the fingers occur in smokers, the differential diagnosis of arterial occlusion related occupational trauma from Buerger's disease is not easy.

Raynaud's phenomenon is a prominant symptom in a group of patients who have arterial occlusion in the hand and fingers that is associated with repeated occupational trauma. The patients with this type of arterial occlusion are labors who frequently use tools that require a squeezing action of the hand or whose hands are subjected to repetitive blunt trauma or the use of vibrating tools. While the hypothenar area suffers the most frequently such an injury[14], the affected region is not necessarily confined to the hypothenar area.

A 41-year-old subway motor man complained of pain, coldness and cyanotic discoloration of the right fourth finger and Raynaud's phenomenon of the right all fingers for about one year. He had to use the tool that required a squeezing action of his right fingers during working every day. Brachial angiography revealed occlusion of the ulnar, the superficial palmar arch, and the proper digital arteries: neither the palmar metacarpal nor the common palmar digital artery for the fourth finger was visualized (Fig. IX-1). Although the arterial occlusion in his right hand and fingers was considered a result of chronic arterial injury due to occupational trauma, it was difficult to differentiate his angiographic apperance from that in Buerger's disease. There was no evidence of occlusive arterial disease elsewhere than in the affected hand, but it was not out of bounds of possibility that ischemic

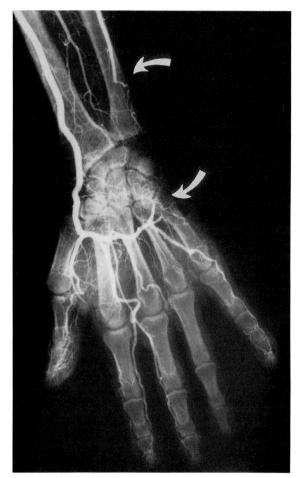

Figure IX-1. Right brachial arteriogram of a 41-year-old man hypothenar hammer syndrome. The ulnar artery and the palmar arch are occluded around the wrist (arrows), and multiple occlusions of the metacarpal and digital arteries are also seen.

symptoms might manifest themselves in the other extremities in the future in this patient,because he was a heavy smoker for about 20 years. Viewing the matter from a different standpoint, it might be imagined that occupational occlusive arterial disease of his right hand might have occurred on the basis of a thromboangiitic lesion. Detecting how trauma could participate in the pathogenesis of Buerger's disease remains an unsolved question, but exposure of the vessels to repetitive mechanical and thermal irritations might have a promoting influence on the development of the arterial occlusive lesion of Buerger's disease.

Necrotic lesions occurred in 72% of the 255 patients with the disease in our series ; to put it the other way around, neither gangrene nor ulceration developed in 28% of all the patients. While smoking produces spectacular disabilities, prohibition of smoking and protection from exposure to cold and injury at early stage may restore the disease process quiet. As "vibration-induced white finger" appears in the foots which are exposed to the percussion of the vibratory tools[15], vasospastic disturbances due to occupational repetitive trauma are not necessarily confined to the hand. In case of occupational occlusive arterial diseases of the hand in smokers, keeping a check on the existence of occlusive arterial disease elsewhere than in the affected extremity and the systemic manifestations of the disease and a follow-up examination of the patients under prohibition of smoking are indispensable to the differential diagnosis from Buerger's disease.

Thoracic outlet symdrome

As a vascular complication of thoracic outlet syndrome, particularly in case of the pressence of a cervical rib, repetitive arterial embolism originated in the damaged intima of the subclavian artery sometimes produces chronic ischemic symptoms of the upper limb bearing resemblance to those in Buerger's disease. Routine roentgenograms should be obtained of the cervical spine, and these should be carefully scrutinized for the presence of cervical ribs, anomalous first thoracic ribs, clavicular exostoses, vertebral abnormalities, and the like[16].

Behçet's disease

In patients with Behçet's disease, peripheral ischemic symptoms of the extremities such as gangrene or Ranynaud's phenomenon sometimes manifest themselves[17]. Angiographic[18] and pathohistologic[19] findings of the occlusive lesions are not always distinguishable from those in Buerger's disease.

Because of abnormal hypersensitive response to various stimuli to the vessel, direct vascular surgery is liable to cause an insuffcient healing of the anastomotic sites and the long-term results of arterial reconstruction including repair of aneurysms has been reported to be poor. Syatemic manifestations such as iritis, aphthous ulceration of the mouth , ulceration of the genitalia, superficial and deep thrombophlebitis, erythema nodosum-like eruption and positive needle reaction of the skin are the main points in view of the differential diagnosis.

Aortitis symdrome

Although the subclavian artery was the most frequently involved, as an old name "pulseless disease" means, the arteries of the lower extremity were rarely affected: the prevalence was 3-7 per cent[20-22]. However, the ischemic symptoms of the affected limb were usually claudication, fatigue or coldness, and no necroic lesions occurred as a rule. In contrast to Buerger's disease, the overwhelming majority of patients with aortitis syndrome is female and the aorta and its main branch arteries are mostly involved. In other words, the stage of the former's operations is the arteries of muscular type; the stage of the latter's operations is the arteries of elastic type.

Vasospastic disorders

In addition to chronic or permanent ischemic signs due to organic occlusion of the vessels, other phenomena which are vasomotor in nature may be associated with Buerger's disease, and it is these that must be differentiated from similar phenomena accompanying Raynaud's disease, erythromelalgia, scleroderma, sclerodactyly, and acrocyanosis. If we do not overestimate the importance of single manifestation of vasomotor irritation, but regard as more significant the clinical course and the symptoms in their totality, we will not fail to separate very clearly in our minds the true vasomotor neuroses from the organic vascular disease attended with vasomotor phenomena, as Buerger exquisitely said[13].

REFERENCES

1. Shionoya S. Buerger's disease (thromboangiitis obliterans). In: Rutherford RB ed. Vascular surgery. Philadelphia: W.B. Saunders, 3rd ed, 1989, pp 207-17.
2. Shionoya S.(I-79).
3. Doerr W. Die Pathologie Virchow's und die Lehre von der Arteriosklerose. Pathologe 1987; 8: 1-8.
4. Hirai M, Shionoya S.(VI-12).
5. Mozes M, et al.(VI-15).
6. Shionoya S, Ohta T, Nishikimi N. Definition der Endangiitis aus klinischer Sicht. In: (II-17), pp 8-10.
7. Inada K, et al.(I-74).
8. Cabezas-Moya R, Dragstedt LR II.(VI-26).
9. Richards RL. Thrombo-angiitis obliterans: clinical diagnosis and classification of cases. Br Med J 1953; 1: 478-81.
10. Theis FV. Thromboangiitis obliterans: a 30-year study. J Am Geriat Soc 1958; 6: 106-17.
11. Samson RH, Scher LA, Veith FJ. Combined segment arterial disease. Surgery 1985; 97: 385-96.
12. Haimovici H. Patterns of arteriosclerotic lesions of the lower extremity. Arch Surg 1967; 95: 918-33.

13. Buerger L.(I-42).
14. Conn J Jr, Bergan JJ, Bell JL. Hypothenar hammer syndrome : posttraumatic digital ischemia. Surgery 1970 ; 68 : 1122-8.
15. Hashiguchi T, Sakakibara H, Furuta M, Yamada S, Horio K, Toibana N. Raynaud's phenomenon in the lower extremities induced by vibration exposure. : report of three cases. JJTOM 1988 ; 36 : 651-7 (in Japanese).
16. Judy KL, Heymann RL. Vascular complications of thoracic outlet syndrome. Am J Surg 1972 ; 123 : 521-31.
17. Mishima Y, Ishikawa K, Ueno A. Arterial involvement in Behçet's disease. Jpn J Surg 1973 ; 3 : 52-60.
18. Matsuo T, Iida T, Tominaga S, Hashimoto T, Shimizu T. Arteriographic findings of the upper extremities in Behçet's syndrome. In : (IV-14), pp 268-72 (in Japanese).
19. Shimizu T, Hashimoto T, Matsuo T, Tominaga S, Iida T, Yoshizawa H. Clinico-pathological studies on vasculo-Behçet's syndrome. Nipponrinsho 1978 ; 36 : 798-807 (in Japanese).
20. Nakao K, Ikeda M, Kimata S, Niitani H, Miyahara M, Ishimi Z, Hashiba K, Takeda Y, Ozawa T, Matsushita S, Kuramochi M. Takayasu's arteritis : clinical report of eighty-four cases and immunological studies of seven cases. Circulation 1967 ; 35 : 1141-55.
21. Tada Y, Ueno A. Five cases of aortitis syndrome with occlusion of the peripheral arteries. In : Inada K, ed. Report of the Ist Meeting of the Aortitis Syndrome Research Committee, the Ministry of Health and Welfare of Japan, 1974, pp 10-6 (in Japanese).
22. Sakuma M, Yasuda K, Tanabe T. Lower extremity arterial reconstruction in aortitis syndrome. In : Mishima Y, ed. Annual Report of the Research Committee on Systemic Vascular Disorders, the Ministry of Health and Welfare, Japan, 1986, pp 44-7 (in Japanese).

CHAPTER X
TREATMENT

Buerger[1] said that patients affected with thrombo-angiitis obliterans did not suffer directly from the disease itself but from the disastrous occlusive thrombosis: a distinct differentiation must be made between the symptoms referable to the malady itself, and to those attributable to the results of vascular occlusion, and therefore due to impoverishment of circulation.[2]

While the incipient lesion of Buerger's disease is an acute inflammatory one, involving the arterial and venous walls, we will expect an occlusive thrombosis as the immediate sequence, and, such a distinct differentiation is impossible as a matter of fact. Therefore, the fundamental policy of the treatment for ischemia due to the disease is the same as that for circulatory insufficiency caused thrombotic occlusion of the vessels. When a case presents itself with features indicative of obstructive vascular lesions, it behooves us first to investigate the extent and locality of the occlusive process. As the arterial occlusive process is accompanied by the development of collateral vessels, the degree of the circulatory insuffciency rests on the compensatory function of the collaterals. Because the cause of Buerger's disease is unknown, there is no causal treatment and all the present treatments are symptomatic ones.

A. Prerequisites for Treatment

There exists no causal treatment, but it is possible to arrest progression and recurrence of the disease.

Tobacco abstinence

The only way to arrest the disease is abstinence from smoking. Any therapeutic procedure not accompanied by a cessation of smoking, including arterial reconstruction, will be unsuccessful in treating the arterial insufficiency.[3,4] The case of a patient with Buerger's disease who had simultaneous quadrilateral gangrene of the digits was reported in 1937.[5] During the 27 ensuing years, he had abstained from smoking, and there has been no reactivation of his disease; he represented the ideal in terms of treatment and response.[6]

The possibilities of disaster resulting from even a few cigarettes a day or an occasional smoke should be emphasized : a reduction in the numbers of cigarette is completely meaningless. The results that the digital pulse volume recorder amplitude decreased significantly in response to both low and high nicotine cigarettes suggest that little is to be gained by switching from high to low nicotine cigarettes.[7] Tabacco in all forms should be considered poison for the patients with Buerger's disease, and the patients must prevent themselves from exposure to the tobacco smoke of smokers in houses, places of work and public facilities. An adverse effect of involuntary smoking deserves much consideration, though further clinical and epidemiologic studies should investigate the effect of involuntary smoking on the course of the disease, using a more refined characterization of smoke exposure.

It is a difficult period for both physicians and patients until the patients realize the imperative significance of prohibition of smoking. It is not seldom that the fiducial relationship between the two is lost. In spite of emphatic advice with regard to cessation of the use of tobacco, it is the actual circumstances that quite a few patients smoke again after healing of necrotic lesions or remission and have a relapse of the disease, and it is also an undeniable fact that some patients with Buerger's disease are addicted to tobacco or so intent on their self-destruction that they continue to smoke either openly or surreptitiously. Treatment of the patients with Buerger's disease is haunted by the problem of smoking, from the beginning to the end.

Corelli[8] named Buerger's disease "cigarette smoker disease," and his principle of treatment for the patients with the disease was thoroughgoing as follows :

The patients must be hospitalized in wards where nobody should be allowed to smoke, including the hospital staff, the patients' visitors and relatives, as well as the other patients suffering from various different diseases, which would not require prohibition of smoking. They had a ward where only patients with the disease or arteriosclerosis were admitted and where smoking was absolutely forbidden, and the vigilance was strict, night and day. The patients with Buerger's disease, who are inveterate smokers and psychologically labile with regards to smoking, must be helped, assisted and led to the firm belief that it is absolutely mandatory to stop smoking.

Corelli rated malariotherapy as the most "broad-spectrum" antiinflammatory agent very high. He publicly declared that surgeons and angiologists, supporters of the surgical treatment, should not touch any more patients with the disease and transfer them to him. Campbell et al.[9] reported that 88 of 128 patients with the disease still used tobacco despite of the repeated admonitions on the follow-up analysis. de Takats[10] told to the patients not to come back to his clinic unless they could say they had stopped smoking, because he would be unable to do anything for them.

General regimen

Patients with Buerger's disease who have rest pain, gangrene or ulceration of the extremities should be treated at a hospital where they can keep quiet mentally and physically in a comfortable environment, can avoid weight bearing and other trauma to ischemic extremities and can bring about a sympathetic understanding between patients, nurses and doctors.

Bed rest alone in healthy surroundings usually results in improvement in symptoms and manifestation of the disease without special therapeutic procedures. Intractable pain of necrotic lesions which has compelled the patient to be addicted to the use of narcotic or analgesic drugs is not infrequently relieved and tolerable without the drugs in one to two weeks. Under careful observation about the clinical course of the disease during this period, spontaneous healing potential of the ischemic lesion may be evaluated and a therapeutical principle will be decided. In case where the patient develops critical ischemia symptom in spite of a rest cure, it suggests an acute aggravating process of the disease due to thrombotic occlusion and an emergency procedure should be under consideration.

B. Conservative Treatment

All the patients with Buerger's disease should be conservatively managed at first, irrespective of manifestation of the disease. In chronic arterial occlusive disease, a number of extremity arteries are spared from obstructive lesions. The goal of medical treatment is to develop flow through the remaining patent vessels and the compensatory collateral network. For this purpose, avoidance of vasoconstriction and provoking of vasodilatation have been taken into account.

It is a matter of course that exposure to cold should be avoided, but it is difficult to inhibit vasoconstriction by drugs. No positive effective influence of vasoactive substances on the vasospastic phenomena has been obtained yet. In order to increase the blood flow through the nutrient vessels to the ischemic region distal to the sites of arterial occlusion, selective vasodilatation of the collateral vessels is necessary. Because there are no vasodilating drugs that can act selectively on these collateral vessels, however, the value of systemically administered vasodilators has been controversial.[11-15] The reasons why the difference in the response to vasodilating drugs between the intact arteries and the collaterals are obscure. As increase in blood flow due to vasodilation in the target area is expected only under the condition with no reduction in the perfusion pressure resulting form the drug. At the present there are two methods to increase flow through the collateral vessels:

exercise and intraarterial infusion of vasodialators to the target area.

Physical method of enhancing the circulation

Buerger[16] said that therapeutic measures should be directed towards the conservation of warmth, enhancement of the circulation, the prevention of traumatism, and the treatment of local conditions.

Buerger[16] suggested that certain passive exercises might be of value in inducing hyperemia or rubor in the affected limb, and therefore, therapeutically beneficial in increasing the blood supply: this method was the logical therapeutic outcome of his method of diagnosticating impairment of circulation of the lower extremities, in that it used the phenomenon of induced rubor, or induced hyperemia in a therapeutic way.

The affected limb is elevated with the patient lying in bed, to from 60° or 90° above the horizontal, being allowed to rest upon a support for from 30 seconds to 3 minutes, the period of time being the minimum amount of time necessary to produce blanching or ischemia. As soon as blanching is established, the patient allows the foot to hang down over the edge of the bed for from 2 to 5 minutes, until reactionary hyperemia or rubor sets in, the total period of time about 1 minute longer than that necessary to establish a good red color. The limb is then placed in the horizontal position for about 3 to 5 minutes, during which time an electric heating pad or a hot water bag is applied, care being taken to prevent the occurrence of a burn. The placing of the limb in these three successive positions constitutes a cycle, the duration of which is usually from 6 to 10 minutes. These cycles are repeated over a period of about one hour, some 6 to 7 cycles constituting a séance. The number of sérances cannot be categorically stated but should vary with the case. In general way they should occupy at least 6 to 7 hours a day, that is every alternate hour during the daytime. He said that if the method was carried out daily for a sufficiently long period, it was of greater value in improving the circulatory conditions and increasing the blood supply, than any of the other mechanical or thermal means that were at their disposal.

Ratschow,[17] a pioneer in the diagnostics and treatment of peripheral arterial occlusive disease, indicated that the development of the collateral vessels was promoted by augmentation of the flow velocity through the collaterals. All the procedures that augment the flow velocity in the target area serve the purpose. To be concrete, the following processes answer the purpose: 1) keeping the reduction of the vascular resistance of the collaterals; and 2) augmentation of the demand for blood supply in the peripheral tissues: pharmacological dilatation of the arteries brings about simultaneously a reduction in systemic blood pressure. In practice, it means to exercise the ischemic extremities, namely, an increase in blood flow is induced by intense reactive hyperemia. Gymnastic exercises originated by Ratschow are to move round the patient's feet or to close and open his hands in the elevated position of the extremities, and have spread throughout the world: the principle of his training is the same as that of "Buerger's exercise."

Schoop[18] has carried on Ratschow's tradition and established the principles of conservative treatment for chronic arterial occlusive disease of the extremities.

He regarded the aim of conservative treatment as follows:

1. Augmentation of blood supply at rest. In case of only peripheral arterial occlusion accompanied with an increased nervous tension of the vessels, blood supply to the periphery may be increased by inhibiting the sympathetic strain.
2. Increase in blood supply in reserve. Flow velocity through the collaterals is increased by ischemic muscle training, and the increased flow velocity dilates the collateral vessels. An intermittent rapid increase in flow velocity is most favorable for the development of the collaterals.
3. Better distribution and utilization of circulatory blood. Trained muscles can fulfil a certain quantity of movement with less blood supply compared to untrained muscles. By muscle training the metabolic activity, particularly its aerobic capacity may be increased: the number and size of mitochondria in the muscle is increased and the efficiency of the use of blood is more improved.
4. Learning of more befitting technique of walking. By repeated walking at a quick pace until occurrence of muscle pain, claudication distance can be prolonged. An effective walking technique appropriate for each person may be acquired by patient walking exercise.
5. Stabilization of cardiovascular system. Without question, blood supply to the periphery rests on the cardiac function and systemic circulatory state.
6. Removal of additional adverse factors. Elimination of additional unfavorable factors is not infrequently more effective therapeutically than increase in blood supply. As improper loading due to unstable equilibrium, painful alteration of the joints and muscles, and chronic inflammatory venous stasis due to insufficient venous return are ready to cause walking disturbances, remission of these lesions improves intermittent claudication.

Carter et al.[19] reported that walking exercise resulted in improved walking distance in patients with intermittent claudication, and they suggested that factors other than increased development of collateral vessels were important in determining walking ability, judging from small pressure changes after training. Together with walking training, gymnastic exercise is indispensable to enhancing circulation. Prevention of atrophy of the muscles and stiffness of the joints and improvement of power of locomotion are the aim of the gymnastic exercise. If the patients with ischemic limbs are not in motion, their capacity for locomotion is on the decrease. Walking training and physical exercise is the treatment of choice for intermittent claudication in Buerger's disease, particularly for foot and arm claudication.

Pharmacologic measures

Because there are no vasoactive substances that can act selectively on the collateral vessels, the only method to avoid the systemic adverse effcts of vasoactive drugs is an intraarterial administration of the drugs to the target area. Although some vasodilating drugs such as reserpine and ATP-preparation had been injected into the artery in the affected limb, intraarterial injection method has been got into the spotlight with the advent of prostaglandins.

Prostaglandins

The discovery of prostaglndins has opened a new field in the treatment of severe ischemia. The first report in 1973 concerning the use of prostaglandin E_1(PGE_1) in arterial occlusive disease described the intrafemoral artery infusion of PGE_1 at a dose of 1 ng/kg/min for about 10 min every hour for 24 to 72 hours in four patients with severe rest pain or ulceration due to arteriosclerosis obliterans.[20] In December 1973, experimental and clinical studies on the application of PGE_1 began in Japan, and the method of the continuous intraarterial infusion of PGE_1 has been established.[21,22]

Degradation of PGE_1 in the pulmonary circulation[23] is both a demerit and a merit : PGE_1 which passed through the target area is almost completely metabolized in the lung and the recirculated drug is in too low concentration to disply an adverse effect on the other organs beside the affected limb. The drug-induced systemic hypotension due to vasodilatation does not occur. Therefore, in case of the intraraterial route, PGE_1 is able to produce maximal vasodilation and inhibition of platelet aggregation action at a minimum of concentration ; its pharmacologic effects are restricted within the target area, causing no systemic influence because of extensive degradation of PGE_1 in the pulmonary circulation.

Continuous intraarterial infusion of PGE_1

From December 1973 through October 1982, 72 patients underwent the continuous intraraterial infusion of PGE_1 at our hospital for the management of intractable necrotic lesion of the ischemic limbs with no indication of surgical treatment : Buerger's disease in 64 patients, arteriosclerosis obliterans in 6, and collagen disease in 2.[24]

There were 67 men and 5 women, ranging in age from 26 to 77 years(mean, 43.2± 10.8 years). As the procedure was repeated 5 times in one, 4 times in one and twice in 7 patients because of recurrence of the necrotic lesion or a new necrotic lesion in another limb, 86 extremities underwent the PGE_1-infusion in all. By means of percutaneous puncture or cutdown, a catheter with 0.5 mm in inner and 1.0 mm in outer diameter was inserted into the main artery of the diseased limb: into the femoral artery in 84 limbs, the peroneal in 1, and the brachial in 1. The catheter was inserted into the deep femoral artery in cases with total occlusion of the superficial femoral artery: it was generally lodged near the entrance to the Hunter's canal and its correct insertion was always certified by angiography. After the catheter was connected with the portable infusion-pump, the catheter was fixed on the chest and abdominal wall with adhesive plaster to prevent its falling.

On the basis of our previous investigation, PGE_1 was infused at a dose of 0.1 ng/kg/min in all the patients at the start: the solution in the infusion-bag consisted of 1) 0.1 ng/kg/min of PGE_1; 2) 1.000 units/day of heparin; 3) 500 mg/day of aminobenzyl penicillin; and 4) saline. The capacity of the bag was 25 ml and 5 ml of the solution was infused per day. When the initial dosage of the drug brought about no good results, PGE_1 was increased in concentration of 0.15 to 0.5 ng/kg/min 1 to 2 weeks after the commencement of the infusion. On the other hand, PGE_1 was decreased in concentration of 0.05 to 0.075 ng/kg/min, when swelling, pain or tenderness was recognized in the neighborhood of the cannula tip, mostly above the knee; these local side effects might be related to hyperpermeability of the vessel wall due to PGE_1. The troubles promptly disappeared after reduction in concentration of the drug.

In 28 of the 86 limbs the necrotic lesions were healed by the infusion for 9 to 135 days (mean: 38.4 ± 27.1 days); in 33 limbs the lesions were noticeably improved by the infusion for 5 to 140 days (mean: 47.7 ± 31.3 days), and in 25 limbs the lesions were unchanged by the infusion for 1 to 94 days (mean: 33.0 ± 22.8 days). Because there was no dose-dependent relationship between the dose of PGE_1 and the clinical response, the dosage of the drug should be determined in accordance with clinical response and side effect individually. Examination of the state of the superficial femoral artery in relation to the clinical response to the drug showed that patency of the artery was associated with a high success rate, whereas the opposite applied when the artery was occluded. The reduced efficacy of the intraarterial infusion of PGE_1 into the deep femoral artery could be attributable to a small fraction of the drug reaching the foot because of collateral vessels with high vascular resistance, together with a steal phenomenon to the well-perfused thigh muscles.[25,26]

At the beginning of this treatment, thrombotic occlusion occurred in 2 cases, bleeding in 1 and infection in 1, in relation to technical failure: by thrombectomy or emergency procedures, the affected limbs were salvaged, but one patient underwent thigh amputation because of serious infection and sepsis. Roentgenograms of 11 patients who received the infusion-therapy for 15 to 95 days from January 1982 through October 1982 did not show cortical hyperostosis of the long bones of the lower extremity which was reported to occur following long-term administration of

PGE_1 in infants with cyanotic congenital heart disease.[27] There was no abnormal variation in laboratory findings during or after the treatment in all cases. The C-reactive protein test was intensified in 29 cases during the infusion, but it returned to normal after completion of the treatment. Eleven of the 25 limbs with a poor clinical response later had to undergo above or below knee amputation because of advanced necrotic lesions of the extremities. Judging from the relationship between the state of the superficial femoral artery and the clinical response, foot ischemia in patients with infrapopliteal arterial occlusion, as most frequently seen in Buerger's disease, seems amenable to the intraarterial PGE_1-infusion.

Out of 255 patients with Buerger's disease in our series, 40 limbs with intractable ulceration, in whom neither arterial reconstruction nor sympathectomy was feasible, underwent continuous intraarterial infusion of PGE_1 in a dose of 0.03 to 0.5 ng/kg/min (mean: 0.17 ng/kg/min). With a 13 to 84 (average: 44) day infusion, ulcers healed in 12 (30%) of 40 extremities, improved in 21 (52.5%), and were unchanged in 7 (17.5%). Four of the 7 extremities with no effect of the infusion had to received above or below knee amputation becasuse of advanced necrotic lesions.

Intravenous drip infusion of PGE_1

In view of the practical advantages of the intravenous over the intraarterial route and because of the recognition of beneficial effects in the contralateral limb during intraraterial infusion of the drug, the efficacy of intravenous injection of PGE_1 for ischemic ulceartion was compared with that of intraarterial administration.[24,28] However, while an intravenous drip infusion of PGE_1, in a dose of 5-10 ng/kg/min, was effective for improvement in ischemic symptoms, the intravenous route was clearly inferior to intraarterial administration in regard to the healing of trophic lesions.

The lesser efficacy of the intravenous infusion of PGE_1 might be attributed to an underdose in the target area. Nevertheless, the intravenous route is prefered to the intraraterial in cases with involvement of the iliofemoral segment because of the difficulty of inserting the catheter into a target artery. In addition, long-term intravascular insertion of the catheter into the deep femoral artery carries the risk of damaging the collateral vessel and is less effective than insertion into a patent superficial femoral artery.

From hemodynamic study on 83 ischemic limbs which received intravenous drip infusion of PGE_1 at a dose of 6.4 to 12.6 ng/kg/min (average: 9.5 ± 1.5) for 60 to 90 min, Hirai et al.[29] obtained the results as follows: 1) significant increase in blood flow at the calf and foot, amplitude of pulse wave at the first toe, velocity at the common femoral, posterior tibial and dorsalis pedis, and skin temperature at the foot and toes; 2) more significant increase in blood flow, velocity and skin temperature in the distal level of the leg than in the proximal level; and 3) insignificant change in segmental blood pressure of the leg and crest time of pulse wave. These findings indicates that PGE_1 dose not cause a selective dilatation of the collaterals, but lowers the resistance in peripheral small vessels with an increase in distal blood flow. If PGE_1 reduces the collateral resistance more than the peripheral arterial resistance, a shortening of crest time and an increase in distal blood pressure should be observed.

An insignificant increase in velocity at the femoral artery and a significant decrease in calf skin temperature without increase in blood flow at the calf might be induced by shunting the blood in the skin of the leg to the foot in patients with arterial occlusion proximal to the popliteal artery. Furthremore they found that 12 out of 66 ischemic limbs showed a decrease in skin temperature at the toe after PGE_1 infusion: 7 of the 36 limbs with suprapopliteal occlusion and 5 of the 30 limbs with infrapopliteal occlusion. The steal phenomenon observed in 18% of all the patients investigated occurred most frequently in the limbs with rest pain and/or gangrene. As no beneficial effect of PGE_1 was expected in patients whose blood flow at the toe was reduced following infusion of the drug, attention must be given to the steal phenomenon in managing critical limb ischemia.

Prostaglandins in the treatment of ischemic limbs

Prostaglandins are exciting substances for angiologist because of their properties of improving peripheral circulation as far as ischemic limbs are concerned, though a possible pharmacological mechanism of therapeutic usefulness of the drug on tissue healing remains to be resolved, and controversy continues regarding of the efficacy of PGE_1 in the treatment of ischemic ulcers.[30,31]

Judging from the observation that no significant increase in distal blood pressure occurred by intraarterial infusion of PGE_1 in patients with peripheral arterial occlusive disease, it was said that mechanism other than vasodilatation and inhibition of platelet aggregation should be considered as for a good effect of PGE_1 on tissue healing.[32] However, measurement of blood flow, blood pressure, oxygen tension and local skin temperature may be not sensitive enough to detect a hardly discernible hemodynamic change in peripheral circulation by pharmacotherapy. The importance of the antiplatelet effects of PGE_1 is also difficult to assess in therapeutic dosage. PGE_1 might act on rheological properties of blood by inhibition of platelet aggregation and other unknown biologic effects such as increasing red cell deformability to improve microvascular circulation in the diseased extremity.[33]

While discovery of prostacyclin(PGI_2), the most powerful inhibitor of platelet aggregation in addition to vasodilator, has enriched the content of prostaglandin therapy in peripheral arterial occlusive disease,[34] its clinical application is restricted because of lack of chemical stability. Various clinical trials on many derivatives of PGE_1 and PGI_2, inhibitors of thromboxane synthetase, and products of eicosapentaenoic scid are in progress now, but it is important to determine which condition will respond well to the vasoactive substances by evaluating the drug-induced hemodynamic changes in the peripheral circulation. Satisfactory clinical results may be expected in only those ischemic lesions with spontaneous healing potential, and the response to the drugs is individually different, probably according to each pathophysiological state. Prostaglandins are not a panacea for arterial insufficiency.

Other medications

Inhibitory influence on the experimental thrombus formation[35] and therapeutic effect on healing of ischemic ulcers of antiplatelet drugs[36] have been reported, but controversy continues regarding its usefulness for improvement in ischemic symptoms of the patients with Buerger's disease[37], though thrombolytic agents with heparin may be indicated in case of acute aggravation due to thrombotic occlusion.

As there is no vasoactive drugs primarily improving the collateral perfusion, the therapeutic effect of changing the rheological properties of blood has been studied, and it has definitely shown that increased red-cell flexibility tended to counteract the effect of increasing blood viscosity by higher hematocrit and increased plasma-fibrinogen concentration. Improvement in rheological abnormalities in the microcirculatory system may be achieved by correction of these risk factors, and the reduced blood viscosity is alleged to bring about the amelioration of ischemic attacks.[38,39] Hemodilution studies carried out under isovolemic and hypervolemic conditions showed an improvement of microcirculation by lowering hematocrit.[40] Patients with Buerger's disease revealed not infrequently an increased hematocrit value, and the procedure lowering the blood viscosity by saline-infusion was reported to be effective for healing of ischemic ulceration in 1913.[41]

Intentional and controllable reduction in fibrinogen concentration down to value of about 70 mg% with a defibrinogenic agent was considered to produce multifactorial improvement of the rheological properties of the blood.[42] In case of hyperfibrinogenemia, the defibrinogenation therapy may be most effective. There are drugs available, such as pentoxifylline, that can lower blood viscosity to a certain degree and positively affect erythrocyte flexibility.[43] At the present time, however, there are no practical methods available to verify an increased effective capillary flow in the target area by pharmacotherapy.

In addition to that, it is to be desired to determine at the beginning which patients will respond well to the drugs by objectively evaluating individually the drug-induced hemodynamic change in the affected limb. Although arterioles in the vascular areas distal to arterial occlusion are maximally dilated, due to the local accumulation of vasodilating metabolites, the blood flow is decreased because of the low driving pressure. Therefore, measures increasing distal blood pressure could be helpful in the treatment of skin ulcers: mineralcorticoid and salt administration induced moderate hypertension enough to improve ischemic symptoms.[44] Clinical application of the drug-induced hypertension is practically problematical, but a Fowler's position is known to be helpful to relieve ischemic pain by increasing the distal perfusion pressure.

Bridging treatment

It is essential that something be done to try to help the patient through the difficult time between the onset of acute symptoms and eventual clinical improvement. The most difficult aspect is the war against intractable pain. Particularly in case of severe ischemic pain, how to alleviate the pain is an urgent problem for both patients and physicians, and it is an important problem to meditate a way out of the most suffering pass for the patients in despair of controlling themselves and fighting the disease.

The "bridging" treatment[45] includes tobacco withdrawal and rest of body and mind as a matter of course, and the epidural nerve block is frequently needed in case of severe pain due to critical ischemia. Epidural anesthesia gives quick relief and a 1 to 2-week administaration via an indwelling catherter provides relief for the patient, who otherwise must keep his leg dependent around the clock. In addition, alleviation of dependent edema speeds healing. Although epidural anesthesia produces sympathectomy-like vasodilation, it will subsequently need to be supplemented by surgical sympathectomy in the more serious cases. Hyperbaric oxygen therapy may also relieve pain and accelerate healing of ischemic ulcers.[46,47]

"Bridging" treatment is the term we use for the appropriate use of epidural anesthesia, PG infusion, antithrombotic agents, or hyperbaric oxygen to help the patient through periods of acute exacerbation. The aim of the bridging treatment is to reduce stasis and sludging in the microvascular system to increase capillary flow and to improve tissue oxidation. In most cases the pain is appeased and most patients calm themselves down. In parallel with the "bridging" treatment, a radical therapeutic plan should be framed, based on the diagnostic result and the course of the disease.

Local treatment

A "trophic" ulcer may be caused by injury, infection, edema, or metabolic malfunction, in addition to lack of nutrition. Trophic ulcers in ischemic limbs should be considered "ischemic" ulcers only if they are caused by an arterial occlusion which critically curtails blood flow at rest. This is relatively rare in chronic arterial occlusive disease when resting blood flows are usually adequate while vascular reserve is abnormally low. Ischemia at rest, however, may then be superimposed by extravascular factors which are preventable or amenable to therapy.[48]

Two rather common examples of such complications are edema and external compression. Either one may be elicited by infections, burns, or mechanical or thermal injury. It may sound paradoxical, but the physician who recognizes the true pathogenesis of such an ulcer located in an ischemic limb can develop a rational treatment plan with little need for concern about the underlying etiology.[48] In the treatment of necrotic lesion in the patients with Buerger's disease, the superimposed extravascular factors on arterial insufficiency should be discerned. An ulcer of primarily ischemic origin is usually located in the digits, and excruciatingly painful.

Controlof edema
Edema in the affected foot is caused mainly by dependency and infection. Culture of any discharge and appropriated testing for sensitivity to antibiotics are indispensable. It reduces tissue perfusion with arterial blood and is frequently seen in patients with ischemic limbs who keep the leg dependent during night and day to relieve rest pain. It is attributable to elimination of edema due to bed rest without dependency of the leg that ischemic ulceration shows a tendency to healing shortly after commencement of the epidural anesthesia.

At the same time, external compression should be prevented by a protecting device which distributes the weight of the foot on the bed over as large a surface as possible to reduce the load on the protruding areas of the affected foot. It is understandable that prohibition of keeping the leg with ischemic ulceration dependent has been instructed to the patients from ancient times, in view of controlling edema. Edema of dependency in the ischemic limb can be adequately controlled by raising the head of the bed by 20 to 25 cm, which may allow the patient to sleep without pain and with minimum edema.

Management of infection
Ulcers may be infected or contaminated, a distinction essential for therapy. They should be treated with systemic antibiotics if cellulitis is present. Local antibiotics are usually not used in patients with Buerger's disease, because of the occasional topical sensitization or irritation of the skin which raises the demand for blood, delays healing, may result in spreading of the infection, or may convert contamination into infection of adjacent tissues or deep structures.[48]

There are several factors that contribute to the unsatisfactory results of use of antibiotics for ischemic necrosis: lack of an adequate blood supply to the necrotic area, and infection with two or more organisms with different sensitivities to antibiotics, including fungal infection.

Sensitized skin does not epithelize well, and the tissues around an ulcer do not contract well if cellulitis is present. The essential ingredients of ulcer healing, granulation, epithelization and contraction can proceed in a contaminated ulcer, but are likely to be interfered with in an infected one.[48]

Medical bath

As attempts to control the infection with antibiotics alone have been disappointing, the local use of an aqueous solution such as iodine solution or an ointment such as collagenase ointment has been reported to be effective for decrease of the inflammation and chemical debridement.[49,50] However, in our clinic tepid saline is used for washing and soaking of the necrotic lesion: a safe upper level is 33°C, and the time for a tepid bath is limited within 5 minutes. The aim of the bath is not to macerate the lesion but to debride tenderly the lesion. It has a favorable impact on the healing of ulcers.

Dry gauze dressings over the ulcerated area are used between foot soaks. The gauze, moistended before removal each time it is changed, acts as a mild mechanical debriding agent. Dry gauze dressings are superior in treating ischemic ulceration than wet dressings. Ulcers between the toes may be treated by separating the toes with thin dry gauze strips.

Debridement

In case where the surface of the ulceration is covered with necrotic tissue or purulent matter, we talk the patient into debriding the wound with the soaked gauze tenderly himself at the time of the saline bath.

If the nonoperative debridement is not effective, surgical debridement is necessary. In that case any mechanical injury to the surrounding ischemic tissue should be avoided with the greatest possible care. When gangrene of the digits shows full demarcation, namely, separation is complete, such gangreneous parts can be removed surgically. Proper timing is of the essence, and viable tissue must not be damaged during this procedure. In patients with gangreneous lesions, a healing with a good scar after complete demarcation is the final end of the treatment. Curettage is effective for development of a granulation rich in vessels, and repeated curettage is frequently needed in many cases.

Patient careful local management is particularly important to promote the spontaneous healing potential of the necrotic lesion even in case of critical ischemia. When ischemic ulceration occurs on the basis of the interdigital fungal infection, oral or local application antifungal products is indicated, but a local adverse effect due to ointment or liquor should be most carefully controlled.

Local surgical debridement is confined to removing the gangrenous tissue. The aim is to remove just the dead tissue to improve drainage and to aid drying and separation.[51] In other words, the aim of debridement is to remove obstacles to the wound healing process, and the procedure be in no hurry. Unless in case of necrotic lesions with no spontaneous healing potential, timely debridement usually brings about a successful outcome. Regardless of local or systemic therapy, strict foot or hand care to reduce skin demand for blood has a favorable impact on the healing of ulcers. This implies daily washing and soaking with lukewarm saline and self-inspection as for the presence of trophic changes.

C. Surgical Treatment

If conservative treatment is not able to prove successful in the improvement of ischemic symptoms or meet the patients' demand, they stand in need of surgical treatment. Surgical treatment mainly consists in regional sympathetic denervation to increase circulation to the skin and procedures designed to restore arterial blood flow.

1. Regional sympathetic denervation

Regional sympathetic denervation produces vasodilatation, prevents vasoconstriction and may be of value in patients with Buerger's disease.

Sympathetic ganglion block with drugs

From old times regional sympathetic block with alcohol had been applied for patients for whom the risk of surgical sympathectomy was deemed excessive or the prognosis for life was foreshortened. Recently phenol injection of the sympathetic chain has widely used instead of alcohol[52]. Fujita and his colleagues[53] considered the disappearance of claudication pain due to destruction of the gray rami as a merit of phenol injection. They found significant increase in muscle blood flow after exercise in the anterior tibial and the gastrocnemius muscles by sympathetic block with phenol.

While we can understand why regional sympathetic denervation is helpful in treating the patients with rest pain or superficial ischemic ulceration, the influence of the sympathetic block with phenol on intermittent claudication seems to require further examination. As intermittent claudication is attributable to shortage of muscle blood flow at movement which is 20-30 times larger than that at rest, does the muscle blood flow increase to such an extraordinary extent by sympathetic denervation?

Sympathectomy

Surgical sympathetic denervation was widely used for the treatment of chronic arterial occlusive disease until the 1960s, because alternative methods of improving limb perfusion were unavailable. With the development of arterial reconstruction techniques, sympathectomy gave the status of optimal surgical therapy in patients with chronic arterial occlusive disease to direct vascularization. However, sympathectomy is now widely used yet for Buerger's disease, because arterial reconstruction is not frequently feasible to the patients of the disease, owing to the peripheral localization of the disease.

In 1926 Osawa[54] reported good results of sympathectomy performed in 8 patients with Buerger's disease: thoracic sympathectomy in one and lumbar sympathectomy in 7 cases. He advised to remove the middle cervical ganglion and ganglion stellatum for sympathetic denervation of the upper extremity and the lumbosacral ganglia within the region from the third lumbar to the third sacral vertebra for sympathetic denervation of the lower extremity. Although Osawa used the anterior route, Stewart[55] recommended the posterior route through the chest for the removal of the inferior cervical and first thoracic ganglia in 1934. As Ito and Asami found no reduction of the muscular tonus after lumbosacral sympathectomy, they set up a question about the doctrine of sympathetic tonic innervation of the skeletal musculature.[56]

On the basis of the postoperative course of 50 patients with Buerger's disease who underwent 136 sympathectomies, de Takats[57] concluded as follows in 1944: Sympathectomy deprived the extremity of its vasoconstrictor tone, and improved circulation in limbs in which blood vessels were occluded but did not influence the course of the disease. The patient who is a candidate for a sympathectomy must demonstrate the presence of an adequate collateral vascular bed and must show that he is in a quiescent stage of the disease, in a state of remission; nor should the disease show too much visceral extension. He told every thing about the value of sympathectomy in the treatment of Buerger's disease.

As preoperative studies he emphasized the importance of the loss of sweating and change in skin temperature after a sympathetic block with drug: the paradox drop of skin temperature of each individual finger or toe meaned that not only would this digit not benefit from sympathectomy, but a rapidly developing gangrene might occur following the operation. He removed sympathetic ganglia at least between the top of the 2nd to the bottom of the 3rd lumbar vertebra through an extraperitoneal anterolateral muscle-splitting incision; the 3rd rib was resected paravertebrally through the dorsal route and the chain was sectioned below the 3rd thoracic ganglion, and the distal end was clipped with a metal clip, the proximal end was implanted into muscle.

In 1951 Toda[58] recommended removal of the 3rd and 4th throacic sympathetic ganalia for denervation of the upper limb; removal of the 2nd and 3rd lumbar for the lower based on sweating examinations after sympathectomy. He, who had succeeded in removal of the occluded segment with vascular transplantation in dogs at that time, expressed the hope that arterial revascularization would relieve the patients from sufferings.

The vasodilatation by lumbar sympathectomy at rest was characterized by a preferred distribution of blood to the skin and to the subcutaneous tissue of the foot and toes.[59] Much of this increased flow was deemed to pass through naturally occuring arteriovenous anastomoses.[60] Limitations in arterial inflow imposed by proximal occlusive lesions may mitigate this increase, and the return of vasomotor tone toward normal with time may further diminish it. Nevertheless, some patients may receive sufficient increase in blood flow to help superficial ischemic ulcers heal or to relieve ischemic rest pain. The nonvascular effects of sympathectomy may also be beneficial in these situation, in changing oxygen demand : supply ratios and in attenuating pain perception.[61]

Sympathectomy is particularly indicated for superficial trophic lesions of the skin or vasospastic symptoms, such as coldness or cold sensitivity. As no significant improvement in muscle circulation occurs after sympathetic denervation,[62,63] it is not indicated for intermittent claudication.[64] Some clinical reports in improvement in walking time among claudicants who underwent sympathectomy may simply reflect the natural history of claudication.

The purpose of sympathetic denervation is to remove vasoconstrictor tone in the peripheral region of the extremity ; it cannot be expected to benefit ischemic limbs with thoroughly dilated vessels lacking in vasospastic reactivity. In critical limb ischemia there is breakdown of the microvascular flow regulating system, namely, vasomotion, with maldistribution of blood flow in the microcirculation, especially the nutritive skin capillaries, and no return of vasomotion in the digital region toward normal is usually recognized after arterial reconstruction : the characteristic skin color change, "rubor," often persisted even after ischemic ulceration had healed.

We usually remove L2,3 and 4 for the lower extremity by extraperitoneal route through pararectal incision and T2,3 and the lower third of the stellate ganglion for upper extremity by transpleural axillary or extrapleural posterior approach sympathectomy : the posterior approach with partial resection of the 2nd and the 3rd rib is advantageous to remove Kuntz's nerve, sympathetic collaterals through the intercostal nerve roots to the stellate ganglion. These are sufficient for maximal effect and avoid loss of ejaculation and Horner's syndrome, respectively.

Sympathectomy was performed in 130 (51%) of the 255 patients with Buerger's disease in the author's series : lumbar in 108 (concomitant with arterial reconstruction in 24) and thoracic in 26 (both lumbar and thoracic in 4). The indications for sympathectomy were gangrene or ulceration in 84 (63%), rest pain in 24 (18%), and coldness or paresthesia in 26 (19%). For the most part of the patients, their ischemic symptoms were improved except a few cases with unchangeable effect. A "borrowing-lending" phenomenon from one extremity to the other seems to be unlikely to occur,[65] but the steal from poorly vascularized to normally vascularized area, "hemometakinesia,"[66] has been reported.[67] It also should not be forgotten that postsympathectomy neuralgia or exsiccation of he skin due to no sweating not rarely bothers the patients for a long time. With distal arterial reconstruction such as femorocrural bypass grafting, concomitant lumbar sympathectomy has been performed with the expectation that there might be an increase in arterial flow through the revascularized segment as the result of reduction in peripheral vascular resistance.[68] Although there have been reports of improved patency rates of small vessel reconstruction by concomitant sympathectomy, controversy continues regarding the significance of sympathectomy as an adjunct to arterial reconstruction.[69,70] However, contraindicated cases for the addition of lumbar sympathectomy were not frequently encountered in our series, though it was difficult to predict the success of sympathectomy.

There is a discord of opinion on the question[59] whether sympathectomy has a beneficial effect on the collateral compensatory circulation of the ischemic limb.[59,64] Postoperative clinical course correlated better with flow velocity in the foot than with distal blood pressure as there was a reduction in toe blood pressure by sympathetic nerve block.[71] While sympathectomy did not change the course of Buerger's disease, the effect of sympathetic denervation on improvement in vasospastic symptoms mostly persisted, as far as complete surgical denervation was carried out.[72]

2. Peripheral nerve division

The history of the war against Buerger's disease may be regarded as the history of a battle against intractable ischemic pain. In 1922 Silbert[73] reported three cases of Buerger's disease in whom the posterior tibial nerve was exposed under local anesthesia and injected with alcohol at the internal malleolus and pain in the foot was relieved. He emphasized that this treatment was palliative and made no claim to cure the disease, but simply eliminated for a time its most distressing symptom.

Smithwick and White,[74] in 1930, were the first to report a technique for alcohol injection of the sensory nerves exposed through the skin incision in the leg in order to render the foot insensitive, in 11 patients with necrotic lesions due to Buerger's disease or arteriosclerosis obliterans. They advocated exposing the nerves low enough in the leg so that the injection did not paralyze the muscles of the leg and sufficiently proximal to the lesion to anticipate a reasonable chance of primary operative wound healing. In 1935 the same authors[75] reported their further experience with peripheral nerve block in 45 cases, and touched the following points. The results were better in the patients with Buerger's disease than in the arteriosclerotic group; patients with pulsation of the popliteal vessels did better than those in which the vessel was obliterated at this level. The nerves might either be injected with alcohol or crushed; the latter method was more simple and equally effective, although the nerves regenerated more rapidly. Besides controlling pain, the circulation to the part might be increased because the anesthetic area was also deprived of its vasoconstrictor nerves.

Laskey and Silbert,[76] in 1933, recommended nerve section with immediate suture in preference to alcohol injection, because it was impossible to be sure that all of the nerve fibers came in contact with the alcohol and alcohol leaking from the nerve into the tissues might cause necrosis. On the basis of the results of 46 patients with necrotic lesions in the lower extremities caused by arteriosclerosis with and without diabetes mellitus and Buerger's disease who were treated by nerve blocking with injection of alcohol and crushing, division, division and sutures, or crushing 2 to 6 mm of the nerve, in 1936, Smith[77] reported that nerve block permitted recovery with fewer major amputations and made it possible to perform minor ones where major ones might primarily had been indicated. In patients with Buerger's disease in his series, he noticed an increase in the local temperature in the anesthetized area to varying degrees, depending upon the degree of arterial occlusion and spasm in the vessel wall. Smith emphasized that peripheral verve block was an anatomic operation which should not be attempted until the operator had familiarized himself with the exact local anatomy : poor wound healing might be attributed to extensive dissection because of lack of anatomic knowledge and failure to appreciate the amount of operative trauma these tissues would tolerate.

In the editorial of the Journal of Cardiovascular Surgery, entitled "Is there a place for peripheral nerve crush ?", Deterling[78] attempted to revive the peripheral nerve division in the treatment of patients with advanced stages of arteriosclerosis obliterans when arterial reconstruction was not feasible, but amputation was not clearly indicated. Alpert et al.[79] performed 12 multisensory peripheral nerve divisions (the sural, superficial and deep peroneal, and posterior tibial nerves) under epidural anesthesia in 10 patients with intractable ischemic foot pain, and they brought forward the two major indications for nerve division, after concluding that revascularization was impossible, as follows : 1) the presence of localized, dry, and contained acral gangrene in patients who were not candidates for a lesser amputation ; and 2) patient or family refusal of a limb amputation.

Unlike the original nerve division 10 cm above the ankle joint, Takao and his colleagues[80] advocated selective blocking technique of these sensory nerves at the level of the ankle joint to achieve a sufficient effect at a minimum area of anesthesia, instead of unnecessarily excessive anesthetic area. Preservation of limb and control of pain become compelling goals in the treatment of patients with Buerger's disease for whom arterial reconstruction is not possible : sympathetic denervation is unlikely to relieve the effects of severe ischemia in these patients. Patients generally prefer anesthesia or hypesthesia to pain, but persistent numbness or paresthesia after nerve division sometimes hurts a patient's feelings. The aim of the sensory nerve division is only to relieve the patient from intractable pain, and not

3. Arterectomy

Leriche, who advocated resection of the obliterated arterial segment on the ground of that an obliterated artery provoked distal vasospasm in the anastomotic network of vessels, reported the follow-up results of 78 arterectomies in peripheral arterial occlusive disease in 1937.[81] Although arterectomy was performed alone or concomitantly with sympathectomy in those days,[82] it is now abandoned.

4. Adrenalectomy

On the basis of hyperplasia of the zona fasciculata with increased lipoid content and atrophy or even disappearance of the zona glomerulosa and of accompanying vasoconstrictive phenomena as a manifestation of hyperadrenalemia in the patients with Buerger's disease, an abnormal activity of the adrenals was considered to cause a widespread peripheral vasoconstriction of the extremities that vascular occlusion would be mad more likely, through disturbances in the interrelated cortical and medullary functions, and adrenalectomy[83] or adrenomedullectomy[84] was regarded to be indicated for the patients with Buerger's disease. On the basis of a follow-up study of 110 patients with the disease who were treated by adrenalectomy and sympathectomy from 1942 to 1962, Kunlin et al[85] concluded that sympathectomy was the most effective vasodilating measure, but the indication of adrenalectomy was doubtful.

While adrenalectomy had been employed mainly in the French-speaking nations,[86] in expectation of controlling the disease progression, the effect of the operation is questionable and adrenalectomy or adrenomadullectomy should not be recommended as the treatment of Buerger's disease.

5. Muscle revascularization by vascular implantation

Direct arterial reconstruction is not often feasible for the patients with Buerger's disease because of the multiple occluded distal arteries. Experiences with many patients without indication for vascular reconstruction encouraged vascular surgeons to pursue a new method of directly providing a significant blood supply to ischemic muscles.

Receiving a hint from the results of myocardial revascularization by implantation of the internal mammary artery into the ventricular myocardium[87] and of vascular connections established by arteries implanted into the lower extremity with plastic sponge as intermediary,[88] we succeeded in revascularization of the hind limb of the dog by vascular implantation into the leg muscle.[89-91]

We implanted the autogenous saphenous vein, leaving 2-3 branches of the implant open, provided with 4-5 mm cauded arteriovenous fistula, into the gastrocnemius muscle of the patients suffering from severe calf caludication for whom no surgical procedure was indicated. Only 5 of 19 implants were patent during 2 months period and no obvious anastomosis between intramuscular vessels and the branches of the implant was recognized in arteriograms. Therefore, this implantation technique has been given up for revascularization of the calf muscles.

6. Omental transplantation

In 1965, from the experimental myocardial revascularization by omental graft without pedicle, Vineberg et al[92] revealed that the detached omental graft formed anastomotic capillary channels with surrounding tissues within 3 days and arteriolar-sized channels within 8 days, and they named the characteristic of the free omental graft "omental trophism." In 1967 Goldsmith[93] showed experimentally that the intact omentum could be lengthened and placed in the leg, resulting in the delivery of an additional source of blood to the extremity.

In 1977 Nishimura and his colleagues[94] reported the excellent results of omental transplantation into the severely ischemic legs because of extensive arterial occlusions distal to the popliteal trifurcation for relief of limb ischemia, by a free omental graft. This technique, which required microsurgical vascular anastomoses, resulted in a high success rate: claudication disappeared in 13 of 16 patients (81%) and rest pain diminished in 15 (94%). Eight of 10 patients in this series had ischemic leg ulcers, which completely healed within 3 months after omental placement into the leg. Objective improvement was further documented using arteriography, radioisotope angiography, thermography, and photoelectric plethysmography. Performance of 133-Xe clearance studies of the anterior tibial muscles demonstrated increased postoperative muscle blood flow during exercise and hyperemia. Angiograms done in 14 patients consistently revealed augmented collateral channels, in spite of finding that the femorogastroepiploic anastomoses had become obstructed in 11 of these patients. This information led the investigators to believe that a functioning anastomosis to a free omental graft was necessary only to maintain its viability for only a relatively short period before neocirculation has been established. They believed that the benefits derived from placing the omentum into an ischemic limb was due to increased muscle blood flow secondary to what they described as "biological bypass revascularization through arteriolar nets on the omentum implanted over the diseased segment."

Goldsmith,[95] who performed brain vascularization by intact omentun in dogs in

1973, carried out revascularization of an ischemic upper extremity of 61-year-old man with occlusion of the right subclavian artery through implantation of the omentum.[96] The omental trophism or biological bypass revascularization is regarded as a fact, but it is a question whether the increased blood flow through the omental graft is enough for relief of severe ischemia.

On the other hand, the angiogram of the omentum showed blood flowing into the leg, but the question arose as to whether the blood went into the deep tissues of the leg or simply returned through the omental veins. On the basis of the experiment that marked radioactivity was detected in less than one minute in the iliac vein blood sample from the leg with omental implantation in dogs, though the contralateral iliac vein blood sample showed a delayed and much reduced level of isotopic activity, Goldsmith[93] suggested that the blood through the omentum crossed into the vascular channels of the leg, producing the intense and early spike of activity noted.

7. Arterial reconstruction

Although it is ideal to restore the circulation with direct arterial reconstruction, wonderful technique is not frequently applicable to the patients with Buerger's disease, because of widespread arterial occlusions at multiple levels with prevalence in the distal extremities. With development of surgical techniques in the reconstruction of small vessels, compared with what the arterial reconstruction was, it has been more frequently performed in the patients with Buerger's disease.

Thromboendarterectomy (TEA)

As thromboendarterectomy is indicated for a localized occlusive lesion of the artery, the procedure is very rarely feasible to the patients with Buerger's disease. Only some cases of suprapopliteal involvement may permit this technique.

In case of aortofemoral bypass grafting, endarterectomy of the proximal segment of the deep femoral artery, in a sense of profundaplasty, is applicable (endarterectomy of the exit flow vessel). In case of occlusion of the superficial femoral artery, endarterectomy of the deep femoral artery improves an inflow into the thigh (endarterectomy of the inflow vessel). With exception of the cases above described, however, there is no indication for thromboendarterectomy in the arm and leg arteries as a rule.

The cause of early failure after thromboendarterectomy seems to be related to the presence of a remnant of the inflammatory lesion in the revascularized segment.[97] Whether the skip lesion, a localized occlusive lesion, could be successfully repaired by thromboendarterectomy remains an unsolved problem. Unlike arteriosclerotic occlusive lesions, it is not easy to find a leavage plane in the media appropriated for thromboendarterectomy in the skip lesion in Buerger's disease. Unless a cleavage plane without the remnant of thromboangiitis is detected in the media, long-term patency of the revascularized segment is unpromising, because of the thrombogenic potential of the rough interior of the residual wall.

As a matter of course, closure of the arteriotomy should be done with a patch graft. Thromboendarterectomy deals not only with the obstruction of the lumen but also with the pathology of the arterial wall. Knowledge of the mural lesions of Buerger's disease and of the location of the leavage planes is essential for the correct performance of thromboendarterectomy.

The external iliac artery is sometimes occluded throughout its entire length in Buerger's disease, but eversion endarterectomy[98] consisting of removing the blocked arterial tree from the body, developing a plane between the adventitia and the central core, and then pulling the adventitia down over the core, seems to have a poor chance of success.

Bypass grafting

Bypass grafting is most frequently employed as a procedure of arterial reconstruction in Buerger's disease. Operative procedures vary according to the sites of arterial occlusions. The key to success in bypass grafting lies in selecting sites of anastomoses that provide the best available arterial inflow and exit vessels that are adequate.

Aortoiliac occlusion

In advanced cases with arterial occlusion in the aortoiliac region, such synthetic graftings as aortofemoral bypass are employed, if there is a runoff vessel suitable to the distal anastomosis in the femoral region. As the external iliac artery is completely occluded throughout its entire length in case of involvement of the iliac arteries with the disease, common ilio-or aortofemoral bypass grafting is usually indicated. Because the superficial femoral artery is much more frequently involved with the occlusive lesion than the deep femoral artery, the operative indication for bypass procedure mainly depends on runoff capacity in the deep femoral artery, and endarterectomy of the proximal segment of the deep femoral artery contributes to marked improvement in the lumen of the exit vessel.[99]

In case of juxtarenal aortic occlusion due to secondary thrombosis on the basis of occlusion of the bilateral iliac arteries, thrombectomy of the infrarenal aortic segment and aortibifemoral bypass grafting is the treatment of choice.[100] As the natural course is frequently eventful and lethal, the juxtarenal aortic occlusion should be surgically reconstructed as soon as possible. The patients with involvement of the aortoiliac region in addition to occlusion of leg arteries in Buerger's disease generally suffer from severe ischemia of the lower extremities, and arterial reconstruction of the inflow vessels to the leg arteries is the first consideration, because it provides the most effective healing of ischemic lesions.[101] However, it is far from reassuring to maintain long-term patency of the revascularized segment, because of poor runoff vessels due to the multiple occluded distal arteries. If the revascularized segment fails after ischemic ulceration had healed, no trophic lesions usually recurred unless the patient resumed smoking, but we should not be optimistic about the future proximal progression of thrombosis in case of the juxtarenal aortic occlusion.

Aortoiliac arterial reconstruction is regarded as an uncommon procedure for the patients even at the advanced stage of Buerger's disease on the whole.

Femoropopliteocrural occlusion

In Buerger's disease, at least one or two infrapopliteal arteries are always occluded and suprapopliteal segment is not infrequently involved through skip or continuous progression. When the popliteal artery remains continuously patent with a crural artery, femoropoliteal bypass is indicated. To an isolated popliteal artery segment, single femoropopliteal[102] or sequential bypass grafting[103] is applicable. In case of complete occlusion of the popliteal artery, femorocrural bypass should be considered (Fig. X-1, 2, and 3). As the peroneal artery most frequently escapes from occlusive lesions among the infrapopliteal arteries and fairly furnishes the foot and toes with blood,[104] peroneal artery revascularization is certainly possible and capable of providing limb salvage.[105]

While synthetic grafts are employable for above and below knee femoropopliteal bypass grafting[106], autogenous vein is the graft of choice for infrapopliteal bypass[107](Fig. X-4). The greater saphenous vein is most suitable for the graft across the knee joint, but it is frequently occluded or of inadequate diameter due to inflammatory changes; the lesser saphenous,[108] the cephalic, or the basilic vein[109] should be used in such circumstances, if at all possible, because autogenous vein is superior to prosthetic grafts for bypasses crossing a joint and will remain patent in spite of poor runoff. It is not easy to evaluate the quality of the vein before operation. Venography[110] is most reliable to preoperative evaluation of saphenous vein suitability in spite of its invasiveness and thrombotic complication. Macroscopic inspection of the vein through the skin frequently misestimates the extensibility of the vessel wall. An inadequate vein graft inevitably causes early failure of the reconstruction.

In case of below knee femoropopliteal or femorocrural bypass, in situ[111] or nonreversed translocated[112] vein graft is said to be superior than reversed vein graft, in view of the hemodynamic advantages of having the larger diameter of the vein proximal and the tapered end distal and the preservation of viability of the graft.[113] However, careful handling and meticulous technique appear to be more

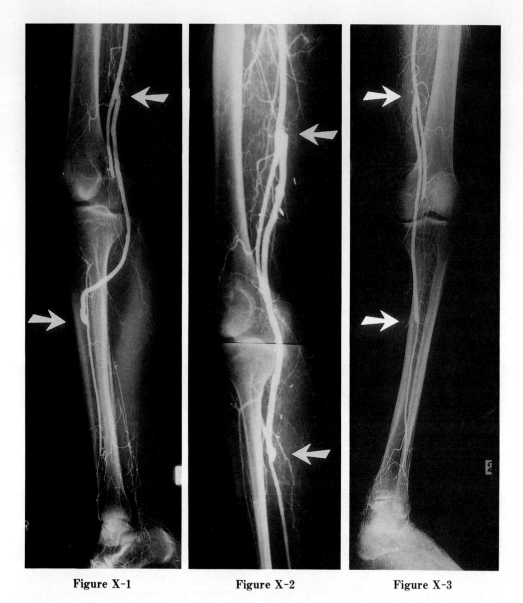

Figure X-1. Right femoral arteriogram of a 37-year-old man with Buerger's disease after femoro-anterior tibial bypass grafting with reversed saphenous vein (arrows).

Figure X-2. Right femoral arteriogram of a 33-year-old man with Buerger's disease after femoro-posterior tibial bypass grafting with in situ saphenous vein (arrows).

Figure X-3. Left femoral arteriogram of a 47-year-old man with Buerger's disease after femoro-peroneal bypass grafting with reversed saphenous vein (arrows).

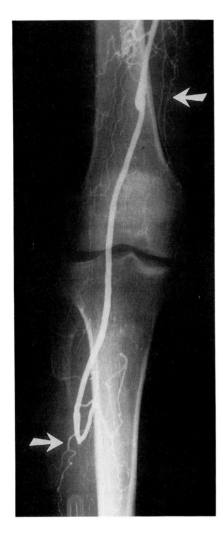

Figure X-4. Right femoral arteriogram of the same patient as in Figure VII-19 five years after femoroperoneal bypass grafting with reversed saphenous vein. The graft remains patent even though the peroneal artery has become occluded for the most part (arrows). (From Shionoya S. In: Rutherford RB ed. Vascular Surgery 3rd ed. W. B. Saunders, 1989, pp 207-17.)

important than the theoretic advantages of preserving the vasa vasorum,[112] and it is not easy to put one thing above the other.

Together with the quality of the vein, the capacity of the runoff vessels is one of the most important factors of early graft failure. While a good visualization of the pedal arch continuously with the infrapopliteal artery is considered to indicate a good condition of the runoff vessel,[114] there is a limited ability to predict physiologic function from anatomic findings.

It is understood that no scheme for grading runoff is perfect, likely to be universally accepted, or will always correlate with early or late graft failure. Nevertheless, a grading scheme that provides some degree of correlation with outcome is desirable and in 1986 an Ad Hoc Committee appointed by the Society for Vascular Surgery and the North American Chapter of the International Society for

Cardiovascular Surgery (Chiarman: R.B.Rutherford)[115] proposed a grading scheme, which might be applied to all levels of distal anastomosis rather than just to femoropopliteal bypass: it grades both the degree of occlusion and the relative contribution to outflow of each vessel from 0 to 3 and combines the two in a decimal system that assigns 1 to a widely patent runoff and 10 to an isolated, blind segment. In this scheme, higher values correspond to higher resistances so that resistances in series and in parallel can be consistently graded.

In 1989 Karacagil et al.[116] evaluated the runoff with a new grading system, based on findings at intraoperative postreconstruction serial angiography. This concept, which takes foot vessel involvement into account in patients with only one patent crural artery, is a modification of the traditional method of runoff assessment. Good runoff was defined as patency of two or three lower leg arteries to the foot or one patent vessel continuous with intact anterior or posterior foot arch. In limbs with no patent vessel or one patent vessel with deficient or occluded foot arches, the runoff was classified as poor. The cumulative primary patency rates at 12 months in groups with good and poor runoff were 81% and 37%, respectively. They concluded that the predictive value of the new method was superior to the standards proposed by the Ad Hoc Committee in USA. This improved prediction can be ascribed to the optimal angiographic technique and selective evaluation of foot runoff.

When the angiographically visualized segment of a crural artery was longer than 12 cm, irrespective of continuous flow with the pedal arches, we performed femorocrural bypass grafting with autogenous vein. In case where the superficial femoral artery appeared intact in arteriograms, the proximal end of the graft was anastomosed with the superficial femoral artery to shorten the length of a graft.[117]

Although intraoperative angiography is the best method for complete visualizing the distal arterial tree, an noninvasive, preoperative evaluation of the runoff is desirable. Preoperative measurement of distal blood pressure and blood flow were not predictive of early graft failure.[118] In an effort to determine whether or not resistance offered by the arteries of the foot (below the ankle) influenced the results of arterial reconstruction, a "distal runoff resistance index" was calculated by dividing the difference in blood pressure between the ankle and the toe by the brachial systolic pressure (A-T gradient). No correlation between the preoperative A-T gradient and graft patency could be demonstrated. Postoperative A-T gradient also did not provide predictive data on late failure of grafts. Although the increase in toe pressure was significantly smaller than that in ankle pressure after the arterial reconstruction, the postoperative toe pressure was of value in predicting healing of ischemic ulcerations: an increase in toe pressure index (TPI) more than 0.1 correlated with healing of the lesion.[119]

Occlusion of arteries of the foot
In case of relatively localized arterial occlusions around the ankle, an autogenous vein bypass grafting from the crural artery to the dorsalis pedis or the plantar artery is rarely feasible.[120,121]

Occlusion of the forearm arteries
For severe ischemia of the upper limb due to extensive occlusions of the arm arteries, autogenous vein bypass grafting is rarely indicated[122](Fig. X-5). In view of active movement of the upper limb, in situ bypass with the cephalic or the basilic vein is superior than bypass grafting with the reversed vein (Fig. X-6 and 7). However, because of inevitably frequent extension and flexion of the elbow joint, it is not easy to maintain a long-term patency of the graft.

Our results of bypass grafting
Bypass graftings were performed in 44 (17%) of 255 patients with Buerger's disease in the author's series : aorto-or iliofemoral bypass in 10, femorofemoral in 2, femoropopliteal above knee in 2, femoropopliteal below knee in 6, femorocrural in 21, popliteocruroal in 4, tibiotibial in 2, axilloradial in 1, brachioradial in 1 and brachioulnar in 2 (seven patients underwent two separate operations). Concomitant lumbar sympathectomy was performed in 24 ; sympathetic denervation had already been carried out in the remaining 18 patients at the author's or at other institutions. The indications for arterial reconstruction were gangrene or ulceration in 28 limbs (55%), rest pain in 10 (20%), claudication in 11 (21%), and graft infection in 2 (4%).

Follow-up ranged from 1 to 12 years : cumulative life-table patency of 12 suprainguinal grafts was 90% at 1 year, 70% at 2 years and 70% at 10 years ; that of 34 infrainguinal grafts was 56%, 48% and 32%, respectively (Fig. X-8). Cumulative life-table patency of 10 femoropopliteal bypass grafts was 70% at 1 year, 60% at 2 years and 60% at 7 years ; that of 24 femorocrural bypass was 50%, 44% and 44%, respectively, and 29% at 10 years (Fig. X-9). Only one of four bypass grafts in the upper limb remained patent at two years.

Although long-term results of arterial reconstruction in the aortoiliac region are almost satisfactory at the presnet, infrainguinal grafting of medium-and small-caliber arteries continues to pose significant problems, not only in Buerger's disease but also in arteriosclerosis obliterans.[123] Early failures (less than 30 days) are due to errors of surgical technique or judgment and ideally should be detected and corrected during operation whereas late failures (more then 2 years), caused by progression of the underlying disease process, may be dealt with attention to risk factors.[124] In contrast, the intermediate failure rate (less than 2 years) is considerably higher. Judging from our follow-up results that 2-year patency rate was almost the same as 10-year patency rate, it is a great problem to mediate a way out of the intermediate pass for the grafts surviving the perioperative period.

Neointimal fibrous hyperplasia (NFH) has been described as the most important

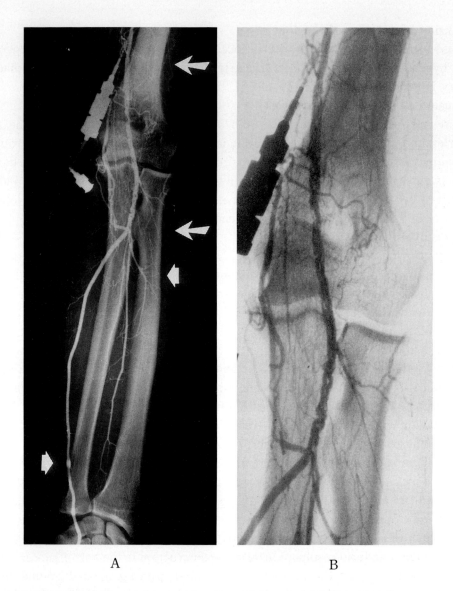

Figure X-5. Left brachial arteriogram of a 46-year-old man with Buerger's disease. A: The radial artery is occluded at its proximal portion (arrow) and the ulnar artery is narrowed above the wrist (arrow); the brachial artery is recanalized after occlusion (arrows). B: Enlargement of the occluded brachial artery.

cause of the intermediate graft failure.[125] NFH develops at the site of endothelial injury where platelets adhere to exposed subendothelial collagen, aggregate and release substances which induce migration and proliferation of fibroblasts and myofibroblasts. This trauma may be directly related to the surgical manipulation during operation or caused by turbulent flow or mechanical mismatch between the

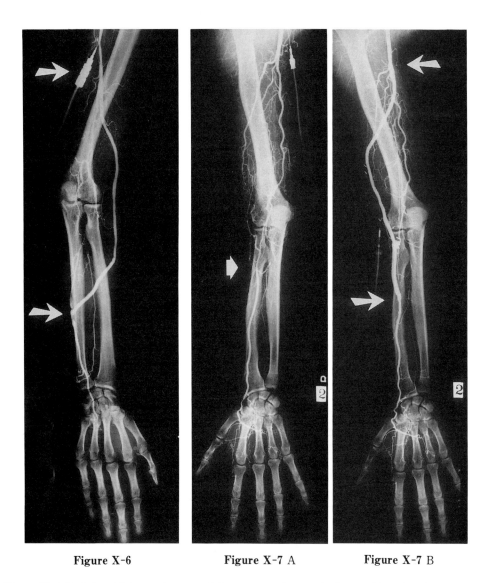

Figure X-6   **Figure X-7 A**   **Figure X-7 B**

Figure X-6. Left brachial arteriogram of the same patient as in Figure X-5 after brachio-ulnar bypass grafting with in situ cephalic vein (arrows).

Figure X-7. Right brachial arteriogram of a 46-year-old man with Buerger's disease. A : The brachial artery and the ulnar artery are occluded, and the radial artery is visualized through collaterals (arrow). B : After brachio-radial bypass grafting with in situ cephalic vein (arrows).

graft and host vessel.[126] While the role of platelet reactivity in this form of intimal hyperplasia seems important, less well established is the direct relation between platelets and NFH, and it remains unsolved whether antiplatelet treatment is effective in preventing these late proliferative changes in vascular grafts and

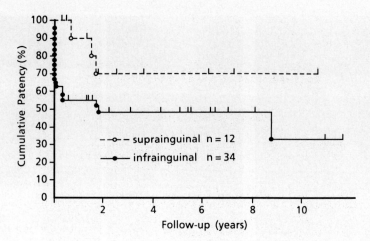

Figure X-8. Comparison of patency curves of suprainguinal and infrainguinal bypass grafts determined by life table method in our series.

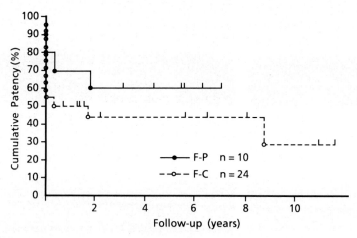

Figure X-9. Comparison of patency curves of femoropoliteal (F-P) and femorocrural (F-C) bypass grafts determined by life table method in our series.

revascularized segments.

As NFH was favored in the autogenous vein graft implanted under poor distal vasculature (runoff),[127] the patients with critical ischemia, namely, with impaired compensatory function of the collateral circulation are placed at a disadvantage. As a three-year multicenter prospective study of effect of ticlopidine, an antiplatelet drug, on arterial reconstruction performance in the lower extremity of the patients with stage III and IV(Fontaine) indicated more superior results in the treated group than in the control group, antiplatelet therapy might be helpful to overcome their handicap.[128]

Patency of vascular grafts is determined by several factors, including the skill of the vascular surgeon, the type and characteristics of the graft material used, persistence of the responsiveness of the transplanted vein grafts to vasoactive substances,[129] and a number of host-related factors such as hemodynamics, graft-host biocompatibility, and thrombogenic potentials of the host. Although many of host-related factors are still poorly understood and difficult or impossible to control, there is ample evidence now that some graft-related factors, especially surface thrombogenicity, can be effectively influenced by certain medications, at least in the early perioperative period.[126]

After femorocrural bypass grafting we usually administer 1,000 units of urokinase/kg/day intravenously, 10,000 units/day of heparin intravenously or subcutaneously (heparin-calcium)[130] and 5-10 ng/kg/min of PGE_1[131] intravenously over 2 hours once or twice daily for about one week. Within one week after operation, urokinase and heparin are changed to 3-5 mg/day of warfarin, with the thrombotest value maintained between 15 and 25%, and antiplatelet drug. The oral antithrombotic therapy will be continued for 2 years. Because of poor runoff, inadequate grafts and progression of the disease, long-term results of arterial reconstruction of the lower extremity in Buerger's disease have been not satisfactory yet.[132,133] While controversy continues regarding the efficacy of antithrombotic treatment on graft survival, it should be remembered that postoperative anticoagulant and antiplatelet therapy will not salvage a poor vascular reconstruction.

As arterial reconstructive procedure does not constitute direct, specific therapy for underlying Buerger's disease, good initial results will give way to recurrence unless the patient abstains from smoking. It is interesting that Lie[134] found an inflammatory occlusive thrombus characteristic of Buerger's disease in the saphenous vein graft in a patient who continued to smoke.

Special measures of arterial reconstruction

Conventional arterial reconstructive procedure is not frequently feasible to patients with Buerger's disease because of the difficulties in harvesting good antogenous vein grafts and the multiple occluded distal arteries, which encouraged vascular surgeons to pursue a method to get over a barrier.

Composite grafting
In order to take a measure to meet the situation of lack of an suitable autogenous vein, composite Teflon or Dacron and vein grafting was devised.[135,136] Yasuda et al.[133] carried out femorotibial composite velour Dacron or Goretex and saphenous vein bypass grafting in four patients with Buerger's disease without adequate vein sufficient for the long bypass: prosthesis in above-knee segment; vein in below-

knee. Patency at one month was 75%, but the remaining two grafts were occluded until 5 months after operation. The high incidence of failure leads to pessimism regarding usefulness of the composite graft for future patients.

A-V shunt procedure

Kusaba[137] contrived a technique for patients with extensive arterial occlusion from the femoral artery to crural arteries. The obstructed superficial femoral artery was reconstructed with an E-PTFE bypass graft and the popliteal artery was recanalized with open endarterectomy and an autovein roof patch graft. During the procedure, thrombi in the orifices of the popliteal branches, such as the descending genicular, the superior genicular, the inferior genicular and the anterior tibial artery were removed as much as possible. Finally, an arteriovenous fistula was created between the end of the recanalized tibioperoneal trunk and the posterior tibial or the peroneal vein, in an end-to-side fashion. Sixty-three extremities have been treated with this technique and remarkable improvement in healing of ischemic ulceration resulted in 72.6% immediately and 57.1% in the follow-up after the surgery.

Crural artery bypass with adjunctive A-V fistula

In 1980s Dardik and his colleagues[138,139] devised distal arteriovenous fistula as an adjunct to maintaing arterial and graft patency for limb salvage. This procedure was indicated for patients with a poor distal outflow.

A longitudinal incision was made on the adjacent wall of the tibial or peroneal artery and the accompanying vein, and the adjacent posterior wall of the incised vessels was sutured to create a common posterior wall. The autogenous vein graft was then anasomosed to the artery and the vein in an end-to-side fashion. Inflowing blood flowed not only into the distal runoff-artery but also into the vein proximal to the fistula, because the vein was ligated just below the fistula. By diversion of the overload on the high-resistance distal vascular bed and augmentation of the inflow, the distal A-V fistula was thought to be effective in maintaining graft and arterial blood flow to a limb that would otherwise require amoutation, without "stealing" of blood from the foot, because the gradient between the proximal inflow site and the distal runoff was so high that reversal of flow at the foot level did not seem likely, no less possible.

They concluded that A-V fistula construction should be limited to the distal third of the leg and it should be abandoned if distal arterial flow was not present to even a minimal degree, because the immediate survival of the limb depended not on retrograde venous flow, i.e., arterialization of the vein, but on the arterial runoff. Kusaba[137] applied the technique to revascularization of severely ischemic limbs, and they considered the procedure as of benefit to some patients with the disease suffering from critical ischemia, though the long term patency rate was not good. Attempts to treat severe ischemia of the lower extremities have been repeatedly tried over a long term of years, and the role of distal arteriovenous fistula as an adjunct to maintaining graft patency and improving foot ischemia remains to be resolved.[140,141]

8. Amputation

Ablation of a limb is the antithesis of all that the vascular surgeon hopes to achieve for his patient, yet it must be done to end the patient's suffering, when an extremity is hopelessly damaged by ischemia. An appropriate rehabilitation with a fit prosthesis may be helpful for the patient to improve the quality of his life.

Judging from the result that necrotic lesions occurred in about 70% of all the patients with the disease in the follow-up period in our series, it is inevitable to snip off the finger or toe through its dead portion at a certain measure of rate, at the utmost a transmetatarsal amputation. Therefore, toe amputation used to be most frequently performed peripheral amputation in patients with Buerger's disease. The circular incision is usually carried out to the bony phalanx, which is divided far enough proximally to permit transverse skin closure without tension. If the blood supply to the amputation stump is considered sufficient, it is seldom necessary to secure haemostasis and only closure required is one or two interrupted sutures. If the primary healing of the stump is questionable, the wound should be left unsutured. If the amputation is to be left open or drained, a simple gauze wick is the drain material preferred. The unsutures or partially open wound will be gradually healed with tender care.

Based on the fact that the ischemic lesions caused by two or three-vessel-occlusions in the lower leg necessitated very seldom a major amputation, Vollmar[142] advocated I-R-A principle in these cases: I-infection-control; R-revascularization (sympathectomy or arterial reconstruction if possible); A-amputation. The latter should be done as the last step of treatment after a period of days or weeks. From a technical point of view he preferred the so-called "borderline-amputation," that meaned removal of the necrotic part of toes or fore-foot without sacrificing healthy tissue. The main advantage of this technique lied in the prevention of infection spreading to a higher amputation level and in the preserving so much as possible of well-nourished tissue of the limb: he has given up completely the exarticulation of a partial necrotic toe in the next proximal joint. After a "borderline-amputation" the spread of infection at a higher level was a very seldom event. He concluded that this form of minor amputation was specially useful in young patients with Buerger's disease and very distal arterial occlusions.

Amputation level determination

Selection of an appropriate level for amputation is of critical importance. Despite the increased risk of failure of healing of a below-knee ampitation compared to that of an above-knee for advanced ischemia, preservation of the knee joint markedly improves the chances of rehabilitation and the quality of life of the amputee, especially in Japanese who sit on one's legs.

Determining the level of amuptation for severe ischemia remains a challenging problem through many years, and must have the cooperation of a surgeon of long experience for its success at the present time. Although several techniques such as segmental blood pressure measurement,[143] skin blood flow measurement with Xe-133 clearance,[144] skin perfusion pressure measurement with ^{131}I-or ^{125}I-antipyrine mixed with histamine,[145] transcutaneous O_2 recording[146] and fluorometric quantification of low-dose fluorescein delivery[147] are now available for this determination: a below-knee amputation was considered to be attempted in limbs with local skin perfusion pressure greater than 20 mmHg,[145] flow values of above 2.4 ml/100 g tissue/min,[144] below-knee blood pressure greater than 70 mmHg,[143] transcutaneous oxygen tension of above 20 mmHg,[146] or dye fluorescence index greater than 42,[147] respectively.

However, because of a transitional zone of decision, wavering in one's judgment, no noninvasive diagnostic method might surely predict the most distal amputation that would heal primarily. Although many factors including the skill of a surgeon influence amputation site healing, adequate cutaneous perfusion at the level of amputation may remain an absolute requirement.

Based on the recent changes in criteria for selecting the level of amputation of the leg that excision of devascularized muscle (even the entire musculature) from a below-knee amputation stump was compatible with normal function of a below-knee prosthesis, a below-knee amputation was considered to be worth doing if the skin appeared viable, though the muscle was ischemic or necrotic.[148] In surgeon's eagerness to wish for a primary healing of the amputation site, the patient should not be deprived of the best opportunity for subsequent ambulation and rehabilitation, because above-knee amputations were related to morbid implications and generalized debility.[149]

In the 255 patients in our series, below-knee amputation was performed in 6 cases and above-knee amputation in 1 at our hospital, for a 2.7 per cent major amputation rate. Six of these seven patients continued to smoke until a decisive moment for their limbs in spite of our advice to abstain from smoking. As long as the patient strictly abstained from tobacco use, the long-term outlook for limb salvage was favorable. Although digital gangrene or ulceration occurred in the majority of patients with Buerger's disease and excising the dry gangrene at a line of demarcation or amputation of a finger or toe was frequently required, no major amputation was inevitable if the disease was detected early enough and was appropriately managed.

9. Selection of patients for treatment

A   Acute stage
    Bridging treatment.
B   Chronic stage
    I   Upper extremities
        Raynaud's phenomenon, coldness and paresthesia:
            Protection from exposure to cold.
        Arm claudication:
            Physical exercise.
        Rest pain:
            Drug treatment.
        Gangrene or ulceration:
            Pharmacotherapy and local treatment. In case of poor spontaneous healing potential, thoracic sympathectomy or arterial reconstruction is indicated.
    II Lower extremities
        Coldness and paresthesia:
        Protection from exposure to cold.
        Intermittent claudication:
            Walking training and physical exercise.
        Rest pain:
            Drug treatment.
            In case of poor response to pharmacotherapy, lumbar sympathectomy or arterial reconstruction is indicated.
        Gangrene or ulceration:
            Pharmacotherapy and local treatment. In case of poor spontaneous healing potential, arterial reconstruction and/or lumbar sympathectomy is indicated.

Conservative treatment may be preferable to surgical treatment at first as a rule. If pharmacological measures are ineffective, surgical procedures should be taken into consideration. Buerger's disease can be controlled, pain relieved, and gangrene arrested by means of strict prohibition of smoking. Contrary to a general concept, major limb amputation is preventable and contraindicated in patients with Buerger's disease, because of good spontaneous healing potential of their necrotic lesions.

REFERENCES

1. Buerger L.(I-45).
2. Buerger L.(I-49).
3. Thomas M. Smoking and vascular surgery. Br J Surg 1981; 68: 601-4.
4. Greenhalgh RM, Laing SP, Cole PV, Taylor GW. Smoking and arterial reconstruction. Br J Surg 1981; 68: 605-7.
5. Littauer D, Wright IS.(VI-35).
6. Ball GV, Wright IS. Thromboangiitis obliterans: simultaneous quadrilateral acute ulcerations in thromboangiitis obliterans. Follow-up studies of a case after 27 years. Am Heart J 1966; 71: 260-4.
7. Lusby RL, Bauminger B, Woodcock JP, Skidmore R, Baird RN. Cigarette smoking: acute main and small vessel hemodynamic response in patients with arterial disease. Am J Surg 1981; 142: 169-73.
8. Corelli F. Buerger's disease: cigarette smoker disease may always be cured by medical therapy alone. Uselessness of operative treatment. J cardiovasc Surg 1973; 14: 28-36.
9. Campbell KN, Harris BM, Coller FA. A follow-up study of patients with thromboangiitis obliterans (Buerger's disease). Surgery 1949; 26: 1003-13.
10. de Takats G. Diagnosis and management of Buerger's disease. Postgraduate Med 1948; 3: 185-91.
12. Bollinger A, Lüthy E. Kompensationsgrad arterieller Verschlüsse und Wirkung intravenös verabreichter vasoaktiver Medikamente. Schweiz med Wschr 1967; 97: 1220-7.
14. Kamiya K, Onogi H, Yamashita F, Kidokoro H, Takeuchi T, Asai S. Vasodilating drugs and peripheral vascular diseases. Rinshogeka 1969; 24: 1535-9 (in Japanese).
11. Gillespie JA. An evaluation of vasodilator drugs in occlusive vascular disease by measurement. Angiology 1966; 17: 280-8.
13. Diaz FV, Casar FP, Alonso JL, Esteban L, Martin E, Salazar JS. Is a new physiopathologic interpretation of obstructive diseases of the arteries possible?: two cases of thromboangiitis obliterans treated with polarizing solution and coronary vasodilators. Angiology 1968; 19: 633-51.
15. Heidrich H. Konservative Therapie peripherer aretrieller Verschluß-krankehiten: Möglichkeiten, Prinzipien und Grundlagen. Münch med Wschr 1978; 120: 23-30.
16. Buerger L.(I-48).
17. Ratschow M. Kritisches zu Ätiologie und Grundlagen einer konservativen Therapie peripherer Durchblutungsstörungen. Langenbech's Arch klin Chir 1959; 292: 188-97.
18. Schoop W. Praktische Angiologie. Stuttgart, Georg Thieme 3rd ed, 1975, pp 154-7.
19. Carter SA, Hamel ER, Paterson JM, Snow CJ, Mymin D. Walking ability and ankle systolic pressures: observations in patients with intermittent claudication in a short-term walking exercise program. J Vasc Surg 1989; 10: 642-9.
20. Carlson LA, Eriksson I. Femoral-artery infusion of prostaglandin E_1 in severe peripheral vascular disease. Lancet; 973; 1: 155-6.
21. Shionoya S, Ban I, Nakata Y, Matsubara J, Shinjo K, Hiari M, Miyazaki H, Kawai S. Continuous intraarterial infusion of prostaglandin for peripheral arterial occlusive disease.

Gekachiryo 1976 ; 34 ; 213-8 (in Japanese).
22. Sakaguchi S, Kusaba A, Mishima Y, Kamiya K, Nishimura A, Furukawa K, Shionoya S, Kawashima M, Katsumura T, Sakuma A. A multi-clinical double blind study with PGE_1 (α-cyclodextrin clathrate)in patients with ischemic ulcer of the extremities. VASA 1978 ; 7 : 263-66.
23. Hammond GL, Cronau LH, Whittaker D, Gillis CN. Fate of prostgalndins E_1 and A_1 in the human pulmonary circulation. Surgery 1977 ; 81 : 716-22.
24. Shionoya S. Clinical experience with prostglandin E_1 in occlusive arterial disease. Inter Angio 1984 ; 3 : 99-103.
25. Nielsen PE, Holstein P, Lielsen SL. Prostglandin E_1 for impending gangrene. Lancet 1977 ; 1 : 192-3.
26. Pardy BJ, Lewis JD, Eastcott HHG. Preliminary experience with prostaglandins E_1 and I_2 in peripheral vascular disease. Surgery 1980 ; 88 : 826-32.
27. Ueda K, Saito A, Nakano H, Aoshima M, Yokota M, Muraoka R, Iwaya T. Cortical hyperostosis following long-term administration of prostagalndin E_1 in infants with cyanotic congenital heart disease. J Pediatr 1980 ; 97 : 834-6.
28. Carlson LA, Olsson AG. Intravenous prostaglandin E_1 in severe peripheral vascular disease. Lancet 1976 ; 2 : 810.
29. Hirai M, Nanki M, Nakayama R. Hemodynamic effects of intravenous PGE_1 on patients with arterial occlusive disease of the leg. Angiology 1985 ; 36 : 407-13.
30. Rhodes RS, Heard SE. Detrimental effect of high-dose prostaglandin E_1 in the treatment of ischemic ulcers. Surgery 1983 ; 93 : 839-42.
31. Schuler JJ, Flanigan DP, Holcroft JW, Ursprung JJ, Mohrland JS, Pyke J. Efficacy of prostaglandin E_1 in the treatment of lower extremity ischemic ulcers secondary to peripheral vascular disease. J Vasc Surg 1984 ; 1 : 160-70.
32. Nielsen PE, Nielsen SL, Holstein P, Poulsen HL, Hansen EH, Lassen NA. Intra-arterial infusion of prostaglandin E_1 in normal subjects and patients with peripheral arterial disease. Scand J clin Lab Invest 1976 ; 36 : 633-40.
33. Yamaguchi H, Furukawa K, Takahashi M. Effects of prostaglandin E_1 on red cell deformability in chronic arterial occlusive disease. Gendaiiryo 1985 ; 17 : 447-50 (in Japanese).
34. Szczeklik A, Nizankowski R, Skawinski S, Szczeklik J, Gluszko P. Gryglewski RJ. Successful therapy of advanced arteriosclerosis obliterans with prostacyclin. Lancet 1979 ; 1 : 1111-4.
35. Weichert W, Pauliks V, Breddin HK. Laser-induced thrombi in rat mesenteric vessels and antithrombotic drugs. Haemostasis 1983 ; 13 : 61-71.
36. Katsumura T, Mishima Y, Kamiya K, Sakaguchi S, Tanabe T, Sakuma A. Therapeutic effect of Ticlopidine, a new inhibitor of platelet aggregation, on chronic arterial occlusive diseases, a double-blind study versus placebo. Angiology 1982 ; 33 : 357-67.
37. Ban I, Shionoya S. Clinical application of Ticlopidine for patients with peripheral arterial insufficiency. Kekkan 1982 ; 5 : 19-27 (in Japanese).
38. Thomas DJ, Du Boulay GH, Marshall J, Pearson TC, Ross Russell RW, Symon L, Wetherley-Mein G. Effect of haematocrit on cerebral blood flow in man. Lancet 1977 ; 2 : 941-3.
39. Nicolaides AN, Bowers R, Horbourne T, Kidner PH. Blood viscosity, red-cell flexibility, haematocrit, and plasma-fbringen in patients with angina. Lancet 1977 ; 2 : 943-5.
40. Rieger H, Köhler M, Schoop W, Schmid-Schönbein H, Roth FJ, Leyhe A. Hemodilution (HD)

in patients with ischemic skin ulcers. Klin Wschr 1979 ; 57 : 1153-61.
41. Koga G. Zur Therapie der Spontangangrän an den Extremitäten. Dtsch Z Chir 1913 ; 121 : 371-82.
42. Ehrly AM. Arwin : Ein neuer Weg zur Behandlung der chronischen arteriellen Verschluß-krankheit. Folia Angiol 1975 ; 23 : 368-72.
43. Angelkort B, Doppelfeld E. Zur Beahndlung der chronischen arteriellen Verschlußkrankheit. Med Klin 1978 ; 73 : 791-7.
44. Krähenbühl B, Holstein P, Neilsen SL, Tonnesen KH, Lassen NA. Induced hypertension as a therapy in Buerger's disease (thromboangiitis obliterans). VASA 1973 ; 2 : 112-6.
45. Eastcott HHG.(II-4), pp 107-8.
46. Kidokoro H. Clinical studies on hyperbaric oxygen therapy for peripheral vascular diseases. Jap J Surg Soc 1968 ; 69 : 429-49(in Japanese).
47. Kobayashi S, Takahashi H, Sakakibara K, Kidokoro H. Clinical experiences of hyperbaric oxygen therapy following non-effective surgery for chronic peripheral vascular obstructive diseases. Jap J Hyperbaric Med 1985 ; 20 : 32-40 (in Japanese).
48. Lippmann HI. Medical management of "trophic" ulcers in chronic arterial occlusive disease. Angiology 1978 ; 29 : 683-90.
49. Altman MA, Richter IH, Kaplan LH. Use of an aqueous triple iodine solution in the treatment of chronic leg ulcers and gangrene. Angiology 1976 ; 27 : 181-7.
50. Beninson J. Medical management of the peripheral vascular ulcer. Angiology 1979 ; 30 : 48-52.
51. Hill GL. A rational basis for management of patients with the Buerger's syndrome. Br J Surg 1974 ; 6 : 476-81.
52. Walker PM, Key LA, MacKay IM, Johnston KW. Phenol sympathectomy for vascular occlusive disease. Surg Gynecol Obstet 1978 ; 146 : 741-4.
53. Fujita T, Kitani Y, Ishizaki K. Phenol sympathetic block for chronic arterial occlusive disease of the extremities. J Jap Soc Clin Anesth 1989 ; 9 : 180-93 (in Japanese).
54. Osawa T. Resection of the sympathetic chain as a therapy for diseases of the upper and lower extremities (lumbo-sacral and cervico-thoracic sympathetic ganglionectomy) Arch Jap Chir 1926 ; 3 : 87-142 (in Japanese).
55. Stewart HH. Sympathetic ganglionectomy for gangrene due to thromboangiitis obliterans. Br Med J 1934 ; 1 : 100-2.
56. Ito H, Asami G. Lumbosacral sympathetic ganglionectomy : its value as a therapeutic measure for thromboangiitis obliterans (with a sidelight upon alledged sympathetic innervation of the tonus of the skeletal muscle). Am J Surg 1932 ; 15 : 26-38.
57. de Takats G. The value of sympathctomy in the treatment of Buerger's disease. Surg Gynecol Obstet 1944 ; 79 : 359-67.
58. Toda H. Sontaneous gangrene. Rinsho 1951 ; 4 : 599-607 (in Japanese).
59. Van der Stricht JP. Effect of lumbar sympathectomy on the lower extremity. J Cardiovasc Surg 1979 ; 20 : 301-6.
60. Cronenwett JL, Zelenock GB, Whitehouse WM Jr, Stanley JC, Lindennauer SM. The effect of sympathetic innervation on canine muscle and skin blood flow. Arch Surg 1983 ; 118 : 420-4.
61. Shannon FL, Rutherford RB. Lumbar sympathectomy : indications and technique. In : (IX-1), pp 764-73.
62. Hirai M, Kawai S, Shionoya S. Effect of lumbar sympathectomy on muscle circulation in dogs

and patients. Nagoya J Med Sci 1975 ; 37 : 71-7.
63. Perry MO. Muscle and subcutaneous oxygen tension. Arch Surg 1978 ; 113 : 176-8.
64. Jacobson JH, Bush HS. Effect of bilateral lumbar sympathectomy on experimentally produced intermittent claudication. Surgery 1963 ; 54 : 617-20.
65. Tice DA, Reed GE, Messina EJ, Clemente E, Redisch W. Lumbsr sympathectomy : effects on vascular responses in the lower extermity of patients with arteriosclerosis obliterans. Arch Surg 1963 ; 88 : 461-3.
66. De Bakey ME, Bursch GE, Ray T, Ochsner A. The "borrowing-lending" hemodynamic phenomenon (hemometakinesia)and its therapeutic application in peripheral vascualr disturbances. Ann Surg 1947 ; 126 : 850-65.
67. de Takats G. Sympathectomy revisited ; dodo or phoenix? Surgery 1975 ; 78 : 644-59.
68. Shanik GD, Ford J, Hayes AC, Baker WH, Barnes RW. Pedal vasomotor tone following aortofemoral reconstruction : a randomized study of concomitant lumbar sympathctomy. Ann Surg 1976 ; 183 : 136-8.
69. Brunner U. Lumbale Sympathektomie bei kruralen Arterienverschlüssen, Besonderheiten der Indikation. VASA 1976 ; 5 : 228-33.
70. Campbell WB. Sympathectomy for chronic arterial ischaemia. Eur J Vasc Surg 1988 ; 2 : 357-64.
71. Nielsen PE, Bell G, Augustenborg G, Paaske Hansen O, Lassen NA. Reduction in distal blood pressure by sympathetic nerve block in patients with occlusive arterial disease. Cardiovasc Res. 1973 ; 7 : 577-84.
72. Nakata Y, Suzuki S, Kawai S, Hiari M, Shinjo K, Matsubara J, Ban I, Shionoya S. Effects of lumbar sympathectomy on thromboangiitis obliterans. J Cardiovasc Surg 1975 ; 16 : 415-25.
73. Silbert S. A new method for treatment of thrombo-angiitis obliterans. JAMA 1922 ; 79 : 1765-6.
74. Smithwick RH, White JC. Elimination of pain in obliterative vascular disease of the lower extremity. Surg Gynecol Obstet 1930 ; 51 : 394-403.
75. Smithwick RH, White JC. Peripheral nerve block in obliterative vascular disease of the lower extermity : further experience with alcohol injection or crushing of sensory nerves of lower leg. Surg Gynecol Obstet 1935 ; 60 : 1106-14.
76. Laskey NF, Silbert S. Thrombo-angiitis obliterans ; relief of pain by peripheral nerve section. Ann Surg 1933 ; 98 : 55-69.
77. Smith BC. Relief of pain by peripheral nerve block in arterial diseases of the lower extremities. Ann Surg 1936 ; 104 : 934-44.
78. Deterling RA. Is there a place for peripheral nerve crush? J Cardiovasc Surg 1962 ; 3 : 329-32.
79. Alpert J, Brief DK, Brener BJ, Parsonnet V. Peripheral nerve division for relentless ischemic foot pain. Arch Surg 1976 ; 111 : 557-60.
80. Takao T, Nakai T, Ooiwa S, Naiki K, Kato R, Fukuta I, Nagata Y, Yano T, Terasawa T. Blocking technique of peripheral sensory nerves for the severe pain of ischemic ulceration and gangrene in the lower limbs. In : (IV-30), pp 340-6(in Japanese).
81. Leriche R, Fontaine R, Dupertuis SM. Arterectomy : with follow-up studies on 78 operations. Surg Gynecol Obstet 1937 ; 64 : 149-55.
82. Kondo H. Statistical review of spontaneous gangrene : with special reference to the relation of the time of beginning of treatment to curative means and their results. Jap J Surg Soc 1942 ;

43 : 543-64(in Japanese).
83. Orban F.(III-20).
84. Kiss T, Degrell S, Kudász J, Sinkó. O. Synergetische Wirkung der lumbalen Sympathektomie und der Adrenomedullektomie. Zbl Chir 1954 ; 37 : 1565-9.
85. Kunlin J, et al.(III-25).
86. Van der Stricht J, et al.(III-26).
87. Vineberg A. Clinical and experimental studies in the treatment of coronary artery insufficiency by internal mammary artery implant. J Interat Coll Surgeons 1954 ; 22 : 503-18.
88. Friedman EW, Lambert PB, Frank HA. Vascular connections established by arteries implanted into the lower extremity with plastic sponge as an intermediary. Surgery 1966 ; 60 : 386-91.
89. Shionoya S, Ban I, Nakata Y, Matsubara J, Miyazaki H, Hirai M, Suzuki S, Tsai WH, Kamiya K. Skeletal muscle revascularization by vascular implantation. J Cardiovasc Surg 1973 ; 14 : 208-14.
90. Tsai WH. Skeletal muscle revascularization by arterial implantation. Jap Circul J 1974 ; 38 : 295-304.
91. Kawai S. Skeletal muscle revascularization by artery implantation with complementary arteriovenous fistula. Folia Angiol 1974 ; 22 : 167-71.
92. Vineberg AM, Shanks J, Pifarre R, Criollos R, Kato Y, Baichwal KS. Myocardial revascularization by omental graft without pedicle : experimental background and report on 25 cases followed 6 to 16 months. J Thoracic Cardiovasc Surg 1965 ; 49 : 103-29.
93. Goldsmith HS. Omental transposition for peripheral vascular insufficiency. Rev Surg 1967 ; 24 : 379-80.
94. Nishimura A, Sano F, Nakanishi Y, Koshino I, Kasai Y. Omental transplantation for relief of limb ischemia. Surg Forum 1977 ; 28 : 213-5.
95. Goldsmith HS, Chen WF, Duckett SW. Brain vascularization by intact omentum. Arch Surg 1973 ; 106 : 695-8.
96. Goldsmith HS. Salvage of end stage ischemic extremities by intact omentum. Surgery 1980 ; 88 : 732-6.
97. Shionoya S, Ban I, Nakata Y, Matsubara J, Hirai M, Miyazaki H, Kawai S. Vascular reconstruction in Buerger's disease. Br J Surg 1976 ; 63 : 841-6.
98. Inahara T. Evalution of endarterectomy for aortoiliac and aortoiliofemoral occlusive disease. Arch Surg 1975 ; 110 : 1458-64.
99. Vänttinen E, Inberg MV. Aorto-iliofemoral arterial reconstructive surgery : with special reference to profunda revascularization. Acta Chir Scand 1975 ; 141 : 600-8.
100. Starrett RW, Stoney RJ. Juxtarenal aortic occlusion. Surgery 1974 ; 76 : 890-7.
101. Ohta T, Ban I, Nakata Y, Matsubara J, Hirai M, Kawai S, Shionoya S. Aortoiliac occlusion in Buerger's disease. Geka 1980 ; 42 : 181-6 (in Japanese).
102. Brewster DC, Charlesworth PM, Monahan JA, Abbott WA, Darling RC. Isolated popliteal segment v tibial bypass. Arch Surg 1984 ; 119 : 775-9.
103. Flinn WR, Flanigan DP, Verta MJ Jr, Bergan JJ, Yao ST Jr. Sequential femoro-tibial bypass for severe limb ischemia. Surgery 1980 ; 88 : 357-65.
104. Hirai M, Ohta T, Shionoya S. The role of the peroneal artery in arterial occlusive disease of the leg. Vasc Surg 1980 ; 14 : 78-83.
105. Dardik H, Ibrahim IM, Dardik II. The role of the peronel artery for limb salvage. Ann Surg

1979 ; 189 : 189-98.
106. Matsubara J, Nagasue M, Hosaka H, Shimizu T. The Dacron EXS graft for femoropopliteal arterial reconstruction. Vasc Surg 1989 ; 23 : 280-5.
107. Hobson RW, O'Donnell JA, Jamil Z, Mehta K. Below-knee bypass for limb salvage. Arch Surg 1980 ; 115 : 833-7.
108. Prenner K, Pendl KH. A new approach for removal of the short saphenous vein as a transplant graft. Vasc Surg 1984 ; 18 : 197-200.
109. Clayson KR, Edwards WH, Allen TR. Dale WA. Arm veins for peripheral arterial reconstruction. Arch Surg 1976 ; 111 : 1276-80.
110. Egan TJ, Nur A, Anderson MC, Corcoran M, O'Driscoll J. Preoperative evaluation of saphenous vein suitability as an arterial graft. Vasc Surg 1984 ; 18 : 229-33.
111. Leather RP. Powers SR, Karmody AM. A reappraisal of the in situ saphenous vein arterial bypass : its use in limb salvage. Surgery 1979 ; 86 : 453-61.
112. Batson RC, Sottiurai VS. Nonreversed and in situ vein grafts. Ann Surg 1985 ; 201 : 771-9.
113. Connolly JE, Stemmer EA. The nonreversed saphenous vein bypass for femoral-popliteal occlusive disease. Surgery 1970 ; 68 : 602-9.
114. O'Mara CS, Flinn WR, Neiman HL, Bergan JJ, Yao JST. Correlation of foot arterial anatomy with early tibial bypass patency. Surgery 1981 ; 89 : 743-52.
115. Rutherford RB, Flanigan DP, Gupta SK, Johnston KW, Karmody A, Whittemore AD, Baker JD, Ernst CB, Jamieson C, Mehta S. Suggested standards for reports dealing with lower extremity ischemia. J Vasc Surg 1986 ; 4 : 80-94.
116. Karacagil S, Almgren B, Bergström R, Bowald S, Eriksson I. Postoperative predictive value of a new method of intraoperative angiographic assessment of runoff in femoropopliteal bypass grafting. J Vasc Surg 1989 ; 10 : 400-7.
117. Yano T, Shionoya S, Ikezawa T, Takurai T, Miyauchi M, Mukaitama H, Nishikimi N. Indication of femorotibial and femoroperoneal bypass for Buerger's disease. Jap J Surg Soc 1989 ; 90 : 1110-6 (in Japanese).
118. Shionoya S, Matsubara J, Hirai M, Kawai S, Seko T, Sakurai T, Ban I. Measurement of blood pressure, blood flow and flow velocity in arterial reconstruction of the lower extremity. Angiology 1983 ; 34 : 244-56.
119. Hirai M, Kawai S, Ohta T, Seko T, Shionoya S. The value of toe blood pressure measurement in arterial reconstruction. Vasc Surg 1981 ; 15 : 380-7.
120. Largiadèr J. Kruro-pedale Rekonstruktionen bei peripherem arteriellem Querschnittverschluss im distalen Unterschenkel(Fallbericht). VASA 1984 ; 13 : 24-31.
121. Sakurai T, Nakata Y, Mukaiyama H, Shionoya S. Two cases with distal tibial bypass below ankle joint. Rinshogeka 1986 ; 41 : 1699-701 (in Japanese).
122. Yano T. Indication of the surgical treatment in Raynaud's phenomenon. Sogorinsho 1989 ; 38 : 3003-5 (in Japanese).
123. Bergan JJ, Veith FJ, Bernhard VM, Yao JST, Flinn WR, Gupta SK, Scher LA, Samson RH, Towne JB. Randomization of autogenous vein and polytetra-fluoroethylene grafts in femoral-distal reconstruction. Surgery 1982 ; 92 : 921-30.
124. Grigg MJ, Nicolaides AN, Wolfe JHN. Detection and grading of femoropoliteal vein graft stenosis : duplex velocity measurements compared with angiography. J Vasc Surg 1988 ; 8 : 661-6.
125. Imparato AM, Bracco A, Kim GE, Zeff R. Intimal and neointimal fibrous proliferation causing

failure of arterial reconstruction. Surgery 1972 ; 72 : 1007-17.
126. Gloviczki P, Hollier LH. Can graft occlusion be prevented by drug? In : Greenhalgh, Jamieson CW, Nicolaides AN eds. Vascular surgery issues in current practice. London, Grune & Stratton, 1986, pp 37-48.
127. Kusaba A, Kina M, Kamori M, Inokuchi K. Hemodynamic study on etiology of late thrombosis of autogenous vein graft. In : (IV-50), pp 344-7 (in Japanese).
128. Shionoya S, Sakurai T, Hirose H, Kusakawa M, Numata M, Sakaguchi S, Tsuchioka H, Ueyama T, Yoshizaki A. Effect of Ticlopidine, an antiplatelet drug, on graft patency after arterial reconstruction in the lower extremity : a three-year multi-center perospective study. In : Strano A, Novo S eds. Advances in vascular pathology 1989. Amsterdam, Excerpta Medica, 1989, pp 1423-8.
129. Yamada I, Shionoya S, Hayakawa A, Kawanishi M, Shimada Y. Physiological changes of the transplanted saphenous veins in dogs. Jap J Smooth Muscle Res 1988 ; 24 : 243-5 (in Japanese).
130. Yano T. Surgical considerations on Buerger's disease. Gekachiryo 1989 ; 61 : 876-80 (in Japanese).
131. Tanabe T, Mishima Y, Shionoya S, Katsumura T, Kusaba A. Effect of intravenous drip infusion of prostaglandin E_1 on peripheral vascular reconstruction. Inter Angio 1984 ; 3 : 63-8.
132. Nakata Y, Kawai S, Matsubara J, Ban I, Shionoya S. Factors influenced on prognosis of reconstructive surgery for peripheral arterial occlusions : comparative study between arteriosclerosis obliterans and thromboangiitis obliterans. J Cardiovasc Surg 1977 ; 18 : 547-53.
133. Yasuda K, Yokota A, Ohta S, Kawakami T, Tanabe T. Femorotibial bypass in the patients with Buerger's disease and arteriosclerosis obliterans. In : (VII-21), pp 317-21 (in Japanese).
134. Lie JT. Thromboangiitis obliterans (Buerger's disease)in a saphenous vein arterial graft. Hum Pathol 1987 ; 18 : 402-4.
135. Dale EA, Pridgen WR, Shoulders HH Jr. Failure of composite (Teflon and vein)grafting in small human arteries. Surgery 1962 ; 51 : 258-62.
136. Linton RR, Wirthlin LS. Femoropopliteal composite Dacron and autogenous vein bypass grafts. Arch Surg 1973 ; 107 : 748-53.
137. Kusaba A. Current status in treatment of the Japanese with chronic arterial occlusive disease of the lower extremities. Inter Angio 1987 ; 6 : 223-31.
138. Ibrahim IM, Sussman B, Dardik I, Kahn M, Israel M, Kenny M, Dardik H. Adjunctive arteriovenous fistula with tibial and peroneal reconstruction for limb salvage. Am J Surg 1980 ; 140 : 246-51.
139. Dardik H, Sussman B, Ibrahim IM, Kahn M, Svoboda JJ, Mendes D, Dardik I. Distal arteriovenous fistula as an adjunct to maintaining arterial and graft patency for limb salvage. Surgery 1983 ; 94 : 478-86.
140. Lengua F, Buffet JM, Kunlin J. Distaler arterio-venöser Bypass zur Vena saphena pedis in der Behandlung schwer ischämischer Syndrome ohne direkte Rekonstruktionsmöglichkeit. VASA 1981 ; 10 : 227-9.
141. Campbell H, Harris PL. Patency of the primary pedal arch, blood flow through a femoro-tibial graft, and the role of a distal arteriovenous shunt. J Cardiovasc Surg 1983 ; 24 : 490-2.
142. Vollmar J. Surgical considerations on the terminology and treatment of the so-called Buerger's disease. J Cardiovasc Surg 1973 ; 5 : 37-9.
143. Barnes RW, Shanik GD, Slaymaker EE. An index of healing in below-knee amputation : leg

blood pressure by Doppler ultrasound. Surgery 1976 ; 79 : 13-20.
144. Moore WS, Henry RE, Malone JM, Daly MJ, Patton D, Childers SJ. Prospective use of Xenon Xe 133 clearance for amputation level selection. Arch Surg 1981 ; 116 : 86-88.
145. Holstein P, Sager P, Lassen NA. Wound healing in below-knee amputations in relation to skin perfusion pressure. Acta orthop scand 1979 ; 50 : 49-58.
146. Knote G, Bohmert H. Zur Bestimmung der Über lebensfähigkeit Nekrosegefährdeter Hautareale. Fortschr Med 1977 ; 95 : 640-4.
147. Silverman DG, Roberts A, Reilly CA, Brousseau DA, Norton KJ, Bartley E, Neufeld GR. Fluorometric quantification of low-dose fluorescein delivery to predict amputation site healing. Surgery 1987 ; 101 : 335-41.
148. Herman BE, Peirce EC. Recent changes in criteria for selecting the level of amputation of the leg. Angiology 1978 ; 29 : 410-2.
149. Huston CC, Bivins BA, Ernst CB, Griffen WO. Morbid implications of above-knee amputations. Arch Surg 1980 ; 115 : 165-7.

Chapter XI
NATURAL HISTORY

The specifity of the disease is derived from its natural history and the results of medical or surgical treatments should be evaluated through the insight into the natural history of Buerger's disease.

There was a 27 year-follow-up study of case whose disease became completely quiescent after cessation of smoking[1], whereas a spectacular case of Buerger's disease with an uninterrupted ingravescence who continued to smoke until his death was reported[2]. The natural history of Buerger's disease is checkered by remission or recurrence according to the patient's renunciation of smoking. An extensive literature now exists on many phases of this malady, but a little is known concerning the natural history of a large number of the patients with Buerger's disease. Particular attention should be directed not only to the ultimate amputation or preservation of the extremities but to the course of ischemic symptoms and complications.

One hundred fifty-one (59%) of the 255 patients with Buerger's disease in our series were followed up at the end of 1989, one to twelve years after their first examination at our hospital, by questionnaire or interviewing about their present status. In the absence of an exact knowledge of etiology, one of the best bases for the understanding of chronic disease is a biologic approach[3]. The important point for the classification of chronic disease is to call attention to the value of the biologic assay in evaluating disease and to the necessity for studying its evolution over more extensive periods than have hitherto been customary.

Present ischemic symptoms

Coldness of the finger or the toe was noticed in 76 (52%) of 151 cases, and paresthesia of the dital region of the extremities in 34 (23%). These two are symptoms of which the patient is conscious and the majority of the patients are worring about the symptoms, though it is difficult to grade its degree. Skin color change was noticed in 76 (50%) of 151 cases; pale in 18 cases; cyanotic in 7; and red in 51. Fifty-six (37%) of 151 cases were troubled with foot claudication, and 50 cases (33%) suffered from calf caludication. However, 29 patients complained of both foot and calf claudication. It might be difficult to decide whether the patient could differenciate the foot claudication from the calf one, though some patients complained of calf claudication in addition to foot pain in walking in case of occlusion of only the infrapopliteal arteries in Buerger's disease.

Rest pain was recognized in 11 (7%) of 145 cases, but we have found ischemic rest pain most difficult to get across to not only patients but also physicians. Gangrene or ulceration remained or recurred in 18(12%) of 151 cases. While necrotic lesions bothered 7 of 32 patients who continued to smoke, the lesions were found only in 11 of 119 patients who stated that they abandoned smoking; the difference in the prevalence of necrotic lesions between smokers and nonsmokers would probably have been greater if an objective test, such as the measurement of urinary cotinine, had been used to evaluate the degree of exposure to tobacco smoke.

The major complications that they informed of were as follows: gastric ulcer in 19 cases; hepatitis in 17; diabetes mellitus in 14; hypertension in 12; myocardial infarction including angina in 6, and cerebral infarction in 6. While high frequency of liver disease was prominent, there was no relationship of the past history that they received blood transfusion at operation with the liver disease. Heart disease was found mainly in patients with fifty years of age or over.

Outcome as to life and limb

During the follow-up period, from 1977 through 1989, five patients died. The causes of death were mesenterial thrombosis in three cases and myocardial infarction in two. All the former three cases had juxtarenal aortic occlusion, and two of them previously underwent arterial reconstruction, i.e., aortofemoral bypass grafting. The age at death was 33, 47 and 60 years, respectively: the presumed time elapsed after the onset of symptoms was 14, 5 and 16 years, respectively. As one patient was not suitable for arterial reconstruction because of occlusion of iliofemoropopliteal segment and another patient had a late graft failure, mesenterial thrombosis might be caused secondary ascending thrombosis based on the juxtarenal aortic occlusion. The latter two cases died at the age of 48 and 51 years, respectively: the presumed time elapsed after the onset of symptoms was 10 and 2 years, respectively. One patient underwent brachioulnar bypass with autogenous vein because of pain of the finger, and the other received femoropopliteal bypass grafting because of calf claudication.

There were six patients who underwent amputation of the extremities at other institutions after they were discharged from our hospital; below-knee in 1; metatarsal foot in 1; and digital in 4. No patients underwent major limb amputation who declared their prohibition of smoking.

In 1960 Juergens et al.[4] reported the follow-up results on 520 nondiabetic patients less than 60 years of age who had a clinical diagnosis of arteriosclerosis obliterans of the lower extremities made at the Mayo Clinic in the period 1939 through 1948, from the standpoint of pathogenesis, prognosis and clinical course of the disease. Ten-year survival rate for patients with aortoiliac occlusion was 46.6% and that for patients with femoral artery occlusion was 57.2% : in approximately three fourths of the patients who died, the cause of death was thought to be disease of the coronary arteries.

Four per cent of the patients required amputation of a leg shortly after the diagnosis of ASO was made at the clinic, and an additional 4.9% per cent subsequently required amputation during the 5-year period following the initial examination. Only 3.0% per cent of patients with intermittent claudication as the only symptom of their disease required an amputation during this period. Eleven and three-tenths per cent of patients who continued to smoke, but none who abstained from smoking, had amputations within 5 years.

In 1963 McPherson et al.[5] reported clinical and prognostic differences between patients with TAO and patients with ASO : both of them were 45 years of age or less when given a diagnosis of chronic occlusive peripheral arterial disease at the Mayo Clinic in the period 1945 through 1949 ; TAO in 45 patients, TAO probable in 104, ASO in 41 and ASO probable in 78. Ten-year survival rate for patients with TAO was 93.6%, that for patients with TAO probable was 89.6%, that for patients with ASO was 66.6% and that for patients with ASO probable was 70.8%. The survival rate of patients with TAO compared with a normal group of persons and was distinctly better than the survival rate of patients with ASO. Five deaths occurred in the TAO group of which 2 (40%) were attributed to coronary heart disease, one to mesenteric vascular occlusion, and 2 to unknown causes. While there were 8 deaths in the probable TAO group, five (62.5%) were attributed to coronary heart disease, one to cerebrovascular disease, and 2 to unknown causes. There were 11 deaths in the probable ASO group, 9 of which (81.8%) were attributed to coronary heart disease, one to cerebrovascular disease, and one to unknown causes. There were 28 deaths in the ASO group, 22 (78.5%) of which were attributed to coronary heart disease, 3 to cerebrovascular disease, one to carcinoma of the lung, and two to unknown causes.

The incidence of amputation of a leg in 32 patients with TAO was 12.6%, that in 71 patients with TAO probable was 7.0%, that in 34 patients ASO probable was 11.8% and that in 62 patients with ASO was 6.4%. Although coronary heart disease alone accounted for almost three fourths of all deaths in this study, it appeared to cause death at an earlier age and with greater frequency in patients with ASO than in patients with TAO. As described in detail in a paragraph of visceral involvement with Buerger's disease, controversy regarding the pathogenesis of coronary lesions in patients with the disease need no repetition here.

In 1980 Nielubowicz et al.[6] found three deaths in 46 patients with TAO who were followed for 2-10 years : 2 of the 3 patients died of pulmonary embolism or sepsis and pneumonia after multiple amputations. Owing to the long survival of the amputated patients and no involvement of the visceral vessels in the autopsied cases, they indicated that the disease might be limited only to the extremities.

The survival rate of patients with TAO in our series compared favorably with that in the Mayo and the Warsaw series. In common with the Nagoya experience, vascular accidents such as coronary or mesenteric thrombosis accounted for the majority of all the deaths of patients with TAO in the Mayo study. The fact that no patients died of malignant tumor in the both series might be owing to an age structure composed of the younger generation. Judging from that patients with TAO had a practically normal survival as compared with a normal population of the same age and sex distribution, it may not be given as a conclusion that coronary thrombosis affects patients with TAO with greater frequency than normal population.

The rate of major amputation in patients with TAO in our series was much lower than that in the Mayo series. The likelihood of survival of digits or legs may depend on the stage of the disease at the first medical examination, prohibition of smoking, and the patient's self-control of avoiding traumatic and cold injury to the ischemic tissues. Because of the difference in the period when the investigation was carried on between the two studies, of course, it is impossible to make a discrimination between them with reference to the rate of limb amputation in patients with TAO.

Employment conditions

One hundred forty (93%) of the 151 cases were on the job and 11 left their job mostly because of an advanced age. According to the previous investigation[7] about the employment conditions of 165 patients with TAO who were treated at our hospital from 1967 through 1979, 148 patients (90%) remained on job. Thirty of the 148 patients had to change types of their occupation because of trophic lesions, paresthesia of digits or intermittent claudication.

As coldness, paresthesia, or intermittent claudication remained in the majority of patients with Buerger's disease even after necrotic lesion of the digitis had healed, these symptoms made the patients unfit for the jobs which necessitated exposure of the digits to cold or long walking and the patients were obliged to take up other employment. All the patients were in the prime of manhood and they must dare to work as the breadwinner of a family in spite of the sequelae of the disease.

Natural history of patients with Buerger's disease

Apart from thrombophlebitis migrans or proximal progression of occlusion of the main artery, it is not always easy to confirm recurrence of the disease process through aggravation of the subjective ischemic symptoms. The aggravation of coldness, paresthesia or pain does not always depend on the worsening of ischemia. The occurrence of ulceration or gangrene in the digits doesn't necessarily mean that the minor tissue loss spontaneously resulted from the exacerbation of critical ischemia : the necrotic lesion may follow mechanical, chemical or thermal trauma regardless of deterioration of ischemia.

Compared with the ischemic symptoms before the treatment, the degree of symptoms was improved in 75 (59%) of 127 cases, unchanged in 40 (32%), and worsened in 12 (9%) in our series. Because complete prohibition of smoking, protecting from traumatic and cold injury and patient walking training have an influence upon the patient's residual symptoms, his natural history is completely under his self-control. The patient's consitutional susceptibility to smoking permanently remains and the disease probably recurs, if he smokes again, but he can live the almost same social life as a healthy person unless he uses tobacco again.

However, every problem about Buerger's disease may be not resolved only by prohibition of smoking. In 1988 Ohta and Shionoya[8], based on the follow-up study on fate of the ischemic limb in the patients with Buerger's disease in our another series, reported that 61 (48%) of the 127 patients who did not abstained from smoking, had recurrence of ischemic ulceration but no necrotic lesions recurred in the remaining 66 patients (52%) ; on the other hand, in 16 (10%) of 162 patients ischemic ulceration recurred though they stated they had abandoned smoking.

Laying aside the question of confirming the truth of the patient's testiononey, there might be some patients with Buerger's disease who were less affected by smoking, and whose use of tobacco was not directly linked with the occurrence of necrotic lesions.

Recurrence of the disease in ex-smokers suggests that smoking might be not the only deleterious factor influencing the natural history of Buerger's disease. However, a high priority for future studies is more reliable measurement of exposure to tobacco smoke in the environment and elucidation of effects of involuntary smoking on the disease process.

REFERENCES

1. Ball GV, Wright IS.(X-6).
2. Cabezas-Moya R, Dragstedt LR.(VI-26).

3. Moschcowitz ELI. A biologic concept of disease. JAMA 1932 ; 99 : 714-7.
4. Juergens JL, Barker NW, Hines EA. Arteriosclerosis obliterans : review of 520 cases with special reference to pathogenic and prognostic factors. Circulation 1960 ; 21 : 188-95.
5. McPherson JR, et al.(VI-20).
6. Nielubowicz J, Rosnowski A, Pruszynski B, Przetakiewicz Z, Potemkowski A. Natural history of Buerger's disease. J Cardivasc Surg 1980 ; 21 : 529-40.
7. Shionoya S, Nakata Y, Hirai M, Kawai S, Phta T, Ban I. Long-term follow-up results of patients with Buerger's disease : with special reference to their return to work. Gekachiryo 1980 ; 43 : 357-63 (in Japanese).
8. Ohta T, Shionoya S. Fate of the ischemic limb in Buerger's disease. Br J Surg 1988 ; 75 : 259-62.

Chapter XII
WHAT IS BUERGER'S DISEASE ?

Buerger's disease has been said to be a disease of misconceptions, though Buerger was the first to point out the thrombotic and inflammatory nature of the process, the involvement of veins as well as arteries and the characteristic clinical phenomena. He incorporated all these concepts in the name which he gave to the disease, thromboangiitis obliterans. Through the irony of chance, however, a splendid clinicopathological term, thromboangiitis obliterans, led to confusion in later ages. The name is precise and convenient enough to be applied to various vascular lesions from the standpoint of pathohistology. As the specificity of the disease is derived from its clinical characteristics, "Buerger's disease" is a better name than "thromboangiitis obliterans," which tends to be associated with impractical histopathologic criteria.

Epidemiology

At the present time no nationwide epidemiological study on Buerger's disease is available except that in Japan. While the percentage of the disease among chronic peripheral arterial occlusive disease is less than 5 per cent in Europe and USA, that is 20 to 30 per cent or more in Asia.

The change in the number of new patients at many institutions by years gives an impression that the number of new patients with Buerger's disease is decreasing in Japan, but the number of patients under the care of a physician remains almost unchanged, because of recurrence of the disease. Its incidence in Japanese is estimated to be about 5 per 100,000 population. As to occupations of the patients, muscular laborers formerly ranked high, but there is now no significant high prevalence in them in Japan.

The percentage of the female patients has been several per cent. According to recent investigations in some countries the percentage seems to be increasing, but it remains unknown whether the increase in prevalence of Buerger's disease among women might be related to their increased use of tobacco or not. Women might have the disease in a much milder form, and the disease might have been overlooked because of the failure of development of typical ischemic symptom.

Etiology

While the cause of Buerger's disease is not yet known, smoking is very closely related with exacerbations and remissions of the disease without doubt. Essentially all patients with Buerger's disease are smokers and it remains an open question whether true nonsmokers develop the disease. Because the incidence is very low, even among heavy smokers, an immunopathogenesis for the disease has been considered probable.

Evidence for this includes an increase in complement factor C4, anti-elastin and anti-collagen antibody, cellular sensitivity to human type I or type III collagen, organ specific autoantibodies and C3 component, non-organ specific antibodies and leukocyte migration inhibition factor against tobacco antigen. Based on HLA analysis in patients with Buerger's disease, it has been speculated that there might be a gene in Japanese controlling susceptibility to the disease, linked to the presence or absence of some HLA antigens. However, the significance of these immunologic findings remains to be resolved. Although a hypercoagulable stats has been observed in association with exacerbations of ischemic symptoms in patients with the disease, its causal significance is unknown. Tobacco smoking, whether it is a direct etiologic factor or only a strongly contributory one, plays a pivotal role in disease development and progression.

Pathology

Buerger's disease is an inflammatory occlusive disease primarily involving the small and medium-sized arteries and veins of the extremity.

At acute stage, the occluded artery appears to be tense or swollen and periarterial tissue edematous. The lumen is obstructed with fresh thrombus in which a focal inflammation, consisting of multinucleated giant cell, epithelioid cells, and leukocytes, in the form of microabscess, is frequently observed. Inflammatory cells, mainly lymphocytes and fibroblasts, infiltrate throughout the media and adventitia, but no necrotizing lesions are found in the media.

At chronic stage, the occluded artery appears to be contracted and indurated. The artery and veins may be bound into a rather firm cord so that they can be separated only with difficulty. The advanced lesion is characterized by some recanalization of the thrombus, a fibrous thickening of the intima, and increased fibrous tissue in the media and adventitia. While the internal elastic membrane is partially destroyed or fragmented, the general architecture of the vessel wall is well preserved. The histopathologic features in involved superficial veins bear a close resemblance to those in the affected artery.

The granulomatous reaction with giant cells lends a characteristic appearance to the thrombotic lesion of Buerger's disease at acute stage; this picture is never seen in thrombi associated with arteriosclerosis obliterans or simple arterial thrombosis. Although there are a number of reports of "generalized" Buerger's disease, the majority of the occlusive lesions outside of the extremities were interpreted as arteriosclerotic or thrombotic in nature.

Pathophysiology

The most characteristic pathophysiologic change in Buerger's disease is stagnation of the peripheral or distal circulation in the extremity principally due to arterial occlusion, i.e., breakdown of the microvascular flow system.

The lack of vasomotion in the microcirculation is characteristic for patients with Buerger's disease, and rubor of the digits is a representative feature of abnormal vasomotion: abnormal vasomotion produces maldistribution of blood flow with some capillaries not perfused or underperfused. In addition vasospasm, local hypercoagulable state and increased blood viscosity participate in the breakdown of microvascular flow regulating system. When the pedal arterial velocity is less than 1.0 cm/sec and toe pressure index is less than 0.3, ischemic ulceration is either imminent or present.

Clinical manifestations

As the disease commences peripherally and the disease may pass unnoticed until the occlusive lesions involve the forearm or crural arteries, it is not surprising that the first clinical manifestations are multifarious, i.e., coldness, paresthesia, skin color changes, intermittent claudication, rest pain, and gangrene or ulceration: necrotic lesions do not always follow claudication and may predece it.

Although foot claudication is a characteristic symptom associated with ischemia of the foot due to infrapopliteal arterial occlusion, calf claudication may be experienced if the desease progresses to the suprapopliteal segment. Recurrent superficial thrombophlebitis develops on the arm, the lower leg, or the foot. Redness of the skin over the affected vein and tenderness usually disappear in 2 to 3 weeks leaving a black-brown pigmentation. "Phlebitis migrans" is a pathognomonic episode characteristic of Buerger's disease (as an angiitis), but its occurrence often escapes the patient's attention.

While the upper extremity is involved in addition to the lower limb in the majority of the patients, ischemic symptoms of the fingers are not always recognized. The accompanying veins of the main crural arteries are often involved in the disease, but as a rule, no disturbance of venous return in the deep vein system is seen. Gangrene and ulceration may occur spontaneously (spontaneous gangrene), but in the majority of cases, the necrotic lesions follow various forms of trauma, including iatrogenic. In our series, 249 of 255 patients with Buerger's disease were men (98%) and 6 were women (2%). The age at the onset of symptoms ranged from 19 to 49 years (average, 35.8±7.7 years). All the patients were smokers.

Clinical course

In the lower extremity, the disease commences in the digital arteries and the small arteries in the foot and then proceeds to involve the crural arteries. After the crural arteries are affected, the pattern of infrapopliteal arterial occlusions is set up, up to a certain point, though there is often further deterioration in the most distal vessel. Further progression of the disease takes one of two forms : 1) continuous progression and 2) skip progression. It is worth notice that independently of occlusion of the toe and foot arteries, the arterial occlusions occur in the branches of proximal arteries such as the muscular branches of the posterior tibial artery and the deep femoral artery or the branches of the internal iliac artery.

The disease may involve segments as far proximal as the external iliac artery. More proximal occlusion is caused by secondary thrombosis or an iatrogenic event, e.g., failure of an aortofemoral bypass. In our series, arterial occlusion was limited to the infrapopliteal segment in 60 per cent of patients at the time of initial evaluation. Arterial occlusion had already progressed to the femoropopliteal segment in 32 per cent, and to the aortoiliac region in 8 per cent. In the upper extremity, the process begins in the digital arteries and the small arteries in the hand, and then proceeds to involve the forearm arteries. In contrast to the lower extremity, involvement of the brachial artery rarely follows affection of the forearm arteries.

From the onset of symptoms to the end of follow-up in our series, gangrene or ulceration occurred in 72 per cent of the 255 patients, thrombophlebitis migrans in 43 per cent, and involvement of the upper extremity in 90 per cent. Two limbs were affected in 17 per cent of all the patients, three in 43 per cent, and four in 40 per cent. If the patient continues to smoke, three- or four-limb involvement might be the regular course of the disease with the lapse of time. Because of the high incidence of necrotic lesions in patients with the disease, removal of the necrotic digits was inevitably performed. As their ischemic ulcers have mostly a good healing potential, however, the minor amputation answered the purpose.

Diagnosis

Our clinical criteria for the diagnosis of Buerger's disease are : 1) smoking history ;

2) onset before the age of 50 years; 3) infrapopliteal arterial occlusive lesions; 4) either upper limb involvement or phlebitis migrans; and 5) absence of atherosclerotic risk factors other than smoking. The clinical diagnosis of Buerger's disease is made when all five requirements are met.

"Migrating" phlebitis and upper extremity involvement are considered to be systemic manifestations of Buerger's disease. In the author's series, both upper limb involvement and phlebitis migrans occurred in 34 per cent. Patients with both involvements were compared to those with either, and no significant difference in clinical course was found between the two groups. Therefore, either upper limb involvement or phlebitis migrans seems sufficient to support the clinical diagnosis of Buerger's disease.

Arteriographic findings such as abrupt or tapering occlusion, "corkscrew" or "rootlike" collaterals, and accordion-like appearance serve as supporting evidence, and characteristic pathohistologic findings corroborate the existence of the disease.

Treatment

The only way to arrest the disease is abstinence from smoking. Any therapeutic procedure not accompanied by a cessation of smoking will be unsuccessful in treating the arterial insufficiency. As, a number of extremity arteries are spared from obstructive lesions at the beginning, the goal of medical treatment is to increase blood flow through the remaining patent vessels and to develop the compensatory collateral network.

No panacea for the disease exists but it is essential that something be done to try to help the patient through the difficult time between the onset of acute symptoms and eventual clinical improvement. The most difficult aspect is the war against intractable pain. "Bridging therapy" is the term we use for the appropriate use of epidural anesthesia, PG infusion, antithrombotic agents, or hyperbaric oxygen to help the patient through periods of acute exacerbation. Walking training and physical exercise is the treatment of choice for intermittent claudication. Because of good natural healing potential of most trophic lesions in Buerger's disease, the digital necrotic lesion should be conservatively managed at first. In case of poor spontaneous healing potential, sympathectomy or arterial reconstruction should be considered, though direct arterial reconstruction is not often feasible because of the multiple occluded distal arteries.

All efforts should be concentrated on the healing of ulceration or successful auto-or surgical amputation of gangrene. Although minor amputation, such as digital, is frequently necessary, "foot salvage" is easily accomplished. "Foot salvage" means retention of a functional foot that allows standing and walking without a prosthesis. In our series, sympathectomy was performed in 130 (51%) of

255 patients and bypass grafting was carried out in 44 (17%): 47 procedures in the lower extremity and 4 in the upper extremity (seven patients underwent two separate operations). Below knee amputation was performed in 6 cases and above knee amputation in one: all the patients except one refused to abandon smoking.

Natural history

The traits characteristic of Buerger's disease are found in the natural history of the disease. One hundred fifty-one (59%) of the 255 patients with Buerger's disease were followed up for a 12-year-period in our series. During the follow-up period, five patients died. The causes of death were mesenterial arterial or venous thrombosis in three cases and myocardial infarction in two: all the former three cases had juxtarenal aortic occlusion, and two of them underwent arterial reconstruction.

Judging from that patients with Buerger's disease had a practically normal survival as compared with a normal population, the involvement of the visceral vessels outside the extremities seems to be rare and it may not be given as a conclusion that coronary thrombosis affects patients with the disease with greater frequency than normal population. While ischemic symptoms such as coldness, paresthesia or intermittent claudication remained in not a few patients, the majority of the patients were on the job, though the residual symptoms necessitated some patients to take up other employment.

The patient's natural history was uneventful, if he absolutely abandoned smoking. On the other hand, any treatment for the disease was ineffective unless he abstained from smoking. If the disease is diagnosed at the early stage and the patients keeps to deny himself the pleasure of smoking the prognosis as to limb and life is favorable, and he can live socially and enjoy life in almost the same way as a healthy person.

Summary

Buerger's disease is characterized by peripheral arterial occlusion of the extremities in young smokers, and true Buerger's lesions outside the extremities seem to be rare. Although the incidence of the disease is low in Europe and the United State, the treatment of patients with the disease is still one of the most important problems of vascular surgery in Asia, because of its high rate among chronic peripheral arterial occlusive disease. The etiology remains unknown, but there is an extremely close relationship between the use of tobacco and the occurrence or recurrence of the disease. If the patient absolutely and permanently abandons smoking, the natural history is uneventful. In spite of a high incidence of digital gangrene and ulceration, a functional foot can almost always be preserved because of the good spontaneous healing potential of the trophic lesions.

As the specifity of the disease is derived from its clinical features characterized with ischemia of peripheral extremities, inflammatory character and self-limited disease process, "Buerger's disease" is a better name than "thromboangiitis obliterans," a pathohistologic term. The diagnosis should be based principally upon knowledge of the natural history of the disease. An understanding of the natural course of the disease not only has prognostic value but also places the role of surgical or conservative treatment in the proper perspective. Surgeons treating patients with Buerger's disease should take note of this and avoid premature and possibly unnecessary surgery. Buerger's disease is now not a disease of misconceptions, and it should be diagnosed and managed on the basis of a clear conception of the true nature of the disease.

INDEX

Page numbers followed by (f) refer to figures ;
page numbers followed by (t) refer to tables.

Abrupt occlusion, 122, 124, 125, 126, 127, 128, 132
Absence of atherogenic risk factors, 5, 19
   among diagnostic requirements, 192
Accordion-like (rippling or corrugated) appearance, 85, 124, 125, 127, 128, 136 (f), 139, 140-143
   incidence and site of, 139, 140
Acute stage, 57-61
Adrenalectomy, 217
   adrenomedullectomy, 217
Adrenocortical disfunction, 40
   17 OHCS and 17 KS excretion, 40
Affection of popliteal artery, 136 (f), 137 (f), 156, 161
Age at onset, 113
   among diagnostic requirements, 190
Allen test, 159
Allergy, 42, 43
   denicotinized tobacco extract, 43, 45, 46
   hypersensitiviness to tobacco, 42, 43
   Prausnitz-Kuster test, 43
Amputation level determination, 232, 233
   by fluorescein delivery, 232
   by segmental blood pressure with Doppler flowmeter, 232
   by skin blood flow with Xe-133 clearance, 232
   by skin perfusion pressure with ^{131}I- or ^{125}I-antipyrine, mixed with histamine, 232
   by transcutaneous O_2 recording, 232
Amputation, 231-233
   above-knee, 232, 233
   amputation level determination, 232, 233
   amputation rate, 233
   below-knee, 232, 233, 243
   borderline-, 232
   I-R-A principle, 231, 232
Aneurysm formation, 74, 75, 137
Anomalous course, 125, 133
Anticoagulant drugs, for bridging treatment, 229
   for portoperative adjunct, 209
Antiplatelet drugs, for healing of ischemic ulcers, 208

   for postoperative adjunct, 229
Aortitis Syndrome, 197
Aortoiliac involvement, 164-171
   in abdominal aorta, 167-171
   in common iliac artery, 167
   in external iliac artery, 164, 165
   in internal iliac artery, 131 (f), 166, 167
   in lumbar arteries, 169, 170
   rate of occlusion of deep femoral artery in, 165
Arterectomy, 217
   Leriche's working hypothesis of, 74
Arteriitis stenosans coronariae, 71, 176
Arteriographic characteristics, 121-148
   abrupt occlusion, 125, 126, 132
   accordion-like appearance, 124, 125, 140-143
   anomalous course, 125
   bridging collaterals, 125, 126, 146
   corkscrew collaterals, 123, 125, 126, 130, 145
   description of arteriographic features, 125, 126
   diffure smooth narrowing, 125, 138, 139
   dilatation, 125, 126, 137
   early venous filling, 125, 126, 142
   fine thread, 126, 140
   irregularity, 125, 126, 135, 136
   kinking, 123, 125
   moth-eaten stenosis, 125, 126
   segmental occlusion, 134
   standards of judgement of normal arteriogram, 121
   stenosis, 125, 126
   tapering occlusion, 34 (f), 125, 132, 133
   tree root collaterals, 123, 125, 126, 140
Arteriographic discrimination from arteriosclerosis, in coeliac and mesenterial arteries, 178, 179
   in extremity arteries, 121, 122
Arteriography, through skin incision, 118, 119
Arteriosclerosis obliterans, 8, 193, 194
Arteriosclerotic (senile) gangrene, 12
Arteriovenous anastomosis, for revascularization of ischemic leg, 13, 72

Arteritis obliterans. See Endarteritis obliterans.
Autogenous vein bypass, in situ, 221, 223, 225
  nonreversed translocated, 221
  reversed, 221, 223
Autoimmune mechanism, anticollagen antibody, 43, 44
  antielastin antibody, 43
  circulating immune complexes, 44
  complement factor, 43, 44
  HLA-antigens, 44, 46, 47
  in pathogenesis, 43-44
  organ specific autoantibodies, 44
A-V shunt procedure, for cases with extensive occlusion, 230

Behçet's disease, 196
Benign type of arteriosclerosis, 70
Billroth, T., 2, 4
Blackfoot disease, 35
Blood flow velocity, in foot, with radioisotopic tracer technique, 81-83
  relation of TPI to, 82-84
  with Doppler flowmeter, 81
Blood viscosity, 89, 90
  increased by polycythemia or hyperfibrinogenemia, 90
  measured by viscometer, 89, 90
  reduction in, by increased erythrocyte flexibility, 208
  reduction in, by saline-infusion, 89, 90, 208
Brachial arteriogram, 119, 123, 128, 129, 148, 160
Brachioradial bypass, 227 (f)
Brachioulnar bypass, 227 (f)
Bridging collaterals, 125, 126, 144, 146, 148
Bridging treatment, 209
  antithrombotic agents, 209
  epidural nerve block, 209
  hyperbaric oxygen therapy, 209
  PG infusion, 209
  rest of body and mind, 209
  tobacco withdrawal, 209
Buerger, L., personal history of, 9, 18
Buerger's disease, summarized, 248-254
  clinical course of, 251
  clinical manifestations of, 250, 251
  diagnosis of, 251, 252
  epidemiology of, 248
  etiology of, 249
  natural history of, 253
  pathology of, 249, 250
  pathophysiology of, 250
  summary of, 253, 254
  treatment of, 252, 253
Buerger's exercise, 202
Bypass grafting, 220-229
  adjunctive treatment in, 229
  autogenous vein, 221, 223, 228
  evaluation of runoff in, 223, 224
  graft failures in, 223-226, 228, 229
  graft materials in, 221
  in aortoiliac occlusion, 220, 221
  in femoropopliteocrural occlusion, 221-224
  in occlusion of arteries of foot, 225
  in occlusion of forearm arteries, 225-227
  indication for, 225
  long-term result of, 225, 226, 228, 229
  sequential, 221
  special measures in, 230, 231

Calf claudication, 94, 95, 156, 161, 162, 242, 243
  incidence of, 115
Carbon monoxide, 47, 49
Carboxyhemoglobin, 47
Cases associated with eosinophilia, 76
Cerebral involvement, 18, 171-174
  granular atrophy, 171-173
  incidence of, 69, 172, 174
  site of cerebral arterial occlusion, 173
  type I of Lindenberg and Spatz, 171-174
  type II of Lindenberg and Spatz, 171, 172
  worm-like vessels, 171, 172, 174
Changes in the blood, 41, 42
  hyprercoagulable state, 42, 48, 88, 89
Chief complaints at first visit, 101, 102, 115
Chronic stage, 61-63
Cigarette smoker disease, 200
Classification of clinical course, 184, 185
Clinical diagnostic criteria, 189
Clinical manifestations, 101-116
  blanching after elevation, 103
  clinical correlations, 112-116
  coldness, 102, 115
  cyanosis, 103, 104
  edema, 104

gangrene and ulceration, 107-109, 115
initial symptom, 101, 102, 115
intermittent claudication, 104, 105, 115
involvement of upper extremity, 110, 111
mental symptoms, 111, 112
pain of ischemic neuropathy, 106
paresthesia, 102, 115
rest pain, 105, 106, 115
skin color changes, 102-104, 115
thrombophlebitis migrans, 106, 107, 115
trophic changes, 110
Cold injury, 2, 30, 31, 38
Coldness, 102, 115, 116, 242, 245
Collagen disease, in view of differential diagnosis, 194
  scleroderma, 194
  systemic lupus erythematosus, 194
Collaterals, direct type of, 125, 144
  in occlusion of anterior tibial artery, 120, 121, 144-147
  in occlusion of aortoiliac region, 119, 148
  in occlusion of femoropopliteal segment, 120, 121, 147
  in occlusion of foot arteries, 121
  in occlusion of forearm arteries, 119, 148
  in occlusion of peroneal artery, 145
  in occlusion of posterior tibial artery, 120, 121, 144-147
  indirect type of, 144
  mechanism of development of, 121, 144, 145
Compensatory endarteriitis, 7
Complications, in follow-up, 243
Composite grafting, for cases lacking in suitable antogenous vein, 230
Conservative treatment, 201-211
  pharmacologic measures, 204-209
  physical method of enhancing circulation, 202-204
Constitutional factor, 46, 47
  HLA-antigens, 46, 47
Corkscrew collaterals, 122, 123, 124, 125, 126, 127, 128, 130, 145, 146, 148
Coronary involvement, 16, 174-176
  incidence of, 69, 174, 175
  pathogenesis of, 175, 176
Correlation between vessel involved and its clinical course, 159-171

  in aortoiliac involvement, 164-171
  in femoropopliteal involvement, 161-164
  in involvement of arteries of upper extremity, 159, 160
  in involvement of foot arteries, 160
Cotinine, 49-52
  salivary cotinine, 50
  urinary cotinine, 50-52
Critical limb ischemia, 80, 81
  microvascular defense system (MDS), 80
  microvascular flow regulating system (MFRS), 80
Crural arterial occlusion pattern and necrotic lesion, 155
Crural artery bypass with adjunctive A-V fistula, for cases with poor runoff, 230, 231
Cyanosis, 103, 104, 115, 242

Debridement, 211
  nonoperative, 211
  surgical, 211
Deep vein thrombosis, 72, 73
Defibrinogenation therapy, 208
Dependent rubor, 84, 87, 102, 103, 250
Dermatomycoses, 39
Description of arteriographic features, 125, 126
Diagnostic points, 189-192
  absence of atherogenic risk factors, 192
  age at onset, 190
  infrapopliteal arterial occlusive lesions, 190, 191
  migrating phlebitis, 191, 192
  sex, 190
  smoking, 189
  upper limb involvement, 191, 192
Differential diagnosis, 193-197
  aortitis syndrome, 197
  arteriosclerosis obliterans, 193, 194
  Behçet's disease, 196
  occupational arterial occlusive disease of hand, 194-196
  thoracic outlet syndrome, 196
  vasospastic disorders, 197
Diffuse smooth narrowing, 124, 125, 138, 139
Dilatation, 65, 124, 125, 126, 137
  associated with stenotic skip lesion, 137
Distribution of arterial occlusive lesions, in lower

extremity, 127
in upper extremity, 127, 128
Distribution of perfusion, with ^{99m}Tc-pertechnetate, 95
with Tl-201, 95-97

Early graft failure, 223, 225
Early venous filling, 124, 125, 126, 127, 128, 142
Eating habits, 31
Edema, 104, 209, 210
control of, 210
Elasticophagic giant cells, 60
Employment condition, in patients, 245
Endarteriitis and endophlebitis, 2
Endarteriitis circumscripta, 5
Endarteriitis obliterans, 2, 4, 181
Epidural anesthesia, for bridging treatment, 209
Ergostism, 39, 40
Erythromelia (erythromelalgia), 9, 13
Essentials of diagnosis, 192, 193
Estrogen excretion, 40, 41
Etiological factors, 38-52
allergy, 42, 43
autoimmune mechanism, 43, 44
changes in the blood, 41, 42
cold injury, 38
ergotism, 39, 40
hyperadrenalinemia, 40
infection, 38, 39
metabolic abnormalities, 40, 41
smoking, 44-52
Extraperipheral arterial involvement, 171-185
cerebral, 171-174
coronary, 174-176
generalized, 182-185
visceral, 176-182

Female patients, arteriographic findings of, 34 (f), 127, 131 (f)
discriminating collagen disease in, 190, 194
in negro, 16
incidence of, 33, 113, 190
ischemic symptoms of, 34, 35
Femoral arteriogram, 119-121, 123, 129, 151-158
Femoro-anterior tibial bypass grafting, 222 (f)
Femoro-posterior tibial bypass grafting, 222 (f)
Femoroperoneal bypass grafting, 222 (f), 223 (f)

Femoropopliteal involvement, 147, 161-163, 164 (f)
clinical types of, 161
incidence of occlusion of deep femoral artery in, 128, 163
rate of proximal progression in, 161, 162
Fine thread, 126, 127, 128, 139, 140 (f)
First case in negro, 16
First femal case in negro, 16
Fontaine's classification, 102
Foot claudication, 90-93, 104, 105, 161, 191
incidence of, 115, 242
Foot salvage, 252

Gangrene and ulceration, 87, 95, 107-109, 246
incidence of, 108, 109, 115, 116, 243
relation of upper limb involvement and/or thrombophlebitis migrans to, 109, 160
General regimen, 201
Generalized involvement, 182-185
Geographical distribution of patients in Japan, 32 (f)
Gross pathology, described by Buerger, 10, 63, 64
arteriosclerosis, 10, 63, 64
periarteritis, 10, 63, 64
thrombotic occlusion, 10, 63
HB virus, 39
Healing potential of ischemic ulceration, 95-97
Hemodilution, lowing blood viscosity, 208
Histology, described by Buerger, 10-12
HLA-antigens, 46, 47
Hyperadrenalinemia, 40
Hyperbaric oxygen, for bridging treatment, 209
Hypercoagulable (prethrombotic) state, 42, 48, 88, 89
Hypertension, drug-induced, as therapy, 208, 209
Hypoplasia of arteries, 15, 114, 133, 134, 146, 168-170
Hypothenar hammer synchome, 195. See also Occupational arterial occlusive disease of hand.

I-R-A principle, 231, 232
Impaired arterial pulsations, 114
Incidence of Buerger's disease, 28-35
in Belgium, 29
in China, 16, 30

in Czechoslovakia, 29
in Females, 33
in France, 29
in Germany, 28, 29
in India, 29, 30
in Indonesia, 30, 31
in Israel, 29
in Italy, 29
in Japan, 31-33
in Korea, 30
in Poland, 29
in Portugal, 28
in Switzerland, 29
in Thailand, 31
in UK, 28, 29
in USA, 28
Infection, as etiological factor, 38, 39
  dermatomycoses, 39
  HB virus, 39
  management of, 210
  rickettsia, 39
  streptococcus, 39
  syphilis, 39
  typhus, 39
Inflammatory arteriosclerosis, 71
Infrapopliteal arterial occlusive lesions, among diagnostic reguirements, 123, 124, 128, 190, 191
  foot claudication due to. See Foot claudication.
Initial pattern of arterial occlusion and clinical course, 158
Initial symptom, 101, 102, 115
Instep claudication, 104, 105
Intermediate graft failure, 225-228
  NFH, as cause of, 225-228
Intermediate stage, 61
Intermittent claudication, in upper limb, 105
Interpretation of pathologic findings, 63-65
Involuntary smoking, 48-52
Involvement of foot arteries, as initial lesion, 63
  incidence of, 160
  relation of ischemic ulceration to, 160
Involvement of muscular branch arteries, 162, 163, 164
  in deep femoral artery, 34 (f), 128, 163, 164 (f)
  in sural artery, 68 (f)

Involvement of upper extremity, 4, 5, 14, 109, 110, 111
  among diagnostic reguirements, 191, 192
  as initial symptom, 111, 113, 115
  as systemic manifestation, 111
  incidence of, 110, 115, 116, 159, 160
  site of arterial occlusion in, 124, 127, 128
Irregularity, 65, 122, 124, 125, 126, 127
Ischemic neuritis, 106
Ischemic ulceration, 95

Japanese specific HLA-antigen, 46
Juxtarenal aortic occlusion, 168-171, 220

Kinking, 125, 127, 128

Late graft failure, 224, 225
Lesions outside extremitis, 69-71. See also Extraperipheral arterial involvement.
Local treatment, 209-211
  control of edema, 210
  debridement, 211
  management of infection, 210
  medical bath, 211

Main stream, 48, 49
Malariotherapy, 200
Malignant thrombophlebitis, 73
Malignant type of arteriosclerosis, 70, 71, 176
Manner and rate of progression of arteiral occlusion, in lower extremity, 151, 156, 157, 162
  in upper extremity, 148
Medical bath, 211
  as chemical debridement, 211
Mental symptoms, 111, 112
Metabolic abnormalities, 40, 41
  17 OHCS and 17 KS excretion, 40
  electrolytes, 41
  estrogen excretion 40, 41
  fat metabolism, 41
  histamine, 41
  protein metabolism, 41
  Thorn test, 40
Microcirculation, in critical limb ischemia, 80, 81
Microvascular defense system (MDS), 80, 81
Microvascular flow regulating system (MFRS), 80, 81

Migrating phlebitis, among diagnostic reguirements, 191, 192. See also Thrombophlebitis migrans
Miliary giant cell foci, in thrombus, 11, 13, 15, 57, 58 (f), 59 (f), 76
Mode of progression of arteriosclerosis, 70, 71, 176
Multinucleated giant cells, around internal elastic membrane, 60
  in media, 60, 61 (f)
  in thrombus, 57, 58 (f), 59 (f), 60
Muscle blood flow measured with Xe-133 clearance, 90-95
  in anterior tibial muscle, 93, 94
  in gastrocnemius muscle, 93, 94
  in plantar muscle, 90-93
  in soleus muscle, 94, 95
Muscle revascularization by vascular implantation, 217-218
  indication for, 218
Myogenic giant cells, in media, 60, 61 (f)

Natural history, effect of smoking on, 242, 246
  of inchemic symptoms, 242, 243, 246
  of life and limb, 243-245
Neointimal fibrous hyperplasia (NFH), as cause of intermediate graft failure, 225-228
Nerve lesions, 73, 74
Nicotine, 43, 49
  nicotine deficiency, 112
Numbering of extremity arteries, 125

Occupational arterial occlusive disease of hand, 111, 159, 194-196
  Raynaud's phenomenon in, 194, 195
  vibration-induced white finger in foot, 196
Omental transplantation, 218, 219
  into lower limb, 218, 219
  into upper limb, 219

Pallor, 104, 242
Paresthesia, 102, 115, 242, 245
Passive smoking. See Involuntary smoking.
Pathological characteristics, 76, 77
  at acute stage, 57-61
  at chromic stage, 61-63
  at intermediate stage, 61

  macroscopic, 10, 57, 61, 63, 64
  microscopic, 64, 65
Pattern of crural arterial occlusion, 152, 153 (t)
  continuous, 154 (f)
  different, 154 (f)
  discontinuous, 155 (f)
  similar, 153 (f)
Peculiar cases associated with eosinophilia, 76
Peripheral nerve division, 215-217
  indication for, 216
  Smithwick's method, 215, 216
Perlschnurarterie. See Accordion-like appearance.
PGE_1, continuous intraarterial infusion of, 204-206
  indication for, 206
PGE_1, intravenous drip infusion of, 206, 207
  steal phenomenon due to, 207
Prausnitz-Kuster test, 43
Prerequisites for treatment, 199-201
  general regimen, 201
  tobacco abstinence, 199-201
Primary involvement of upper limb, 14, 111, 160
Principles of conservtive treatment, 203
Progression of arterial occlusion and trophic lesion, 157
Prostaglandins, 204-208
  continuous intraarterial infusion of PGE_1, 204-206
  in bridging treatment, 209
  in treatment of ischemic limb, 207, 208
  intravenous drip infusion of PGE_1, 206, 207

Quadrilateral extremities involvement, 113, 114, 115

Ratschow's exercise, 202, 203
Raynaud's phenomenon, 103, 104, 116
  as systemic manifestation, 111
  in occupational arterial occlusive disease of hand, 194-196
  secondary, 84, 85
Rest pain, 95, 105, 106, 243
Rickettsia, 39
Rubor, 9, 14, 84, 87, 102, 103, 242. See also dependent rubor.
Runoff vessels, 156, 223

evaluation of, 223, 224

Salivary cotinine, 50
   in children, 50
Segmental occlusion, 123, 124, 134
Selection of patients for treatment, 233, 234
Sensitivity to smoking, 45, 46, 158
Sex, 113
   among diagnostic requirements, 190. See also Female patients.
Site of arterial occlusion, in lower extremity, 151, 152 (t)
   in upper extremity, 128, 129
Site of initial lesion, 60, 61, 63
   arteriographic, in aortoiliac region, 129, 130, 131
   arteriographic, in lower limbs, 128, 129, 130, 163
   arteriographic, in upper limbs, 128, 129
Skip lesion, 65-68, 135, 136, 137, 141 (f), 156
   definition of, 136, 137
   in popliteal artery, 66 (f), 136 (f)
   in sural artery, 68 (f)
   incidence of, 135, 162
   site of, 135, 136, 162, 163
Smoking, among diagnostic requirements, 189
   as etiological factor, 44-52
   effect on endothelial cells of, 47, 48, 49 (f)
   effect on PGs of, 47, 48, 50
   effect on vessel wall of, 46
   vasoconstricting effect of, 45
Soleus claudication, 94, 95
Spontaneous gangrene, 1, 2, 4-9
Standards of judgement, of normal arteriogram, 121
   of nomal venogram, 143
Stenosis and irregularity, 124, 125, 126, 128, 135, 136
   incidence of, 135
   localized, 124, 125 (f), 126 (f)
   moth-eaten, 126 (f)
Streptococcus, 39
Sympathectomy, borrowing-lending phenomenon (hemometakinesia) due to, 214

concomitant lumbar, 215
   indication for, 214
Sympathetic ganglion block, with alcohol, 212
   with phenol, 212
Syphilis, 39

Tapering occlusion, 34 (f), 122, 124, 125, 127, 128, 132, 133, 136 (f)
Thromboangiitis obliterans, history of, 12-24
Thromboendarterectomy, 219, 220
   eversion endarterectomy, 220
Thrombopblebitis migrans, 12, 13, 72, 73, 106, 107
   as initial symptom, 115
   as systemic manifestation, 111, 191
   incidence of, 106, 115, 116
Thrombophlebitis saltans, 72
Tobacco sensitiveness. See Sensitivity to smoking.
Tracer technique, with ^{99m}Tc-pertechnetate, 81 -83
Tree root collaterals, 123, 124, 125, 126, 128, 140, 144, 146, 148
Trench foot, 30
Type of progression of arterial occlusion. See also skip lesion.
   continuous progression, 65, 135, 156, 161
   skip progression, 65, 135, 136, 156, 161
Typhus, 39

Urinary cotinine, 50-52
   criteria for judging involuntary smoking, 51

Vasomotion, 86, 87
Vasospasm, 84, 85
Venous filling time, 103
Venous involvement, 71-73, 143
Visceral involvement, 176-182
   in coeliac and mesenteric arteries, 177-181
   in pulmonary artery, 181, 182
   in renal artery, 176, 177

Wallerian degeneration, 73, 74
Winiwarter, F., personal history of, 2-4